On behalf of Burroughs Wellcome Co., it is a pleasure to provide you this copy of "Acute Respiratory Care of the Neonate."

This book provides a thorough overview of neonatal respiratory care including the latest developments in ventilator care and lung surfactant replacement therapy. We hope the information provided on the physiology and treatment of the infant in acute respiratory distress will prove useful to the care of your patients.

Over the last one hundred years, the tradition of quality pharmaceutical research at Burroughs Wellcome Co. has resulted in the discovery of many medicines for the treatment of acute and chronic diseases. Five scientists associated with Wellcome have been awarded the Nobel Prize in Medicine or Physiology: Sir Henry Dale (1936); Sir John Vane (1982); Sir James Black (1988); Dr. George Hitchings (1988); and Dr. Trudy Elion (1988).

It is only through top quality research that important advances in the care of newborn infants are achieved. The challenge of eliminating perinatal morbidity and mortality is immense but eminently worth pursuing.

As part of Burroughs Wellcome's commitment to research and innovative medicines, it has been my privilege to be associated with the clinical development of a unique synthetic lung surfactant invented by Dr. John Clements of the University of California and licensed by Burroughs Wellcome Co., Exosurf® Neonatal™ (colfosceril palmitate, cetyl alcohol, tyloxapol) for Intratracheal Suspension. Surfactant replacement therapy represents a breakthrough in neonatology that is substantially reducing the morbidity and mortality of respiratory distress syndrome.

I hope you find this book worthwhile.

With best wishes,

Walker A. Long, MD
Clinical Research Division
Burroughs Wellcome Co.

Acute Respiratory Care of the Neonate

A Self-Study Course

Edited by
Jan Nugent, RNC, MSN

Neonatal Network®

Neonatal Network®
191 Lynch Creek Way, Suite 101
Petaluma, CA 94954-2313
(707) 762-2646

Book design and composition by:

First Impressions
Marsha Godfrey

Cover illustration by
Jeri J. Johnston

ISBN: 0-9622975-3-4

TABLE OF CONTENTS

CONTRIBUTING AUTHORS:

Karen Braune, RNC, MSN
University of Alabama at Birmingham
Birmingham, Alabama

V. L. Cassani III, RNC, MS, NNP
William Beaumont Army Medical Center
El Paso, Texas

Louis Gluck, MD
University of California
Irvine, California

M. Susan Inwood, RN
Mount Sinai Hospital
Toronto, Ontario, Canada

Tracy B. Karp, RNC, MS, NNP
Primary Children's Medical Center
Salt Lake City, Utah

Kathleen Koszarek, RNC, MSN
Ochsner Foundation Hospital
New Orleans, Louisiana

Donna Lee Loper, RN, MS
San Francisco General Hospital
San Francisco, California

Anne McCormick, RN, MS
Perinatal Nursing Consultant
Lincolnwood, Illinois

Jan Nugent, RNC, MSN
Ochsner Foundation Hospital
New Orleans, Louisiana

Susan Orlando, RNC, MS
Ochsner Foundation Hospital
New Orleans, Louisiana

Barbara S. Turner, RN, DNSc, FAAN
Madigan Army Medical Center
Tacoma, Washington

Introduction

The field of neonatology, especially the area of newborn pulmonary disorders and neonatal ventilation, is developing at a rapid pace. Today the NICU nurse is challenged to care for a diverse range of respiratory disorders, each with its own specialized technology. The blending of physiology, pathophysiology, and technical and nontechnical caring interventions is critical to provide skilled neonatal nursing. This book pays thoughtful attention to the role of technology in the care of the high-risk neonate in respiratory distress. The authors have carefully combined nursing care activities and technical assessment and procedures.

Morbidity and mortality result from improper and unskilled use of technology. Nurses bear the responsibility of maintaining their knowledge of "state of the art" nursing practice. As the primary caregiver for infants and families in crisis, the nurse is the stabilizing factor, the coordinator of care who ultimately provides for optimal outcome. The challenges in providing high-risk newborn care are numerous and ongoing. The intent of this book is to assist in meeting these challenges.

Jan Nugent, RNC, MSN
Unit Director/Clinical Specialist—NICU
Ochsner Foundation Hospital

1 Physiologic Principles of the Respiratory System

Donna Lee Loper, RN, MS
San Francisco General Hospital
San Francisco, California

In order to provide effective and appropriate nursing interventions to sick neonates, it is necessary to understand the disease process and its usual course as well as to appreciate the various treatment modalities. The foundation for this understanding and awareness is a strong knowledge base of the normal growth, development, and function of the fetus and neonate. This chapter provides the basis for this foundation. It discusses the embryological development of the lung and the role of lung fluid and fetal breathing movements in that development as well as surfactant synthesis and secretion. First breath events and the concomitant changes in pulmonary perfusion are presented, along with a discussion of lung physiology. These provide the basis for understanding the chapters that follow.

EMBRYOLOGIC DEVELOPMENT

Anatomic

Prenatal lung growth occurs in four stages: the embryonic, pseudoglandular, canalicular, and terminal air sac stages. The embryonic stage begins with conception and ends with the fifth week of gestation. Around day 24 a ventral diverticulum (outpouching) can be seen developing from the foregut. This groove extends downward and is gradually separated from the future esophagus by a septum. Between 2 and 4 days later, the first dichotomous branches can be seen. At the end of this stage, three divisions are evident on the right and two on the left (lobar and segmental bronchi).

From 5 to 17 weeks, a tree of narrow tubules forms. New airway branches arise through a mixture of cell multiplication and necrosis.[1] These tubules have thick epithelial walls made of columnar or cuboidal cells. This morphology, along with the loose mesenchymal tissue surrounding the tree give the lungs a glandular appearance, hence the name, "pseudoglandular stage."

By 16 weeks, branching of the conduction portion of the tracheobronchial tree (trachea to terminal bronchioles) is established. These preacinar airways can from this point forward increase only in length and diameter, not in number.[2,3] Toward the end of the pseudoglandular period, the rudimentary forms of cartilage, connective tissue, muscle, blood vessels, and lymphatics can be identified.[4]

The epithelial cells of the distal air spaces (future alveolar lining) flatten sometime between weeks 13 and 25, signaling the beginning of the canalicular stage.[5] A rich vascular supply begins to proliferate, and with the changes in mesenchymal tissue the capillaries are brought closer to the airway epithelium. Primitive respiratory bronchioles begin to form during this stage, delineating the acinus (gas exchanging section) from the conducting portion of the lung.

This development continues until 24 weeks gestation, when terminal air sacs appear as outpouchings of the terminal bronchioles. As the weeks progress, the number of terminal sacs increases, forming multiple pouches off a common chamber (the alveolar duct). The surface epithelium thins considerably as vascular proliferation increases. The latter stretches and thins the epithelium that covers them even more, bringing the capillaries into close proximity to the developing airways.[2] Eventually this leads to fusion of the basement membrane between the endothelium and the epithelium, thus creating the future blood-gas barrier.[1] At term, shallow indentations in the saccule walls can be detected. These primitive alveoli will deepen and multiply postnatally.

Lung structures and cells are differentiated to the point that extrauterine life can be supported around 26 to 28 weeks. Although the normal number of air spaces has not developed, the epithelium has thinned enough, and the vascular bed has proliferated to the point that oxygen exchange can occur.

The respiratory portion of the lung has a continuous epithelial lining composed mainly of two cell types, Type I and Type II pneumocytes. The Type I pneumocyte (squamous pneumocyte) covers approximately 95 percent of the alveolar surface via its long cytoplasmic extensions.[6,7] The thinnest area of the alveolus is composed of these extensions, and it is here that gas exchange occurs most rapidly.

The Type II pneumocyte (granular pneumocyte), although more numerous than the Type I, occupies less than 5 percent of the alve-

FIGURE 1 ▲ Composition of pulmonary surfactant

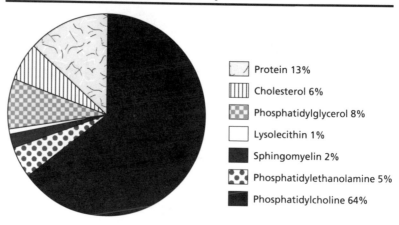

- Protein 13%
- Cholesterol 6%
- Phosphatidylglycerol 8%
- Lysolecithin 1%
- Sphingomyelin 2%
- Phosphatidylethanolamine 5%
- Phosphatidylcholine 64%

From: Farrell PM, and Ulane RE: The regulation of lung phospholipid metabolism, *in* Monset-Couchard M, and Minkowski A, eds., Physiological and Biochemical Basis for Perinatal Medicine, New York, S. Karger, 1981, p. 31. Reprinted with permission.

olar surface.[6] Osmiophilic, lamellated bodies are characteristic of these cells, and it is here that surfactant is thought to be produced and secreted. The first Type II cells are seen during the terminal sac stage, between 20 and 24 weeks. Surfactant secretion is detectable between 25 and 30 weeks gestation, although the potential for alveolar stability does not occur until later, between 33 and 36 weeks.[8,9]

Functional

The functional development of the lung revolves around the biochemistry of surfactant. The lung does, however, secrete other substances and has its own particular macrophage function.

Larger particles (bacteria) not swept away by ciliary action are thought to be removed and destroyed by pulmonary macrophages. Foreign material, once identified, is engulfed by the macrophage. Lysosomes then release enzymes into the space, which results in the destruction of the particle. These cells are critical to the health and continued function of the lung because they contribute to maintaining the sterility of its environment. They are most likely involved in removing surfactant from the alveolar surface as well.

TABLE 1 ▲ Surfactant Composition

% Composition by Weight		
Phospholipids		85
Saturated phosphatidylcholine	60	
Unsaturated phosphatidylcholine	20	
Phosphatidylglycerol	8	
Phosphatidylinositol	2	
Phosphatidylethanolamine	5	
Sphingomyelin	2	
Others	3	
Neutral lipids and cholesterol		5
Proteins		10
Contaminating serum proteins	8	
Surfactant Protein 35 (32–36,000 daltons)	~1	
Lipophilic proteins (6–12,000 daltons)	~1	

From: Jobe A: Questions about surfactant for respiratory distress syndrome (RDS), in Mead Johnson Symposium on Perinatal and Developmental Medicine, Evansville, Indiana, Mead Johnson, 1987, p. 43. Reprinted with permission.

Surfactant is of major importance to the adequate functioning of the lung. Figure 1 diagrams the composition of pulmonary surfactant. It is a lipoprotein with 90 percent of its dry weight composed of lipid.[10] The majority of the lipid (approximately two-thirds) is saturated phosphatidylcholine (PC), of which dipalmitoyl phosphatidylcholine (DPPC) is the most abundant (Table 1). The latter is the component responsible for decreasing the surface tension to almost zero when compressed at the surface during inspiration. Phosphatidylglycerol (PG) accounts for another 8 percent of the phospholipids encountered in surfactant. This is a substantial quantity and is unique to lung cells, broncho-alveolar fluid, and amniotic fluid—making PG a good marker for surfactant. The rest of the compound is involved in intracellular transport, storage, exocytosis, adsorption, and clearance at the alveolar lining.[6,10,11]

The biosynthesis of surfactant is discussed in detail in several publications.[6,10] Surfactant synthesis entails a series of biochemical events that include synthesis and integration of surfactant components in the membranes of the smooth and rough endoplasmic reticulum and multivesicular bodies of the Type II pneumocyte.[6,10] Once assembled, surfactant is transported intracellularly to the Golgi apparatus and then onto the lamellar bodies.[12]

Prior to being physiologically functional, surfactant undergoes a chemical change, becoming a lattice shaped structure known as tubular myelin. This structural change enhances spreadability and adsorption. Once surfactant is synthesized and transformed, it is stored in the lamellar body. Secretion occurs by exocytosis; however, surfactant must migrate to the surface of the liquid layer in order to be physiologically functional.[6,12,13]

Two unique proteins have been identified in the surfactant structure. One has an affinity for phospholipids, especially PG, and is thought to improve its functioning. Phosphatidylglycerol improves the adsorption of DPPC, as does PI (phosphatidylinositol). The combination of PG and protein has an additive effect on DPPC. Therefore, the presence of component

FIGURE 2 ▲ Pathways for phosphatidylcholine synthesis

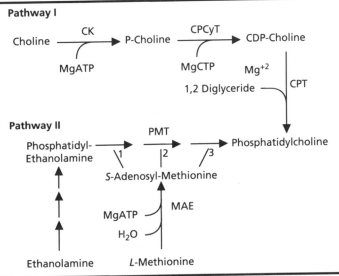

From: Farrell PM, and Ulane RE: The regulation of lung phospholipid metabolism, *in* Monset-Couchard M, and Minkowski A, eds., Physiological and Biochemical Basis for Perinatal Medicine, New York, S. Karger, 1981, p. 31. Reprinted with permission.

FIGURE 3 ▲ Biosynthesis of phospholipids

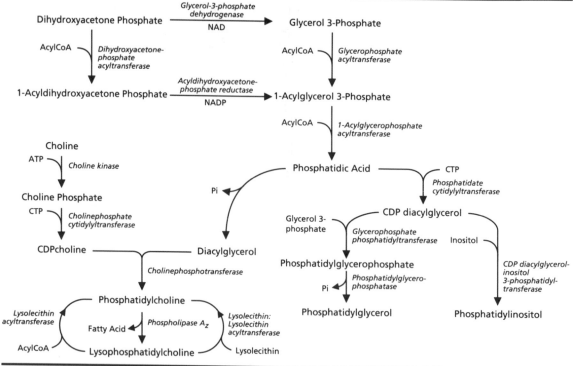

From: Jobe A: Questions about surfactant for respiratory distress syndrome (RDS), *in* Mead Johnson Symposium on Perinatal and Developmental Medicine, No. 30, Evansville, Indiana, Mead Johnson, 1987, p. 13. Reprinted with permission.

parts is not enough; it is the way in which they are transformed by each other that maximizes lung functioning.

There are two major pathways for phosphatidylcholine synthesis (Figure 2). Key precursors for PC synthesis include glycerol, fatty acids, choline, glucose, and ethanolamine.[11] The major pathway is the cytidine diphosphate choline system, which provides the biochemical maturity necessary for alveolar structural integrity and stability.

The other pathway—the methyltransferase system—leads to phosphatidylethanolamine (PE) formation. This pathway has minor significance in the adult lung and seems to play a relatively insignificant role in fetal lung development.[11] This may be due to the ability of choline to be incorporated more effectively into PC than methionine. It has been suggested that the ability of the human fetus to synthesize PC by N-methylation of PE early in

gestation may contribute to survival of infants who are delivered prematurely. Further investigation is needed to elucidate the physiologic contribution of this pathway.

Figure 3 depicts the biosynthesis of phosphatidylcholine, phosphatidylinositol, and phosphatidylglycerol and demonstrates the dependency of the system upon the biosynthesis of phosphatidic acid. The increased production of phospholipids seen in late gestation depends on the increased synthesis of this acid. The majority of phospholipid produced is PC; Figure 4 represents the biosynthesis and remodeling of this critical phospholipid.[10,11]

Figure 4 demonstrates the interaction of the choline pathway and the diglyceride synthesis mechanisms that yield increased PC synthesis during late gestation. Although this interaction yields increased quantities of PC, it is not the highly saturated version identified in the final surfactant compound. The remodeling of PC that occurs in the phosphatidylcholine-lysophosphatidylcholine cycle provides the dipalmitoyl-PC required for surfactant.[11]

As gestation advances, phospholipid content increases, as does the level of saturation. This is accompanied by an increase in osmiophilic inclusion bodies within the Type II pneumocytes. Choline incorporation, which is low in early gestation, has been reported to increase abruptly in rhesus monkeys when 90 percent of

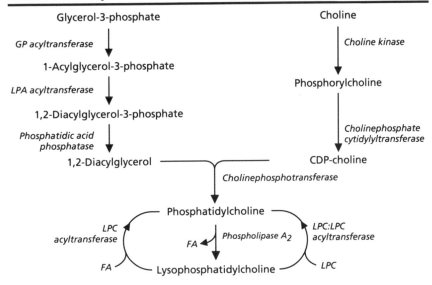

FIGURE 4 ▲ Biosyntheses and remodeling of phosphatidylcholine

From: Farrell PM, and Ulane RE: The regulation of lung phospholipid metabolism, *in* Monset-Couchard M, and Minkowski A, eds., Physiological and Biochemical Basis for Perinatal Medicine, New York, S. Karger, 1981, p. 33. Reprinted with permission.

gestation is completed.[5] This suggests that pathway regulatory mechanisms are modified/enhanced in order to meet postnatal needs. Figure 5 demonstrates the changes in glycerophospholipids in response to system maturation during gestation.

Enzymatic changes in the phospholipid synthesis pathway are discussed in several review articles.[10,11,14] The correlation of these changes to the surge in saturated PC and increase in PG with concomitant decrease in PI (see Figure 5) is not yet

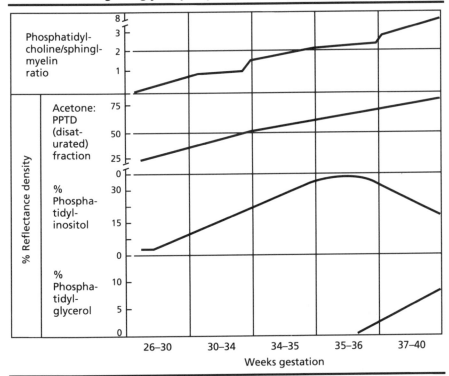

FIGURE 5 ▲ Changes in glycerophospholipids during gestation

From: Merritt TA: Respiratory distress, *in* Zidi M, Clarke TA, and Merritt TA, eds., Assessment of the Newborn: A Guide for the Practitioner, Boston, Little, Brown, 1984, p. 177. Reprinted with permission.

understood. Whether it is a change in concentration of enzyme or substrate, adjustment in catalytic efficiency, change in substrate affinity, or activation of latent enzymes is not entirely known and is currently being investigated.

In addition to enzymes, hormonal regulation of surfactant biosynthesis and secretion have been (and continue to be) investigated. Those hormones that have been implicated include glucocorticoids, adrenocorticotropic hormone, thyroid hormone, estrogens, prolactin, thyrotropin-releasing hormone, catecholamines, insulin, fibroblast pneumocyte factor, prostaglandins, and epidermal growth factor. Only glucocorticoids, thyroid hormone, insulin, and catecholamines are reviewed here.

Glucocorticoids

Glucocorticoids are probably the best known of the hormones affecting surfactant. Liggins' observations in 1969 set off a flurry of research in the area of hormonal control of fetal lung development that has continued to the present.[15] Glucocorticoids accelerate the normal pattern of fetal lung development by increasing the rate of glycogen depletion and glycerophospholipid biosynthesis.

The depletion in glycogen leads to direct anatomical changes of the alveolar structures, thinning the interalveolar septa while increasing the size of the alveoli (air space). Morphologic changes include an increase in the number of Type II pneumocytes and an increase in the number of lamellar bodies within those cells. This occurs in conjunction with a functional maturation of these cells, leading to an accelerated synthesis of surfactant phospholipid.[10,16–19]

Glucocorticoids act by binding to specific receptors within the cytoplasm. This complex interacts with deoxyribonucleic acid (DNA) to produce a specific messenger ribonucleic acid (RNA) that translates its protein code to the ribosomes. The identity of these proteins is currently unknown. Dexamethasone and betamethasone have a higher affinity for the glucocorticoid receptor than do the natural corticoids (cortisol and cortisone), which explains the use of betamethasone during preterm labor.[18]

The question of whether it is the triggering of protein synthesis mechanisms that accounts for the increase in fatty acid synthetase, phosphatidic acid phosphatase, and choline-phosphate cytidyltransferase activity is yet to be answered. There is conflicting evidence that suggests that glucocorticoids could promote the synthesis of an enzyme activator or may influence the production of the heavier of the surfactant apoproteins.[20–24]

Several other questions have yet to be answered as well. It is evident that glucocorticoid action is centered on synthesis, not secretion, and that it affects more than surfactant synthesis. Acting directly on lung tissue, glucocorticoids increase the number of beta-adrenergic receptors and enhance elastin and collagen production, which improves lung compliance.[25]

What is not evident is whether glucocorticoids act independently or in conjunction with other compounds, or whether glucocorticoids directly affect Type II pneumocytes or mediate their action through other lung cells (fibroblasts). Smith suggests that rather than having a direct impact on Type II cells, glucocorticoids may act upon fibroblasts (increasing the production of fibroblast pneumocyte factor), which then affect surfactant production.[26] Of course, it may not be strictly one or the other but some combination of these actions.

Thyroid Hormones

The idea that hormones may work in conjunction with other compounds or hormones is reinforced by observations of the actions of thyroid hormones. Thyroxine (T_4) and tri-iodothyronine (T_3) have been shown to increase the rate of phospholipid synthesis.[10,23,27,28] Thyroid hormones, like glucocorticoids, enhance production of phosphatidylcholine through choline incorporation. They do not, however, increase phosphatidylglycerol synthesis or stimulate the production of surfactant specific proteins.[16,29] While glucocorticoids increase, thyroid hormone seems to decrease fatty acid synthetase activity.[30] These differences suggest different sites of action for these hormones as well as the need for action in conjunction with other hormones.[16]

Low T_3 and T_4 levels have been associated with respiratory distress syndrome, although exact mechanisms are unclear.[11,14,17,31] Ballard and associates have shown that the effects of thyroid hormones are mediated by a specific thyroid receptor to which T_3 has a higher affinity, as well as being a more potent phospholipid synthesis stimulator.[32]

Clinical application of this information is aimed at maximizing beneficial effects through the delivery of hormones or hormone-activating substances without direct contact with the fetus. Naturally occurring thyroid hormones do not readily cross the placenta unless concentrations far exceeding normal levels are achieved. However, thyrotropin-releasing hormone does cross the placenta and stimulates the fetal pituitary gland to produce thyroid-stimulating hormone, resulting in increased production of PC.[17,33] The use of DIMIT, a synthetic thyroid analogue, appears to produce similar results.[17]

Continued investigation of the precise mechanisms of thyroid hormone action is essential. There seems to be little doubt that a synergistic interaction between glucocorticoids and thyroid hormones occurs, apparently at the level of messenger RNA.[16] Significant increases in PC production occur in a shorter period of time when these two hormones are used together (versus individually).[27,28,32] These findings may have significant clinical implications and modify future therapeutic interventions.

Catecholamines

While glucocorticoids and thyroid hormones play a role in enhancing the synthesis of phospholipids, catecholamines stimulate the secretion of surfactant into the alveolar space. This appears to be a direct action of adrenergic compounds on Type II cells.[34] The response is prompt, occurring in less than an hour.

Further research has shown that there is an increase in surfactant and saturated phosphatidylcholine in lung fluid and improved lung stability. This is demonstrated in an increased lecithin-to-sphingomyelin ratio. An added benefit is the inhibition of fetal lung fluid secretion and possible reabsorption of the fluid within the alveoli at the time of delivery. These two effects (increase in surfactant and decrease in lung fluid) work together in preparing the fetus for respiratory conversion.[17,34–37]

Insulin

The development of surfactant appears to be inhibited in neonates born to diabetic mothers who are not well controlled. Whether this is caused by hyperglycemia, hyperinsulinemia, or both is unclear, and research continues to provide conflicting answers. Maturation of surfactant synthesis occurs at the same time glycogen is depleted from the lungs and liver. Insulin inhibits glycogen breakdown, thereby decreasing the substrate available for PC synthesis as well as altering the natural anatomical changes that occur with glycogen depletion.[10,16]

Smith found that the effect of cortisol on choline incorporation was reduced by insulin, even though the cortisol effects on cell growth were not.[38] Gross and co-workers documented no insulin influence and no antagonistic action on the usual dexamethasone response.[39] Mendelson and associates, on the other hand, reported a synergistic effect when cortisol and insulin were combined.[40]

Recent *in vivo* studies have shown hyperglycemia to be the culprit; tissue cultures implicate hyperinsulinemia.[38,39,41] The mechanism remains unclear, although it has been suggested that insulin may antagonize glucocorticoids at the fibroblast level, affecting the production of fibroblast pneumocyte factor.[42] Clinically, the incidence of respiratory distress syndrome has decreased as the need for stricter control of maternal glucose levels has been recognized and monitoring has been made easier.

At present, there seems to be a complex interaction of several hormones and factors that control surfactant synthesis. There continues to be much to learn about surfactant, its synthesis and removal. However, it is apparent that normal lung function is dependent upon the presence of surfactant, which permits a decrease in surface tension at end-expiration and an increase in surface tension during lung expansion. This prevents atelectasis at end-expiration and facilitates elastic recoil on inspiration. Surfactant provides the lung with the stability required to maintain homeostatic blood gas pressures while decreasing the work of breathing.

Pulmonary Vasculature

Pulmonary vessel development occurs in conjunction with the branching of the bronchial tree.[43–45] The arteries have more branches than the airways, and the veins develop more tributaries. The preacinar region has an arterial branch (conventional artery) that runs along each conducting airway branch; supernumerary arteries feed the adjacent alveoli. The preacinar arteries are all present by 16 weeks gestation. If for any reason there is a decrease in the number of airways, there is a concomitant decrease in conventional and supernumerary arteries.[1,44] From 16 weeks on, the preacinar vessels increase in length and diameter only.[4]

As development progresses into the canalicular and terminal air sac stages, intraacinar arteries appear and will continue their development during the postnatal period.[4,44,45] The conventional arteries continue their development for the first 18 months of life. Supernumerary arteries continue to be laid down for the first 8 years.[1,45] These latter vessels are smaller and more numerous, servicing the alveoli directly.[4] If blood flow is reduced or blocked through the conventional arteries, the supernumerary arteries may serve as collateral circulation, thereby maintaining lung function during periods of ischemia or increased pulmonary vascular resistance.[9] Postnatally, the intraacinar vessels multiply rapidly as alveoli appear.[4]

The pulmonary veins develop more slowly, after the arteries. By 20 weeks, however, preacinar veins are present.[45] The development of the veins parallels that of the arteries and conducting airways, although supernumerary veins outnumber supernumerary arteries. Interestingly, both types of veins appear simultaneously.[4] The development of additional veins, as well as the lengthening of existing veins, continues postnatally.

Further development of the pulmonary circulation is related to changes in muscle wall thickness and extension of muscle into arterial walls. The pulmonary artery wall is quite thick at birth, as a result of the low oxygen tension encountered intrauterinely. The wall thins as oxygen tension rises at birth, and the medial layer elastic fibrils become less organized. The pulmonary vein, on the other hand, is found to be deficient in elastic fibers at birth and progressively incorporates muscle and elastic tissue during the first two years of life.[45]

The intrapulmonary arteries have thick walls as well. The smaller arteries have increased muscularity and dilate actively with the postnatal increase in oxygen tension.[44] There is a concomitant fall in pulmonary vascular resistance.[4] Between 3 and 28 days postnatally, these vessels achieve their adult wall thickness to external diameter ratio. The larger arteries take longer, achieving adult levels after 4 to 18 months.[45]

The arteries of the fetus are more muscular than those of the adult or child. The muscle thickness to external diameter ratio decreases postnatally.[4] Muscle distribution changes following birth (with the muscle extending peripherally) continue during the first 19 years of life.

Lung Fluid

Lung fluid is secreted from the beginning of the canalicular stage. This fluid is thought to be derived from alveolar epithelial secretions, however the site and specific mechanism of formation is unclear. It is known that lung fluid is not an ultrafiltrate of plasma or amniotic fluid, nor is it a mixture of the two. Active transport is required to achieve the ion concentrations encountered and is probably derived from active transport of chloride, with sodium following passively. The water flux can be attributed to the osmotic force of sodium chloride.[46]

Osmolarity, sodium, and chloride levels are lower in amniotic fluid than in tracheal fluid; pH, glucose, and protein are higher.[47] The secretion rate is approximately 2–4 ml/kg/minute in lambs, which in term infants is equal to approximately 250 cc/day.[48,49]

Some lung fluid is swallowed, and some moves into the amniotic fluid, although the contribution to the latter is not significant when compared to the volume secreted by the kidneys. The volume of fluid is approximately equal to the functional residual capacity. At term this means there are 10 to 25 cc/kg body weight of liquid that must be either expelled or absorbed.[48,50]

The alveolar fluid is continually secreted and completely turned over every ten hours in the lamb at term.[47] Although its functional importance is not entirely known, lung fluid does play an important part in cell maturation and development, as well as determining the formation, size, and shape of the developing air space. Alterations in fluid dynamics affect pulmonary cell proliferation and differentiation.

Alcorn and associates demonstrated (based on the assessment of Type II cells) that fetuses whose tracheae were ligated had relatively large but immature lungs. Fetuses whose lungs were drained had thick alveolar walls, smaller lungs, and more abundant Type II cells.[51] This was confirmed by Perlman and associates, who found reduced numbers of alveoli in human infants who experienced amniotic fluid leakage.[52]

Therefore, reduced lung fluid production or leakage of amniotic fluid places the fetus at risk for lung hypoplasia.[8] On the other hand, chronic tracheal obstruction leads to hyperplasia with an increase in the number of alveoli, although they are functionally immature.[9]

At the time of birth, the lungs must move from secretion to absorption of lung fluid, or the infant will rapidly succumb, drowning in his own secretions. Normally, secretion ends with birth, and ventilation of the lungs leads to liquid dispersion across the pulmonary epithelium during the absorptive period. At this time the pulmonary epithelium undergoes a reversible increase in solute permeability, leading to a rapid transfer of lung liquid solutes.[49] This is confirmed clinically as the interstitial spaces and lymphatics become distended during the first five to six hours of life, and pulmonary lymph flow increases.[53]

Along with this increase in absorption, there seems to be a decrease in the rate of secretion. The administration of epinephrine to lambs leads to a decrease in fluid secretion. This effect is mediated by beta-adrenergic receptors in the alveolar epithelium and may either suppress the chloride pump or activate a second pump that triggers the absorption process.[49,54] Avery and coworkers suggest that resorption is a sodium pump dependent mechanism because an amiloride infusion can modify the process.[55] This supports the second pump theory.

It is known that the absorption rate increases as gestation progresses, and this can be correlated to an increase in catecholamine levels.[56] Fetal adrenal glands are probably not able to produce sufficient amounts of catecholamines to trigger this mechanism; labor, however, provides sufficient stimulus to release enough epinephrine to stimulate the switch from secretion to absorption.[49] The catecholamine surge that occurs with delivery probably is the final mechanism to assure that this change is completed.[47]

The drop in pulmonary vascular resistance with aeration and the rise in oxygen tension increase the number of alveolar capillaries perfused, resulting in an increase in blood removal capacity. Between the increased lymphatic flow and the dramatic change in the pulmonary blood flow, lung fluid is dispersed within the first few hours following delivery.

Fetal Breathing Movements

Fetal breathing movements can be seen as early as 11 weeks gestation on ultrasound.[57] They are rapid and irregular, occurring intermittently early in gestation. As gestation progresses, their strength and frequency increase, until they occur between 40 and 80 percent of the time, at a rate of 30–70 breaths per minute.[47,57–59] Large movements (gasping) occur 5 percent of the total breathing time, 1–4 times per minute.[57]

This rapid and irregular respiratory activity may contribute to lung fluid regulation, thereby influencing lung growth. The diaphragm seems to be the major structure involved, with minimal chest wall excursion (4–8 mm change in transverse diameter).[60] Movement of the diaphragm is necessary for the chest wall muscles and diaphragm to gain adequate strength for the initial breath.[59]

Diaphragm movement also influences the course of lung cell differentiation and proliferation. Bilateral phrenectomy results in altered lung morphology, with an increase in Type II over Type I cells. Presumably, the innervated diaphragm increases the size of the thorax and thereby increases tissue stress, affecting morphology. Beyond this, however, hypoplastic lungs are found in those situations where fetal breathing movements do not occur.[61]

Fetal breathing movements vary significantly from fetus to fetus. Initially, they are infrequent, increasing with gestational age and becoming more organized and vigorous.[47] Even with these gestational changes, tracheal fluid shifts are negligible, the pressure generated being no more than 25 mmHg.[61] Fetal maturation leads to the appearance of cycles, with an increase in fetal breathing movements during daytime hours.[57,62] Patrick and associates report that fetal breathing movements peak in late evening and reach their nadir in the early morning hours.[63]

Abnormal breathing patterns can be seen during periods of hypoxia. Mild hypoxemia decreases the incidence of fetal breathing movements; severe hypoxemia may lead to their cessation for several hours. The onset of asphyxia leads to gasping that persists until death.[64] Interestingly, the onset of mild hypoxemia (as with umbilical artery occlusion of short duration) may lead to quiet sleep, which for the fetus decreases activity, energy expenditure and oxygen consumption.[57] Although paradoxical in nature, this conservation mechanism may save the fetus while cardiac output is redistributed toward the placenta.

The reduction and cessation of fetal breathing movements seen during labor coincide with the increase in prostaglandin E concentrations seen during the last days before delivery. These findings suggest that prostaglandin metabolism may play a role in respiratory conversion at birth.[65] It remains unknown why irregular fetal breathing movements lead to the sustained respirations of postnatal life.

TRANSITIONAL EVENTS
Respiratory Conversion

At term, the acinar portion of the lung is well established, although "true" alveoli are only now beginning to develop. The pulmonary blood vessels are narrow; only 5–10 percent of the cardiac output perfuses the lungs to meet cellular nutrition needs. This low volume circulation is, in part, due to the high pulmonary vascular resistance created by constricted arterioles.

At term, the lung holds approximately 3 cc/kg of fluid. Lung aeration is complete when this liquid is replaced with an equal volume of air, and a functional residual capacity (FRC) is established. A substantial amount of air is retained with the early breaths. Within an hour of birth, 80–90 percent of the FRC is created. The retention of air is due to surfactant and a decrease in surface tension. Surfactant decreases the tendency toward atelectasis, promotes capillary circulation by increasing alveolar size (which indirectly dilates precapillary vessels), improves alveolar fluid clearance, and protects the airway.[6] Therefore, the concentration and adsorption properties of surfactant must be sufficient to react during the short first breaths (one to ten seconds). Exactly how all this happens is not known.[49]

The gas tension levels that characterize the fetal state would result in significant hyperventilation postnatally; this indicates a diminished responsiveness of the respiratory centers to chemical stimuli in the blood during intrauterine life. Postnatal breathing is responsive to stimuli from arterial and central chemoreceptors (oxygen and carbon dioxide tension in the blood), the chest wall and lungs, musculoskeletal system, and skin, as well as emotions and behavior. The changes that take place at birth and the increase in aerobic metabolism are not only rapid but irreversible. Within a few hours of birth, the neonate is responsive to hypoxia and hypercapnia in much the same manner as an adult.[49]

The actual mechanics of respiratory conversion begin with the passage of the fetus through the birth canal. The thorax is markedly depressed during this passage, with external pressures of 160–200 cm H_2O and intrathoracic pressures of 60–100 cm H_2O being generated.[47,66–68] When the infant's face or nares are exposed to atmospheric pressure, variable amounts of lung fluid are expressed.[67] As much as 28 cc of fluid have been expelled during the second stage of labor, leading to the creation of a potential air space.[47] Recoil of the chest to predelivery proportions allows for passive "inspiration" of variable amounts of air. This initial step helps reduce viscous forces

that must be overcome in order to establish an air-liquid interface in the alveoli.[67]

The forces that must be overcome during the first breaths include the viscosity of the lung fluid column, the tissue resistive forces (compliance), and the surface tension forces at the air-liquid interfaces. The viscosity of lung fluid provides resistance to movement of fluid in the airways. The maximal resistance is at the beginning of the first breath, and the greatest displacement occurs in the trachea.[67,69] The dissipation of tracheal fluid during the vaginal squeeze reduces the amount of pressure that must be generated to move the liquid column down the conducting airways.

As the column progresses down the conducting branches, the total surface area of the air-liquid interface decreases as the bronchiole diameter is progressively reduced. The surface tension, however, increases.[47] It is the surface tension forces that are the hardest to overcome during the first breath events. The maximal forces are encountered where the radii curvature of the airways is smallest (terminal bronchioles)—here the viscous forces are at their nadir.[47,67] In this vicinity the intraluminal pressure must be at its peak in order to prevent closure by tension in the intraluminal walls (LaPlace relationship).[8] If these smaller airways were filled with fluid only (no air-liquid interface), the pressures needed would be considerably less. But this would make alveolar expansion more difficult. Surface tension forces drop again once air enters the terminal air sacs.[47]

Tissue resistive forces are unknown at birth. However, the fluid within the terminal air sacs enhances air introduction, possibly by modifying the configuration of the smaller units of the lung. The fluid enlarges the radius of the alveolar ducts and terminal air sac, thereby facilitating expansion (LaPlace relationship). The lung fluid also reduces the possibility of cellular debris obstructing the small ducts.

During the interval between recoil and the

generation of first breath pressures, the infant may generate a positive pressure within the mouth by glossopharyngeal "frog breathing."[47,67] Another possible contributor to lung expansion is the small increase in pulmonary blood flow that may occur during this time. This flow may lead to capillary erection as pulmonary capillaries uncoil and may increase transpulmonary pressure and lung stability.[67,68] Like "frog breathing," this is not a significant enough pressure to produce lung expansion, though it may contribute modestly to air entry.

The first diaphragmatic inspiration has been reported to begin within nine seconds of delivery and to generate very large positive intrathoracic pressures (mean of 70 cm H_2O). Air enters as soon as the intrathoracic pressure begins to drop with mean inspiratory pressures of 30–35 cm H_2O.[2,47,70]

The large transpulmonary pressure generated by the diaphragm lasts only 0.5–1 second, pulling in 10–70 ml of air.[71] The layer of fluid at the alveolar lining becomes established after the first breath, allowing the molecules of surfactant to reduce the surface tension during expiration.[67] The first expiration is also active, leaving behind a residual volume of up to 30 cc. The magnitude of the expiratory pressure contributes to FRC formation, even distribution of air, and elimination of lung fluid.[47] The second and third breaths are similar to the first but require less pressure because the small airways are open, and surface-active forces are diminished.[67] Lung expansion augments surfactant secretion, providing alveolar stability and FRC formation.

By 10 minutes of age, the FRC is equal to 17 cc/kg; at 30 minutes, it is equal to 25–35 cc/kg.[72] The return of muscle tone after the first breath helps maintain FRC by providing chest wall stability.[47,66]

Lung compliance is four to five times greater by day one and continues to increase gradually over the first week of life. Flow resistance decreases by one-half to one-fourth during this

time and the distribution of ventilation is as even after day one as it is on day three or four.[47]

According to Haworth and Hislop, structural changes in the pulmonary circulation occur in three overlapping phases:[73]

1. Digitation and recruitment occur during the first 24 hours of life in non-muscular and partially muscular arteries. The external diameter of these vessels increases, and the swollen endothelial lining cells flatten. These endothelial cells may play a role in the relaxation of smooth muscle cells by metabolizing substances such as acetylcholine.

2. Reduced muscularity occurs during the first two weeks of life. During this time partially muscular and wholly muscular vessels become nonmuscular and partially muscular, respectively.

3. A growth phase begins after the first two weeks. Muscle tissue begins to reappear in the acinus and continues to develop slowly during childhood. The initial phases allow for the functional adaptation necessary for extrauterine life, and the third phase brings about structural remodeling. This growth creates the relationships seen in the mature system between the external vessel diameter and muscle wall thickness.

In conjunction with the local vascular changes in the pulmonary bed, there are major reorganizational changes within the cardiovascular system. The first breath events and cardiovascular events cannot be separated; they are interdependent and must occur for transition to be successful.

Cardiovascular Conversion

In the fetus, oxygenated blood returns from the placenta via the umbilical vein with an arterial oxygen tension (PaO_2) of 35 mmHg. The blood enters the liver, where a small percentage feeds the liver microcirculation, and ends up in the inferior vena cava. The major portion of the returning blood is shunted directly into the inferior vena cava via the ductus venosus.

The inferior vena cava enters the right atrium, where the majority of its blood flow (approximately 60 percent) is deflected across the right atrium and through the foramen ovale into the left atrium. Here it mixes with the unoxygenated blood returning from the fetal lungs, drops into the left ventricle, and is ejected into the ascending aorta to feed the cerebral arteries and upper extremities.

The remainder of the right atrium blood mixes with the unoxygenated superior vena cava blood returning from the upper body and enters the right ventricle. This mixed blood is ejected through the pulmonary arteries toward the lungs. The high pulmonary vascular resistance allows only 5–10 percent of the blood to enter the lungs, the majority being shunted across the ductus arteriosus into the thoracic aorta, which services the lower segments of the body.

With clamping of the umbilical cord, the placenta, which is a low resistance organ (contributing to the low systemic vascular resistance found in the fetal state) is unavailable. The net result is an increase in pulmonary blood return to the heart and a decrease in systemic blood return. These changes modify the pressures within the atria. Left atrial pressure increases above the right and leads to functional closure of the foramen ovale. The increase in PaO_2 and decrease in prostaglandin levels facilitate functional closure of the ductus arteriosus. These modifications in blood flow and pressures indicate the change from "in series" to parallel circulation and herald cardiovascular conversion.

Once the first breath is taken and cardiovascular conversion is initiated, the infant must be able to attain sustained rhythmic respirations. This requires the central nervous system to be "turned on" so it can take over the regulation of respiratory activity.

RESPIRATORY PHYSIOLOGY
Control of Respiration

The goal of respiration is to meet the oxygen and carbon dioxide metabolic demands of the organism by extracting oxygen from the atmosphere and removing carbon dioxide produced by the organism. The respiratory center is responsible for matching the level of ventilation to the metabolic demand. The assessment of metabolic needs and alteration of ventilation are accomplished by the chemoreceptors.

The peripheral chemoreceptors (carotid and aortic bodies) sense oxygen and carbon dioxide tension; the central chemoreceptors (medullary) are sensitive to PCO_2/[H+] in the extracellular fluid of the brain. When the PaO_2 falls below the acceptable range, the chemoreceptors increase the efferent neural activity to the respiratory center (brain), which brings about an increase in ventilation. At birth, the fetal PaO_2 of 25 mmHg (sufficient for intrauterine growth) increases to 50 mmHg with the first few breaths and then to 70 mmHg in the first hours.[74] This increase in oxygen tension exceeds the fetal demands for oxygen, resulting in relative "hyperoxia" at birth.

This change in oxygen tension causes the chemoreceptors to become inactive and to remain so for the first few days of life.[75] Thus fluctuations in oxygen tension levels may not lead to a chemoreceptor response during these early days of neonatal life.[59] After this lag time, however, the chemoreceptors reset, becoming oxygen-sensitive and playing a major role in the control of respiration.[76,77]

Sustained hyperventilation efforts during hypoxia cannot be maintained by the neonate. Studies in infants and animals demonstrate that an initial hyperventilatory response is followed by a subsequent fall in ventilation and oxygen tensions.[57,78] The reasons for this lack of sustained response are unknown. Davis and Bureau speculate that it may be due to the feeble chemoreceptor output, the central inhibitory effect of hypoxia on ventilation, or changes in pulmonary mechanics.[59]

The neonate's response to carbon dioxide, though more mature than his response to hypoxia, is also limited during the early neonatal period. Neonates can increase ventilation by only 3 to 4 times their baseline ventilation in comparison to the 10 to 20-fold increase adults can achieve.[79,80] Along with this, the threshold of tolerance for carbon dioxide is higher initially, progressively declining over the first month of life.[79] This, too, may be due to the increased arterial carbon dioxide tension ($PaCO_2$) levels found in the fetal state (45–50 mmHg) and the need to reset chemoreceptors.

Modification of ventilatory patterns is dependent upon inspiratory muscle strength, rib cage rigidity, airway resistance, and lung compliance. The status of these factors and the performance of the respiratory pump are controlled through specific reflex arcs.[59]

Chemoreceptors provide information about the metabolic needs of the infant, mechanoreceptors provide information about the status of the respiratory pump, and the central respiratory center integrates this information and establishes the ventilatory pattern that efficiently meets the infant's needs. Each respiratory cycle during a stable state (such as quiet sleep) is uniform in amplitude, duration, and wave form. Behavioral influences as well as active sleep states (REM sleep) alter the regularity of breathing. The information received from the various receptors helps determine the inspiratory time, the expiratory time, the lung volume at which the breath should occur (FRC), the rate of inspiration, and braking of the expiration.[81] The recruitment and adjustment of the various respiratory muscle groups result in the predetermined lung volume being achieved.[59]

The Respiratory Pump

The movement of gas in and out of the lungs is based on the functioning of the respiratory pump, which is composed of the rib cage and respiratory muscles. The pump must move sufficient oxygen and carbon dioxide into and out of the lungs to replace the oxygen consumed and wash out the carbon dioxide that accumulates in the alveoli. Ventilatory efforts in the neonate depend on the strength and endurance of the diaphragm; when these are insufficient, the neonate requires ventilatory assistance.[59]

Diaphragm

The diaphragm inserts on the lower six ribs, the sternum, and the first three lumbar vertebrae. It is innervated bilaterally by the phrenic nerves and expends its work on the lung, the rib cage, and the abdomen. For the diaphragm to work optimally, the intercostal muscles must stabilize the rib cage, and the abdominal muscles should stabilize the abdomen.[60,82] In the term infant, the coordination of these efforts is almost nonexistent, and in the preterm infant, such coordination is even less effective. During REM sleep (the predominant sleep state in the neonate), the intercostal and abdominal muscles are ineffective, contributing to respiratory instability.[82]

The composition of the muscle fibers in the neonate differs from that of the adult. The neonatal diaphragm and intercostal muscles have a lower proportion of fatigue-resistant (Type I) fibers (20 percent as compared to 60 percent in the adult).[59,82,83] Type I fibers increase in number from 24 weeks gestation, when they comprise 10 percent of total fiber content, to reach the adult proportion at 8 months postnatal age.[82] Because of this developmental pattern, the neonate is particularly vulnerable to diaphragmatic muscle fatigue—especially when the work of breathing is increased.[59,82] This vulnerability is potentiated with decreasing gestational age.

The infant's diaphragm is attached to a chest wall that is more pliable than that of the adult. This can lead to distortion of the lower portion of the chest wall during contraction, especially if the contraction is forceful. The decreased efficiency of the contraction and reduced tidal volume can make ventilation less effective and require adjustments in the respiratory pattern.[59]

FIGURE 6 ▲ Lung volumes in the infant and adult

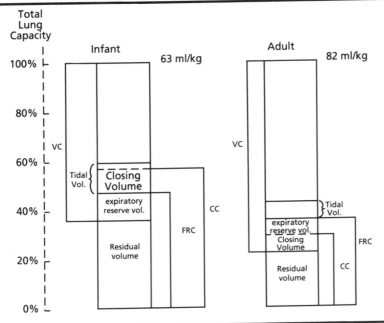

From: Nelson NM: Respiration and Circulation after birth, *in* Smith CA, and Nelson NM, eds., The Physiology of the Newborn Infant, Springfield, Massachusetts, Charles C. Thomas, 1976, p. 207. Reprinted with permission.

Rib Cage and Chest Wall Muscles

The muscles of the rib cage consist of the external intercostal muscles (used during inspiration), the internal intercostal muscles (used during expiration), and the accessory muscles, including the sternocleidomastoid, pectoral, and scalene. The major role of these muscles is to fixate the chest wall by tonic contraction during diaphragmatic excursion. If they are unable to accomplish this goal, collapse and distortion of the chest wall are likely to occur during inspiratory efforts.

If these muscles are able to provide the stability needed, the contraction of the inspiratory muscles of the rib cage can contribute to the thoracic volume. During sighing, the increase in tidal volume is due largely to increased chest wall excursion.[84]

Rib Cage Compliance

The chest wall in the infant is cartilaginous, soft, and pliable. This design allows for compression during passage through the birth canal

without rib fractures and then for further growth and development.[43,85,86] Nelson describes the infant's chest wall as a loose fitting glove surrounding the neonatal lung.[67] The high compliance dictates that for any given change in volume there is almost no change in pressure.[86] This increased compliance is highest in the preterm infant, but it is significant in the term infant as well.

The clinical implications of this highly compliant chest are related to the ease with which lung collapse is possible in the neonate. The low elastic recoil pressure of the neonatal lung and the high compliance of the thorax result in the majority of tidal breathing in the infant being done close to the closing capacity of the lung (Figure 6). This contributes to the possibility of collapse and affects gas distribution.

The mechanical liabilities of a highly compliant chest wall after delivery include a compromised ability to produce large tidal volumes, which necessitates the generation of larger pressures. This requires the infant to perform more work to move the same amount of tidal volume.[86] This is especially true in preterm infants with lung diseases associated with decreased lung compliance. Lung disease increases the respiratory drive in an attempt to generate stronger contractions with high inspiratory pressures that will expand stiff, noncompliant lungs.

The diaphragmatic force and the pliable chest wall lead to chest distortion.[87] Therefore, a portion of the energy and force of the contraction is wasted. Retractions are the clinical signs of these distortions and are indications of the degree of rib cage inward collapse during forceful diaphragmatic contraction.[86] This increase in the work of breathing can lead to fatigue and eventually apnea.

Chest wall compliance combined with lung compliance affects the closing volume, closing capacity, expiratory reserve volume, and functional residual capacity. For the neonate this means a high closing volume and capacity combined with a low expiratory reserve volume and low functional residual capacity—and a propensity toward lung collapse.[67]

MECHANICAL PROPERTIES OF THE RESPIRATORY SYSTEM
Lung Compliance

The pressure gradient necessary to overcome the elastic recoil force in the lung depends on tidal volume and lung compliance. Compliance is the measurement of the elastic properties opposing a change in volume and change in volume (ml) per unit of change in pressure (cm H_2O) (Hooke's law). This can be demonstrated in a curve that relates lung volume to the change in the alveolar-to-intrapleural pressure gradient (transpulmonary pressure). The slope of the curve is the compliance. The flatter the curve, the stiffer the lung.[86] (See Chapter 2, Figure 3.)

Lung compliance depends on the tissue elastic characteristics of the parenchyma, connective tissue, and blood vessels as well as the surface tension in the alveoli and the initial lung volume before inflation. When the lung must be inflated from a very low volume, the required pressure gradient is greater.

Lung compliance in the healthy preterm infant is similar to that in the term infant. The change in lung compliance is sensed by the stretch receptors of the lung. Coupled with the muscle spindle fibers from the respiratory muscles, information is transmitted to the respiratory center in order to modify the drive necessary to maintain ventilation. Lung disease usually leads to a decrease in lung compliance, which translates to a reduced volume change for a given pressure change.

The most significant determinant of elastic properties is the air-liquid interface. When molecules are aligned at an air-liquid interface, they lack opposing molecules on one side. This means the intermolecular attractive forces are unbalanced, and the molecules tend to move away from the interface. This reduces the internal surface area of the lung and augments elastic recoil.

Surfactant varies surface tension, allowing for high surface tensions at large lung volumes and low tensions at low volumes. Surfactant forms an insoluble folded surface film upon compression and thereby lowers surface tension. This tends to stabilize air spaces of unequal size and prevent their collapse. Without surfactant, the smaller alveoli tend to empty into the larger ones, resulting in microatelectasis alternating with hyperareation.

Alveolar collapse occurs in a number of diseases, the most notable being respiratory distress syndrome. In this condition, surfactant deficiency is directly related to developmental immaturity of the lungs and gestational age. Surfactant synthesis also depends on normal pH and pulmonary perfusion. Therefore, any disease or event that interferes with these processes (such as asphyxia, hemorrhagic shock, or pulmonary edema) may lead to surfactant deficiencies.[2,88,89]

Lung Resistance

Lung resistance depends on the (1) size and geometric arrangements of the airways, (2) viscous resistance of the lung tissue, and (3) proportion of laminar to turbulent airflow. Resistance varies inversely with lung volume—that is, the greater the lung volume the less resistance, and vice versa. This is because airway diameter increases with the expansion of the parenchyma.

In neonates and children less than five years of age, the peripheral airways contribute most to airway resistance. This is secondary to the decreased diameter of airways, especially in the periphery. The distal airway growth in diameter and length lags behind proximal growth during the first five years of life. Therefore, a small decrement in airway caliber can lead to a very large increase in peripheral airway resistance.[90] This is seen in the early onset of clinical signs when disease is encountered in the neonate.

Resistance increases with decreasing gestational age and with specific lung diseases that are more prominent in low-birthweight infants (such as respiratory distress syndrome and bronchopulmnary dysplasia [BPD]). The increased resistance is sensed by respiratory muscles, which leads to an increase in ventilatory drive. In the infant with BPD, this may lead to a change in pleural pressure to as much as 20–30 cm H_2O pressure. Changes in the caliber of the larynx or trachea because of edema (e.g., in infants who have repeated intubation for meconium aspiration) or as a result of intubation also increase resistance. This effect may be quite pronounced because the resistance is generated in the large airways, where resistance should be lowest.

Time Constants

A time constant measures the product of lung resistance and compliance and is the time needed for a given lung unit to fill to 63 percent of its final capacity. The alveoli with shorter time constants fill faster than those with longer time constants. Nichols and Rogers observe that if the resistance and compliance are equal in two adjacent lung units, the time constant will be the same, and there will be no redistribution of gases between the alveoli.[86] If the time constant of one unit is longer but the compliances remain equal, the two alveoli will eventually reach the same volume. The longer the time constant, however, the slower the filling will be because of increased resistance.

The time constant can also be lengthened when compliance is increased but resistance remains the same. In this circumstance, the less compliant alveoli will fill faster than its adjacent, more compliant neighbor. This is due to the decreased volume of the alveoli that is less compliant. Redistribution of gas will occur if inflation is interrupted prematurely because of the increased pressure in the less compliant alveoli as compared to the adjacent lung unit.[86]

This redistribution of gases in the lung is not a major factor in the normal lung, in that the alveoli are relatively stable and do not change much in size because of the effect of surfactant upon the lung.[86]

VENTILATION

Dead Space Ventilation

A variable portion of each breath is not involved in gas exchange and is therefore wasted: This is considered "dead space ventilation." There are two types of dead space: (1) Anatomic dead space is that volume of gas within the conducting airways that cannot engage in gas exchange. (2) Alveolar dead space is the volume of inspired gas that reaches the alveoli but does not participate in gas exchange because of inadequate perfusion to that alveoli. The total (anatomic plus alveolar) dead space is termed physiologic dead space. Physiologic dead space is usually expressed as a fraction of the tidal volume, approximately 0.3 in infants and adults.[91] Patients experiencing respiratory failure have elevated dead space to tidal volume ratios, which result in hypoxia and hypercarbia unless counteracted by an increase in the amount of air expired per minute.[86]

Pleural Pressure

The differences in pleural pressure within the lung play a significant role in determining the distribution of gases. During spontaneous breathing, a greater proportion of gas is distributed to the dependent regions of the lung.[92] It is assumed that subatmospheric (negative) intrapleural pressure at the base versus the apex is the reason for this distribution pattern. Interestingly, alveolar pressure remains constant in all regions of the lung. Subse-

FIGURE 7 ▲ Effect of changes in pleural pressure in the lung

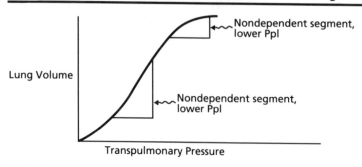

From: Nichols DG, and Rogers MC: Developmental physiology of the respiratory system, *in* Rogers MC, ed., Textbook of Pediatric Intensive Care, vol. 1, Baltimore, Williams & Wilkins, 1987, p. 88. Reprinted with permission.

quently, the transpulmonary distending pressure in the dependent regions is decreased, leading to a reduced lung volume in these areas. As Nichols and Rogers point out, the smaller alveoli in the dependent lung regions lie on the steeper slope of the transpulmonary pressure-to-lung volume curve (Figure 7), resulting in a greater portion of the tidal volume being directed to the dependent alveoli during normal breathing.[86] A greater portion of the pulmonary perfusion goes to the dependent regions as well, thereby matching ventilation and perfusion more closely.

Pleural pressure increases from the apex to the base of the lung, so alveoli become smaller at the base. Smaller alveoli are on the steep portion of the pressure-volume (compliance) curve; thus a given change in transpulmonary pressure produces a greater increase in volume in the smaller alveoli.

Closing Capacity

During quiet breathing in the neonate (especially the preterm infant), it is possible for lung volumes to be reduced below FRC, with dependent regions of the lung being closed to the main bronchi (closing capacity). When the closing capacity exceeds the FRC, the ventilation-to-perfusion ratio drops, and hypoxia and hypercarbia can be seen. If total atelectasis ("white out") exists,

then closing capacity exceeds not only FRC but also tidal volume, and these portions of the lung are closed during expiration and inspiration. The use of end-expiratory pressure in the form of positive end-expiratory pressure or continuous distending pressure (CDP) is designed to raise FRC above closing capacity.[86] This is used in the neonatal population when chest wall compliance leads to marked distortion and altered lung volumes as well as during disease states associated with alveolar collapse (such as respiratory distress syndrome).

The greater closing capacity seen in children under 6 years of age and in adults over 40 is probably due to decreased elastic recoil in the lung.[89,93] Elastic recoil is the property that allows the lung to retract away from the chest wall, creating a subatmospheric pressure in the intrapleural space. The decrease in elastic recoil leads to an increase in subatmospheric pressure in the intrapleural spaces and airway closure in dependent regions.[86]

LUNG VOLUMES
Functional Residual Capacity

Functional residual capacity is established during the first breaths, forming the alveolar reservoir at end expiration, allowing for continuous gas exchange between respiratory efforts, and stabilizing PaO_2. FRC normally comprises 30–40 percent of the total capacity of the lung and may change in volume from breath to breath.

Immediately following birth, FRC is low, but it increases rapidly with successive breaths. In preterm infants, FRC will stay low until lung disease resolves. The goal is to keep FRC above the passive resting volume of the lung (reached after a totally relaxed expiration). The neonate's pliable chest wall, which lends itself to a low FRC, makes this difficult.

FRC's role in the energy expenditure of the respiratory musculature is crucial. It minimizes the work of breathing while optimizing system compliance and maintaining a gas reservoir during expiration.[59]

Perfusion

Alveolar ventilation is dependent upon the airways and pulmonary vasculature. Pulmonary vascular muscle thickness is a function of gestational age, the preterm infant having less well developed smooth muscle. This incomplete development results in a drop in pulmonary vascular resistance much sooner after delivery, predisposing the preterm infant to a faster onset of congestive heart failure and left-to-right shunting.[86] This relatively rapid reduction in pulmonary vascular resistance, combined with the potential for fluid overload, can result in the opening of extrapulmonary shunts, leading to hypoxia and further respiratory deterioration.

Pulmonary Blood Volume

Posture seems to be the major determinant of pulmonary blood volume. In the supine position, pulmonary blood volume is increased secondary to the shift of blood from dependent portions of the body to the central circulation.[86] This may be a transient shift, with return to baseline after a prolonged period of time.[94] Whether this holds true in the infant is unclear; effects of supine positioning in the preterm have not been explored.

Vascular Pressures and Resistance

There are three categories of intravascular pressure associated with the pulmonary circulation: pulmonary artery pressure, perfusion pressure, and transmural pressure. The interaction and relationships between these pressures affect the flow of blood in the lung and are implicated in the distribution of that blood flow.

Pulmonary artery pressure measures the systolic, diastolic, and mean arterial pressures in the pulmonary artery in reference to atmo-spheric pressure at the level of the heart. After birth, the pulmonary artery pressure falls with lung inflation.[95] However, adult pressures are not achieved until several months have passed. Normal systolic, diastolic, and mean pressures in the adult are 22, 8, and 15.[67,86]

Transmural pressure is the difference between the pressures inside and outside the vessel. This is measured differently, depending on the level of the measurement: At upper levels, it is the gradient between pulmonary artery pressure and pleural pressure; at the pulmonary capillaries, it is the difference between pleural pressure and alveolar pressure.[96]

Capillary transmural pressure provides the hydrostatic pressure that tends to force fluid out of the capillaries into the pulmonary interstitium. This is counterbalanced by oncotic pressure forces. The greater the capillary transmural pressure, the more distended the vessel, the greater the flow.

Perfusion pressure is the pressure gradient between two points in the circulation (downward flow). This cascade is needed for blood to flow appropriately. In the pulmonary circulation, this is measured as the difference between pulmonary artery pressure and left atrial pressure.

Perfusion pressure divided by pulmonary blood flow provides a calculated value for pulmonary vascular resistance. An increase in flow, as occurs with activity, produces a drop in pulmonary vascular resistance secondary to the recruitment of additional pulmonary capillaries.[97,98]

Normal Pulmonary Blood Flow

The majority of pulmonary blood flow is distributed to the dependent regions of the lungs because of gravitational forces. In zone 1 (apex of the lung), the alveolar pressure is greater than the pulmonary artery and venous pressures. As a result , the pulmonary vessels collapse, and there is concomitant loss of gas exchange and wasted ventilation.[99]

In zone 2 (middle of the lung), pulmonary artery pressure exceeds alveolar pressure, and blood flow resumes. The perfusion pressure increases as blood flows downward, which results in a linear increase in blood flow. Slowing of blood occurs when the pulmonary venous and alveolar pressures are equal.[99]

In zone 3 (base of the lung), pulmonary venous and pulmonary artery pressures increase, exceeding alveolar pressure. In the more dependent regions of this zone, the transmural pressure increases (with resultant dilation of the vessels), and blood flow increases.[99]

Posture differences between the upright adult and supine-lying infant probably explain pulmonary blood distribution in the infant, but this has not been explicated. The general principles probably still apply but perhaps to a lesser extent. Wasted ventilation in the apices due to lack of perfusion is probably much less likely in the supine position, helping to balance some of the limitations of the neonatal lung.

Abnormal Distribution of Pulmonary Blood Flow

Numerous factors may influence the distribution of pulmonary blood flow in the lung. One of the most significant for the neonate is hypoxia. Vasoconstriction results from alveolar hypoxia. If diffuse, hypoxia may result in an increase in intravascular pulmonary artery pressure, which is more intense in infants than adults.[89,100]

Ventilation-Perfusion Matching

Efficient gas exchange in the lungs requires matching pulmonary ventilation and perfusion. Mismatching of them is the most common reason for hypoxia and a frequent result of the neonatal respiratory system liabilities. The interaction between ventilation and perfusion is expressed as a ratio and reflects the relationship between alveolar ventilation and capillary perfusion for the lung as a whole.

Air space ventilation should be adequate to remove the carbon dioxide delivered to it from the blood, and air space perfusion should be no greater than that which allows oxygenation and complete saturation of the blood in its brief passage through the alveolar capillaries. Ideal efficiency would occur if ventilation were perfectly matched to perfusion, yielding a ratio of 1.

In the healthy adult, capillary blood spends 0.75 seconds in the alveolus, and oxygen-carbon dioxide exchange occurs across the 0.5 micron alveolar-capillary membrane. As the blood leaves the alveolus, the blood gas tensions are identical with those of the alveolar gas. The gas tensions achieved at equilibrium are dependent upon the following factors:[101–104]

1. ventilation rate
2. membrane thickness
3. membrane area
4. capillary blood flow
5. venous gas tensions
6. inspired gas tensions

The ability to achieve equilibrium rapidly depends on the area of exchange being large enough to allow the blood to be spread thinly over the vessel wall and the blood and gas being actively mixed together.[101]

Matching of ventilation to perfusion depends largely on gravity. Both ventilation and perfusion increase with further distance down the lung, perfusion increasing more than ventilation. The right ventricular pressure is inadequate to fully perfuse lung apices. Lung weight leads to a relatively greater negative intrapleural pressure at the apex than at the base. "Therefore, apical alveoli are better expanded and receive a smaller portion of each tidal volume than those at the bases."[102] Along with this, there is reduced perfusion in the apices, creating a high ventilation-to-perfusion ratio $(\dot{V}_A/\dot{Q}_C)$.[87,104]

A ventilation-to-perfusion ratio of zero indicates a shunt. In this situation, no ventilation takes place during the passage of blood through the lungs. The pulmonary capillary blood would arrive in the left atrium with the same gas tensions it had when it was mixed with venous blood. Examples of shunts include the perfusion of an atelectatic area, venoarterial shunts, the right-to-left heart shunts seen in patients with cyanotic congenital heart disease, and right-to-left shunts secondary to persistant pulmonary hypertension of the newborn.

High $\dot{V}_A/\dot{Q}_C$ ratios are the result of increased dead space and occur if the blood is spread in an extremely thin film over a very large surface area or if blood is vigorously mixed with large volumes of air. In these circumstances, equilibration occurs, but a large amount of ventilation is required.[101] There is wasted ventilation either in anatomical conducting airways and/or poorly perfused alveoli (alveolar dead space). Thus a large amount of ventilation is wasted on a relatively small amount of blood without significantly changing the oxygen content. This inefficient gas exchange will eventually result in carbon dioxide retention.

Alveolar under ventilation will result in low $\dot{V}_A/\dot{Q}_C$ ratios. In this situation, ventilation is low in relation to perfusion but not entirely absent. This is the normal state for the lung bases in an erect position. It is also found in persons with disease in which airway obstruction reduces ventilation-to-alveolar units (such as asthma or cystic fibrosis).

The blood perfusing the under ventilated alveoli is not completely oxygenated, and a smaller amount of carbon dioxide is removed. These partial venoarterial shunts contribute this blood to the arterial stream (this is termed venous admixture). This is reflected in an elevated $PaCO_2$ and decreased PaO_2.

Abnormalities of $\dot{V}_A/\dot{Q}_C$ may be secondary to (1) too much or too little ventilation to an area with blood flow being normal, (2) too much or too little blood flow with ventilation being normal, or (3) some combination of the two. Whatever occurs, the lung's regulatory mechanisms work to achieve and maintain the ideal. In areas where $\dot{V}_A/\dot{Q}_C$ is high and carbon dioxide levels are low, local airway constric-

tion reduces the amount of ventilation going to the area. When the opposite occurs, the airways dilate to increase ventilation to the area and improve carbon dioxide exchange. Where oxygenation is also affected and low alveolar oxygen concentrations are found, the lung reduces blood flow to the region. These mechanisms are finite, however.

In the newborn, most of the ventilated areas are well perfused, and there is little dead space. But significant amounts of perfusion are wasted on unexpanded air spaces (intrapulmonary shunts). The newborn's lower PaO_2 demonstrates the widened alveolar-to-arterial oxygen tension gradient, reflecting the increased venous admixture. Although perfusion of unexpanded air spaces may play a significant role in venous admixture, the continued right-to-left shunting through transitional circulatory circuits contributes to the situation. Because of developmental immaturity, the premature infant is at even greater risk for shunting and venous admixture.[105,106]

Shunting and wasted ventilation are normal features of the newborn lung, the latter resulting from the transition from fluid-filled to air-filled lungs, where alveoli are underventilated but normally perfused. These effects begin to dissipate after one or two hours of air breathing. During the first few days of life, the neonatal lung has a greater shunt component and a larger proportion of low $\dot{V}_A/\dot{Q}_C$ areas when compared to the adult lung, although tidal volume, alveolar volume, and dead space volume/breath are similar (when expressed in ml/kg).

SUMMARY

Although the newborn's respiratory system is not fully developed at birth, he does demonstrate capabilities and strategies to achieve sustained respirations. Beyond this, he is capable of achieving gas tension and acid-base homeostasis and of employing compensatory mechanisms to maintain that balance in disease states.

Transition must be seen as an event that takes several days to achieve, with initial responses being aligned with the fetal state. Knowledge of these differences and the progression toward extrauterine stability can guide therapeutic interventions and determine clinical assessment.

Recognizing that the infant has prepared throughout his gestation for this transition can provide us with an appreciation of the accomplishment. The respiratory muscles have exercised and trained to take over the function of the respiratory pump itself, although fatigue may develop quite quickly. Intercostal muscles can stabilize the chest wall, so effective ventilation can be achieved.

Difficulties arise when disease or immaturity are encountered. There is little reserve to increase ventilatory efforts. Sustaining increased respiratory activity may also be limited. The ability to recruit accessory muscles, the use of laryngeal braking (grunting), and the recruitment of new alveoli help improve gas exchange and increase the pulmonary surface area.[59]

For those infants greater than 28 weeks gestation, these mechanisms may be employable, though to what degree and efficiency we do not know. Each infant responds uniquely to the process of transition and to pathology. The development of refined clinical skills and further research may give us more clues as to when and how the respiratory system prepares for and achieves its sustained activity.

REFERENCES

1. Reid LM: Structural development of the lung and pulmonary circulation, *in* Ravio K, et al., eds., Respiratory Distress Syndrome, London, 1984, Academic Press, pp. 1–18.

2. Bucher U, and Reid L: Development of the intrasegmental bronchial tree: The pattern of branching and development of cartilage at various stages of intra-uterine life, Thorax 16, 1961, pp. 207–218.

3. Emery JL: The postnatal development of the human lung and its implications for lung pathology, Respiration (supplement) 27, 1970, pp. 41–50.

4. Inselman LS, and Mellins RB: Growth and development of the lung, Journal of Pediatrics 98, 1981, pp. 1–15.

5. Wessels NK: Tissue Interactions and Development, Menlo Park, California, 1977, Benjamin Cummings.

6. Hallman M: Development of pulmonary surfactant, *in* Ravio K, et al., eds., Respiratory Distress Syndrome, London, 1984, Academic Press, pp. 33–50.

7. Meyrick B, and Reid LM: Ultrastructure of alveolar lining and its development, *in* Hodson WA, ed., Development of the Lung, New York, 1977, Marcel Dekker, pp. 135–214.

8. Bryan AC, and Bryan MH: Control of respiration in the newborn, Clinics in Perinatology 5, 1978, pp. 269–281.

9. Thurlbeck WM: Postnatal growth and development of the lung, American Review of Respiratory Diseases 111, 1975, pp. 803–844.

10. Bleasdale JE, and Johnston JM: Developmental biochemistry of lung surfactant, *in* Nelson GH, ed., Pulmonary Development: Transition from Intrauterine to Extrauterine Life, New York, 1985, Marcel Dekker, pp. 47–73.

11. Farrell PM, and Ulane RE: The regulation of lung phospholipid metabolisms, *in* Monset-Couchard M, and Minkowski A, eds., Physiological and Biochemical Basis for Perinatal Medicine, New York, 1981, S. Karger, pp. 11–31.

12. Milner AD, Saunders RA, and Hopkin IE: Effects of delivery by caesarean section on lung mechanics and lung volume in the human neonate, Archives of Disease in Childhood 53, 1978, pp. 545–548.

13. Smith BT: Biochemistry and metabolism of pulmonary surface-active material, *in* The Surfactant System and the Neonatal Lung, Mead Johnson Symposium on Perinatal and Developmental Medicine, No. 14, Evansville, Indiana, 1979, Mead Johnson, pp. 12–16.

14. Van Golde LMG: Metabolism of phospholipids in the lung, American Review of Respiratory Disease 114, 1976, pp. 977–1000.

15. Liggins GC: Premature delivery of fetal lambs infused with glucocorticoids, Endocrinology 45, 1969, pp. 515–523.

16. Kresch MJ, and Gross I: The biochemistry of fetal lung development, Clinics in Perinatology 14, 1987, pp. 481–507.

17. Ballard PL: Hormonal regulation of the surfactant system, *in* Monset-Couchard M, and Mikowski A, eds., Physiological and Biochemical Basis for Perinatal Medicine, New York, 1981, S. Karger, pp. 42–53.

18. Hitchcock KR: Hormones and the lung: I, Thyroid hormones and glucocorticoids in lung development, Anatomical Record 194, 1979, pp. 15–40.

19. Kitterman JA, et al.: Prepartum maturation of the lung in fetal sheep: Relation to cortisol, Journal of Applied Physiology 51, 1981, pp. 384–390.

20. Brehier A, et al.: Corticosteroid induction of phosphatidic acid phospatase in fetal rabbit lung, Biochemical and Biophysiology Research and Communication 77, 1977, pp. 883–890.

21. Pope TS, and Tooney SA: Effects of glucocorticoid and thyroid hormones on regulatory enzymes of fatty acid synthesis and glycogen metabolism in developing fetal rat lung, Biochemical Biophysica Acta 918, 1987, pp. 141–148.

22. Rooney SA, et al.: Glucocorticoid stimulation of cholinephosphate cytidyltransferace activity in fetal rat lung: Receptor-response relationships, Biochemica Biophysica Acta 888, 1986, pp. 208–216.

23. Ballard PL, et al.: Transplacental stimulation of lung development in the fetal rabbit by 3, 5 dimethyl-3-iso-propyl-L-thyronine, Journal of Clinical Investigation 65, 1980, pp. 1407–1417.

24. Whisett JA, et al.: Induction of surfactant protein in fetal lung: Effects of cAMP and dexamethasone on SAP-35 RNA and synthesis, Journal of Biological Chemistry 262, 1987, pp. 5256–5261.

25. Fiascone J, et al.: Differential effect of betamethasone on alveolar surfactant and lung tissue of fetal rabbits, Pediatric Research 20, 1986, p. 428A.

26. Smith BT: Lung maturation in the fetal rat: Acceleration by injection of fibroblast-pneumocyte factor, Science 204, 1979, pp. 1094–1095.

27. Gonzales LW: Glucocorticoids and thyroid hormone stimulate biochemical and morphological differentiation of human fetal lung in organ culture, Journal of Clinical Endocrinology and Metabolism 62, 1986, pp. 678–691.

28. Gross I, and Wilson CM: Fetal lung in organ culture: IV, Supra-addictive hormone interactions, Journal of Applied Physiology 52, 1982, pp. 1420–1425.

29. Ballard PL, et al.: Human pulmonary surfactant apoprotein: Effects of development; culture and hormones on the protein and its mRNA, Pediatric Research 20, 1986, p. 422A.

30. Pope TS, and Rooney SA: Opposing effects of glucocorticoid and thyroid hormones on the fatty acid synthatase activity in culture fetal rat lung, Federal Proceedings 46, 1987, p. 2005.

31. Cuestas RA, Lindall A, and Engel RR: Low thyroid hormones and respiratory distress syndrome of the newborn: Studies on cord blood, New England Journal of Medicine 295, 1976, pp. 297–302.

32. Ballard PL, Hovey ML, and Gonzales LK: Thyroid hormone stimulation of phosphatidylcholine synthesis in cultured fetal rabbit lung, Journal of Clinical Investigation 74, 1981, pp. 898–905.

33. Rooney SA, et al.: Thyrotropin-releasing hormone increases the amount of surfactant in lung lavage from fetal rabbits, Pediatric Research 13, 1979, pp. 623–625.

34. Dobbs LG, and Mason RJ: Pulmonary alveolar Type II cells isolated from rats: Release of phosphatidylcholine in response to beta-adrenergic stimulation, Journal of Clinical Investigation 63, 1979, pp. 378–387.

35. Corbet AJ, et al.: Effect of aminophylline and dexamethasone on secretion of pulmonary surfactant in fetal rabbits, Pediatric Research 12, 1978, pp. 797–799.

36. Hayden W, Olson EB, and Zachman R: Effect of maternal isoxsuprine on fetal rabbit lung biochemical maturation, American Journal of Obstetrics and Gynecology 129, 1977, pp. 691–694.

37. Walters DV, and Over RE: The role of catecholamines in lung liquid absorption at birth, Pediatric Research 12, 1978, pp. 239–242.

38. Smith BT: Insulin antagonism of cortisol action on lecithin synthesis by cultured fetal lung cells, Journal of Pediatrics 87, 1975, pp. 953–955.

39. Gross I, et al.: The influence of hormones on the biochemical maturation of fetal rat lung in organ culture: II, Insulin, Pediatric Research 14, 1980, pp. 834–838.

40. Mendelson CR, et al.: Multihormonal regulation of surfactant synthesis by human fetal lung *in vitro*, Journal of Clinical Endocrinology and Metabolism 53, 1981, pp. 307–317.

41. Gewolb IH, et al.: Delay in pulmonary glycogen degradation in fetuses of streptozotocin diabetic rats, Pediatric Research 16, 1982, pp. 869–873.

42. Sosenko IRS, Hartig-Beecken I, and Frantz ID: Cortisol reversal of functional delay of lung maturation in fetuses of diabetic rabbits, Journal of Applied Physiology 49, 1980, pp. 971–974.

43. Agostoni E: Volume pressure relationships of the thorax and lung in the newborn, Journal of Applied Physiology 14, 1959, pp. 909–913.

44. Harned HS: Respiration and the respiratory system, *in* Stave U, ed., Perinatal Physiology, New York, 1978, Plenum, pp. 53–101.

45. Hislop A, and Reid LM: Formation of the pulmonary vasculature, *in* Hodson WA, ed., Development of the Lung, New York, 1977, Marcel Dekker, pp. 37–86.

46. Strang LB: Uptake of liquid from the lungs at the start of breathing, *in* DeReuck AVS, and Porter R, eds., Ciba Foundation Symposium: Development of the Lung, London, 1967, J.A. Churchill, pp. 348–391.

47. Milner AD, and Vyas H: Lung expansion at birth, Journal of Pediatrics 101, 1982, pp. 879–886.

48. Mescher EJ, et al.: Ontogeny of tracheal fluid, pulmonary surfactant, and plasma corticoids in the fetal lamb, Journal of Applied Physiology 39, 1975, pp. 1020–1021.

49. Strang LB: Pulmonary circulation at birth, *in* Neonatal Respiration, Physiological and Clinical Studies, Oxford, 1977, Blackwell Scientific Publications, pp. 111–137.

50. Burgess WR, and Chernick V: Respiratory Therapy in Newborn Infants and Children, New York, 1982, Thieme-Stratton.

51. Alcorn D, et al.: Morphological effects of chronic tracheal ligation and drainage in fetal lamb lung, Journal of Anatomy 123, 1977, pp. 649–660.

52. Perlman M, Williams J, and Hirsch M: Neonatal pulmonary hypoplasia after prolonged leakage of amniotic fluid, Archives of Disease in Childhood 51, 1976, pp. 349–353.

53. Weibel ER, and Gil J: Structure-function relationships at the alveolar level, *in* West JB, ed., Bioengineering Aspects of the Lung, New York, 1977, Marcel Dekker, pp. 1–81.

54. Zapletal A, Paul T, and Samanek M: Pulmonary elasticity in children and adolescents, Journal of Applied Physiology 40, 1976, pp. 953–955.

55. Avery ME, Fletcher BD, and Williams·RG: The Lung and its Disorders in the Newborn Infant, Philadelphia, 1981, W.B. Saunders.

56. Liggins GC, and Kitterman JA: Development of the fetal lung, *in* The Fetus and Independent Life, Ciba Foundation Symposium, London, 1981, Pitman, pp. 308–330.

57. Marchal F: Neonatal apnea, *in* Stern L, and Vert P, eds., Neonatal Medicine, New York, 1987, Masson pp. 409–427.

58. Chernick V: Fetal breathing movement and the onset of breathing, Clinics in Perinatology 5, 1978, pp. 257–281.

59. Davis GM, and Bureau MA: Pulmonary and chest wall mechanics in the control of respiration in the newborn, Clinics in Perinatology 14, 1987, pp. 551–579.

60. Mantell CD: Breathing movements in the human fetus, American Journal of Obstetrics and Gynecology 125, 1976, pp. 550–553.

61. Avery ME, and Taeusch WH: Schaffer's Diseases of the Newborn, 5th ed., Philadelphia, 1984, W.B. Saunders.

62. Boddy K, Dawes GS, and Robinson J: Intrauterine fetal breathing movements, *in* Gluck L, ed., Modern Perinatal Medicine, Chicago, 1975, Year Book Medical Publishers, pp. 381–389.

63. Patrick JE, et al.: Human fetal breathing movements and gross body movements at weeks 34–35 gestation, American Journal of Obstetrics and Gynecology 130, 1978, pp. 693–699.

64. Patrick J: Measurement of human fetal breathing movements, Mead Johnson Symposium on Perinatal and Developmental Medicine, No. 12, Evansville, Indiana, 1977, Mead Johnson.

65. Kitterman J, and Liggins GC: Fetal breathing movements and inhibitors of prostaglandin synthesis, Seminars in Perinatology 4, 1980, pp. 97–100.

66. Milner AD, Saunders RA, and Hopkin IE: Effects of delivery by caesarean section on lung mechanics and lung volume in the human neonate, Archives of Disease in Childhood 53, 1978, pp. 545–548.

67. Nelson NM: Respiration and circulation after birth, *in* Smith CA, and Nelson NM, eds., The Physiology of the Newborn Infant, Springfield, Illinois, 1976, Charles C. Thomas, pp. 117–262.

68. Karlberg P: The adaptive changes in the immediate postnatal period, with particular reference to respiration, Journal of Pediatrics 56, 1960, pp. 585–589.

69. Jaykka S: A new theory concerning the mechanism of the initiation of respiration in the newborn, Acta Paediatrica Scandinavica 43, 1954, pp. 399–410.

70. Gruenwald P: Normal and abnormal expansion of the lungs of newborn infants obtained at autopsy, Laboratory Investigation 12, 1963, pp. 563–567.

71. Karlberg P, et al.: Respiratory studies in newborn infants: II, Pulmonary ventilation and mechanics of breathing in the first minutes of life, including the onset of respiration, Acta Paediatrica Scandanavica 51, 1962, pp. 121–136.

72. Klaus M, et al.: Alveolar epithelial cell mitochondria as a source of the surface-active lung lining, Science 137, 1962, pp. 750–751.

73. Haworth SG, and Hislop AA: Normal structural and functional adaptation to extrauterine life, Journal of Pediatrics 98, 1981, pp. 915–918.

74. Strang LB: Neonatal Respiration: Physiological and Clinical Studies, London, 1978, Mosby.

75. Blanco CE, Hanson MA, and McCooke HB: Studies *in utero* of the mechanisms of chemoreceptor resetting, *in* Jones CT, and Nathanielsz PW, eds., The Physiologic Development of the Fetus and the Newborn, London, 1985, Academic Press, pp. 639–642.

76. Bureau MA: Postnatal maturation of the respiratory response to O_2 in awake newborn lambs, Journal of Applied Physiology 52, 1985, pp. 428–433.

77. Girard F, Lacaisse A, and Dejours P: Le stimulus O_2 ventilatoire a la periode neonatale chez l'homme, Journal of Physiology, Paris 52, 1960, pp. 108–109.

78. Albersheim S, et al.: Effect of CO_2 on the immediate response to O_2 in preterm infants, Journal of Applied Physiology 41, 1976, pp. 609–611.

79. Davis GM, and Bureau MA: Pulmonary and chest wall mechanics in the control of respiration in the newborn, Clinics in Perinatology 14, 1987, pp. 551–579.

80. Guthrie RD, et al.: Development of CO_2 sensitivity: Effects of gestational age, postnatal age, and sleep state, Journal of Applied Physiology 50, 1981, pp. 956–961.

81. Widdicombe JG: Nervous receptors in the respiratory tract, *in* Hornbein TF, ed., Regulation of Breathing: Part I, New York, 1981, Marcel Dekker, pp. 429–472.

82. Escobedo MB: Fetal and neonatal cardiopulmonary physiology, *in* Schreiner RL, and Kisling JA, eds., Practical Neonatal Respiratory Care, New York, 1982, Raven Press, pp. 1–18.

83. Keens DH, and Ianuzzo CD: Development of fatigue-resistant muscle fibers in human ventilatory musculature, American Review of Respiratory Diseases (supplement) 119, 1979, pp. 139–141.

84. Thach BT, and Taeusch HW: Sighing in newborn human infants: Role of the augmenting reflex, Journal of Applied Physiology 41, 1976, pp. 502–507.

85. Avery ME, and Cook CD: Volume pressure relationship of lungs and thorax in fetal, neonatal, and adult goats, Journal of Applied Physiology 16, 1961, pp. 1034–1038.

86. Nichols DG, and Rogers MC: Developmental physiology of the respiratory system, *in* Rogers MC, ed., Textbook of Pediatric Intensive Care, vol. 1, Baltimore, 1987, Williams & Wilkins, pp. 83–111.

87. Bryan AC, Mansaell AL, and Levinson H: Development of the mechanical properties of the respiratory system, *in* Hodson WA, ed., Development of the Lung, New York, 1976, Dekker, pp. 445–468.

88. Henry JN: The effect of shock on pulmonary alveolar surfactant, Journal of Trauma 8, 1968, pp. 756–773.

89. Said SI, et al.: Pulmonary surface activity in induced pulmonary edema, Journal of Clinical Investigation 44, 1965, pp. 458–464.

90. Hogg JC, et al.: Age as a factor in the distribution of lower airway conductance and in the pathologic anatomy of obstructive lung disease, New England Journal of Medicine 282, 1970, pp. 1283–1287.

91. Polgar G, and Weng TR: The functional development of the respiratory system, American Review of Respiratory Diseases 120, 1979, pp. 625–695.

92. Rehder K, et al.: Ventilation-perfusion relationship in young healthy awake and anesthetized-paralyzed man, Journal of Applied Physiology 47, 1979, pp. 745–753.

93. Mansell A, Bryan C, and Levinson H: Airway closure in children, Journal of Applied Physiology 33, 1972, pp. 711–714.

94. Hirasuna JD, and Gorin AB: Effect of prolonged recumbency on pulmonary blood volume in normal humans, Journal of Applied Physiology 50, 1981, pp. 950–955.

95. Dawes GS, et al.: Changes in the lung of the newborn lamb, Journal of Physiology 121, 1953, pp. 141–147.

96. Boyden EA: Development and growth of the airways, *in* Hodson WA, ed., Development of the Lung, New York, 1977, Dekker, pp. 3–35.

97. Robotham JL: A physiologic assessment of segmental bronchial atresia, American Review of Respiratory Disease 121, 1980, pp. 533–540.

98. Macklem PT: Airway obstruction and collateral ventilation, Physiological Reviews 51, 1971, pp. 368–436.

99. West JB, Dollery CT, and Naimark A: Distribution of blood flow in isolated lung: Relation to vascular and alveolar pressures, Journal of Applied Physiology 19, 1964, pp. 713–724.

100. James LS, and Rowe RD: The pattern of response of pulmonary and systemic arterial pressures in newborn and older infants to short periods of hypoxia, Journal of Pediatrics 51, 1957, pp. 5–14.

101. Marshall BE, and Marshall C: Continuity of response to hypoxic pulmonary vasoconstriction, Journal of Applied Physiology 49, 1980, pp. 189–196.

102. Krauss RV: Ventilation-perfusion relationship in neonates, *in* Thibealut DW, and Gregory GA, eds., Neonatal Pulmonary Care, Menlo Park, California, 1979, Addison-Wesley, pp. 54–69.

103. Farhi LE: Ventilation-perfusion relationship and its role in alveolar gas exchange, *in* Caro CG, ed., Recent Advances in Respiratory Physiology, Baltimore, 1966, Williams & Wilkins, pp. 148–197.

104. West JB: Regional differences in blood flow and ventilation in the lung, *in* Caro CG, ed., Recent Advances in Respiratory Physiology, Baltimore, 1966, Williams & Wilkins, pp. 198–254.

105. West JB: Ventilation, Blood Flow, and Gas Exchange, 2nd ed., Oxford, 1970, Blackwell Scientific Publications.

106. Koch G, and Wendel H: Adjustment of arterial blood gases and acid base balance in the normal newborn infant during the first week of life, Biology of the Neonate 12, 1968, pp. 136–141.

2 Pathophysiology of Acute Respiratory Distress

Susan Orlando, RNC, MS
Ochsner Foundation Hospital
New Orleans, Louisiana

Neonatal respiratory disorders account for the majority of admissions to intensive care units and result in significant morbidity and mortality. Considering the complex series of cardiorespiratory changes that occur at birth, it is not surprising that the transition to extrauterine life does not always proceed smoothly.

Once the infant shows signs of respiratory distress, prompt diagnosis is essential. Respiratory distress may be related to structural problems, such as poor lung development, or chest wall or diaphragmatic defects. Biochemical and physical immaturity may exist. Abnormalities in the central nervous system may cause alterations in the respiratory regulatory apparatus. Perfusion abnormalities may impair gas exchange. Aspiration and infection can also occur.

Not all infants with respiratory distress have a respiratory disease (Table 1). In some cases, congenital heart disease may be difficult to distinguish from primary lung disease. Labored breathing may result from a metabolic problem. The coexistence of other factors, such as cold stress and polycythemia, may compound respiratory distress.

Most neonatal respiratory problems are treated medically, but surgical intervention may be required for a number of conditions that pre-

TABLE 1 ▲ Differential Diagnosis of Respiratory Distress in the Newborn Period

Presentation with ± cyanosis, ± grunting, ± retractions, ± tachypnea, ± apnea, ± shock, ± lethargy						
Respiratory			**Extrapulmonary**			
Common	*Less Common*	*Rare*	*Heart*	*Metabolic*	*Brain*	*Blood*
Respiratory distress syndrome (hyaline membrane disease)	Pulmonary hemorrhage	Airway obstruction (upper), e.g., choanal atresia	Congenital heart disease	Metabolic acidosis	Hemorrhage	Acute blood loss
Transient tachypnea	Pneumothorax			Hypoglycemia	Edema	Hypovolemia
Meconium aspiration			Patent ductus arteriosus (acquired)	Hypothermia	Drugs	Twin-twin transfusion
				Septicemia	Trauma	
Primary pulmonary hypertension (persistent fetal circulation)	Immature lung syndrome	Space-occupying lesion, e.g., diaphragmatic hernia, lung cysts, etc.			Hyperviscosity	
Pneumonia, especially group B streptococcus		Hypoplasia of the lung				

Modified from: Klaus, MH, Fanaroff, AV, and Martin, RJ: Respiratory Problems. *in* Klaus, MH, and Fanaroff, AV, eds., Care of the High Risk Neonate, Philadelphia, W.B. Saunders Co., 1979; from: Polin RA, and Burg FO: Workbook in Practical Neonatology, Philadelphia, 1983, W.B. Saunders, p. 103. Reprinted with permission.

TABLE 2 ▲ Risk Factors for Development of RDS

Prematurity
Male sex
Maternal diabetes
Perinatal asphyxia
Second-born twin
Familial predisposition
Cesarean section without labor

sent with respiratory distress. Institution of appropriate therapy requires an accurate diagnosis. Knowledge of pathophysiology of neonatal pulmonary diseases is essential to ensure comprehensive management. This chapter discusses the pathophysiology of the most common pulmonary disorders that present as acute respiratory distress in the newborn period.

RESPIRATORY DISTRESS SYNDROME (HYALINE MEMBRANE DISEASE)

Respiratory distress syndrome (hyaline membrane disease, RDS) is the major pulmonary problem occurring in the neonate. This syndrome affects approximately 40,000 infants annually in the United States. Nearly 65 percent of these infants are born at gestational ages of 30 weeks or less.[1] An infant of 37–40 weeks gestational age will rarely develop RDS. The prematurity rate is the major reason RDS remains a major neonatal problem: The frequency of RDS increases inversely with gestational age and primarily affects preterm infants less than 35 weeks of age. However, susceptibility to RDS appears to depend more on the neonate's stage of lung maturity than on precise gestational age.

Despite significant advances in understanding the pathophysiology of the disease, RDS remains a major cause of neonatal death. Advances in the development of preventive therapy, such as pharmacologic acceleration of pulmonary maturity, have not significantly impacted the total incidence of RDS among all infants who are at risk. In a national collaborative study testing antenatal steroid treatment, significant reduction in the incidence of RDS

occurred only among singleton female infants. White male infants received no benefit.[2] Most infants with RDS do not die from primary lung disease but from complications directly associated with RDS such as air leak syndrome, intraventricular hemorrhage, pulmonary hemorrhage, and extreme prematurity.[3] Age at death is usually about 72 hours or less, except in some infants who die of complications of the disease later in the neonatal period.[4]

Risk factors known to predispose the neonate to developing RDS are listed in Table 2. Other factors thought to produce a sparing effect or to lessen the severity of the disease in the at-risk population include toxemia, prolonged rupture of the membranes, chronic intrauterine stress leading to fetal growth retardation, and maternal heroin addiction. Stress appears to be the mechanism that accelerates lung maturity in the fetus. Chronic fetal stress increases production of endogenous corticosteroids and results in accelerated lung maturity. Similarly, antenatal administration of glucocorticoids accelerates fetal lung maturity by enhancing surfactant production in some infants.

Clinical Presentation

Infants with RDS develop typical signs of respiratory distress immediately after birth or within the first six hours. The usual presentation includes a combination of grunting, intercostal retractions, cyanosis, nasal flaring, and tachypnea. In the very small infant, the disease usually manifests itself as respiratory failure at birth. The presence of apnea in the early stage of the disease is an ominous sign usually indicative of hypoxemia and respiratory failure; it may also reflect thermal instability or sepsis.

The clinical course is variable in terms of severity. There is usually a pattern of increasing oxygen dependence and poor lung function, which normally peaks during the first 48 to 72 hours and coincides with resumption of surfactant production and diuresis.

Infants with RDS are predisposed to devel-

FIGURE 1 ▲ **AP view of the chest in infant with respiratory distress syndrome (hyaline membrane disease).** Note the reticulogranular appearance of the lung fields and the extension of air bronchograms.

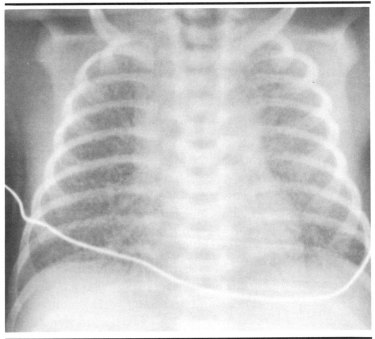

a prolonged recovery phase and ventilator dependency. Surgical intervention becomes necessary for these infants.

Radiographic Findings

The radiologic features of RDS are characteristic (Figure 1). Both lung fields show a fine reticulogranular pattern and marked underaeration leads to a small lung volume. The most distinguishing finding is peripheral extension and persistence of air bronchograms.[6] Prominent air bronchograms represent aerated bronchioles superimposed on a background of nonaerated alveoli. Granularity is attributed to the presence of distended terminal airways (alveolar ducts and terminal bronchioles) seen against a background of alveolar atelectasis.

oping symptomatic patent ductus arteriosus (PDA)—left-to-right shunting through the ductus arteriosus causing compromised cardiovascular or pulmonary function relative to the magnitude of the shunt. The incidence in infants less than 30 weeks gestational age with RDS is 75–80 percent.[5] In infants with the most severe RDS, a large left-to-right shunt may be present on the first day of life without the characteristic ductal murmur.

A significant degree of shunting through the patent ductus results in diminished blood flow to the lower aorta and systemic hypoperfusion. Most of the left ventricular output is diverted back to the lungs. The brain, gut, kidneys, and myocardium may not receive adequate perfusion. Tissue mottling, diminished capillary filling, acidemia, and oliguria may result and mimic the clinical picture of septicemia, intracranial hemorrhage, or a metabolic disorder. In a very small infant, pharmacologic measures may fail to close the PDA and result in

Treatment with positive pressure ventilation commonly results in a more coarse appearance of the lung fields. Granularity is replaced by a pattern of small bubbles. This finding reflects overdistention of the terminal airways. Upon expiration, these bubbles can empty and a "whiteout" effect may be seen. This pattern occurs because alveoli that are not distended result in failure to build a functional residual volume.

In the recovery phase, alveolar aeration occurs, and granularity disappears as surfactant production resumes. The lung fields clear from peripheral to central and upper to lower. The lungs become large and radiolucent and frequently appear hyperaerated.[7]

Etiology and Pathophysiology

Normal postnatal pulmonary adaptation requires the presence of adequate amounts of surface-active material to line the air spaces. In the normal lung, surfactant is continually

FIGURE 2 ▲ The pathophysiology of RDS.

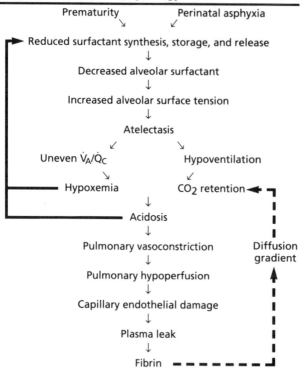

From: Fanaroff AA, and Martin RJ, eds., Neonatal-Perinatal Medicine: Diseases of the Fetus and Infant, 4th ed., St. Louis, 1987, C.V. Mosby, p. 582. Reprinted with permission.

formed, oxidized during breathing, and replenished. Surfactant provides alveolar stability by decreasing the forces of surface tension and preventing alveolar collapse at expiration. This allows more complete gas exchange between the air space and capillary blood. Additional advantages of surfactant include increased lung compliance, decreased work of breathing, decreased opening pressure, and enhanced alveolar fluid clearance. (A more detailed discussion of surfactant can be found in Chapters 1 and 9.)

The development of RDS is thought to begin with surfactant deficiency (Figure 2). This deficiency may be due to insufficient quantity, abnormal composition and function, or disruption of surfactant production. A combination of these factors may be present. The phospholipid composition of surfactant changes with gestational age. (Chapter

1 discusses the physiology of surfactant production and function.)

Inability to maintain a residual volume of air in the alveoli on expiration results in extensive atelectasis. The reduced volume at the end of expiration requires the generation of high pressures to reexpand the lung with each breath (Figure 3).

Infants with RDS will have ventilation-perfusion relationship abnormalities. Hypoxia results from right-to-left shunting of blood through the foramen ovale, causing significant venous admixture of arterial blood. The ductus arteriosus relaxes in response to hypoxia, allowing left-to-right shunting of blood. In addition, intrapulmonary shunting occurs as blood is directed away from areas of the lung that are ventilated (Chapter 1). Hypercarbia results from maldistribution of perfusion in areas of the lung where the alveoli are underperfused with respect to ventilation. Acidemia, hypercapnea, and hypoxia result in increased pulmonary vasoconstriction.

The development of alveolar pulmonary

FIGURE 3 ▲ Pressure-volume curves of normal newborn lung and RDS lung. In the RDS lung, there is very little increase in lung volume with high inflation pressure. The lung collapses to subnormal volume with expiration.

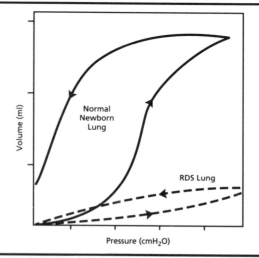

From: Harris TR, Physiologic Principles in Goldsmith JP, and Karotkin EH, eds., Assisted Ventilation of the Newborn, 2nd ed., Philadelphia, 1988, W.B. Saunders, p. 34. Reprinted with permission.

edema adds to the compromised lung function as protein-rich fluid fills the alveolar air spaces. In the preterm infant, a larger amount of fetal lung fluid is present at birth, which contributes to early alveolar flooding. When ventilation is initiated, distal lung units tend to remain fluid filled and undistended while the more proximal airways dilate to accommodate the ventilatory volume. With expiration, the fluid moves to the proximal airways as the lung collapses. The cylic movement of fluids results in erosion of the bronchiolar epithelium. As erosion progresses, hyaline membranes are formed from fibrin and other plasma proteins.

Treatment

Therapy for infants with RDS is directed at providing support for respiratory and cardiovascular insufficiency. Immediate appropriate therapy can be life saving. Preventing alveolar atelectasis, hypoxia, and hypercarbia are the main goals of therapy. General supportive measures must also be maximized. (See Chapter 3 for a detailed discussion of nursing care.) In addition to meticulous nursing care, efforts should be directed at maintaining adequate oxygenation and acid-base balance.

Oxygen must be carefully administered to provide adequate tissue oxygenation without risk of oxygen toxicity. (See Chapter 6 for a detailed discussion of complications of therapy.) An arterial oxygen tension (PaO_2) between 50 and 70 torr is satisfactory for most infants. A very high inspired oxygen concentration may be required to maintain the arterial oxygen tension within an acceptable range. Frequent or continuous monitoring of arterial blood gases is essential during the acute phase of the disease. Transcutaneous oxygen monitors and pulse oximeters provide a noninvasive means of obtaining immediate information on the infant's oxygenation status.

The decision to initiate ventilator therapy should be made individually for each infant. Variables that must be considered include birth-weight, gestational age, postnatal age, results of chest radiograph, progression of disease, and blood gas values, More immature and smaller infants, who will have a greater incidence of fatigue and apnea, generally require mechanical ventilation even when oxygen requirements are low. Some larger infants may be managed with continuous positive airway pressure (CPAP) and will not require intubation and ventilator therapy.

The goal of ventilator therapy is to provide the most effective gas exchange with the least risk of lung damage. Complications such as barotrauma, air leaks, oxygen toxicity, subglottic stenosis, pulmonary infections, cerebral hemorrhage, and retinopathy of prematurity are known to occur.

New therapeutic modalities used in the prevention and treatment of RDS are undergoing clinical trials. Combination therapy utilizing tocolytic agents and antenatal steroid therapy has been shown to reduce mortality, morbidity, and RDS in infants weighing less than 1,000 gm.[8] Advances in high-risk obstetrics such as tocolytic therapy and home monitoring of uterine activity, as well as educational programs for early detection of premature labor, may impact the prematurity rate. Surfactant replacement therapy offers hope in reducing the severity of RDS and, in some cases, eliminating it (Chapter 9).[9] High-frequency ventilation and extracorporeal membrane oxygenation (ECMO) have been tried in cases where conventional ventilator therapy has failed (See Chapters 7, 8, 10).[10,11]

TRANSIENT TACHYPNEA OF THE NEWBORN

Transient tachypnea of the newborn (TTN), also called "wet lung disease" and Type II respiratory distress syndrome, represents one of the most common causes of respiratory distress in the immediate newborn period. Full-term and near-term infants usually present with an increased respiratory rate and mild cyanosis. In

FIGURE 4 ▲ AP view of the chest in infant with transient tachypnea of the newborn. There is a typical pattern of streaky perihilar densities representing resorption of fluid through the pulmonary veins and lymphatics. The lungs are overaerated.

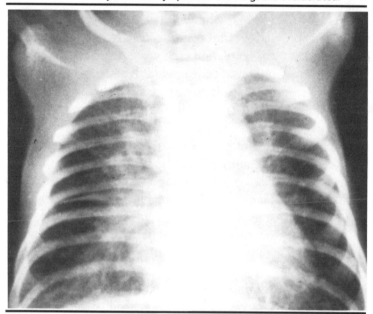

most cases, there is no history of asphyxia. Substernal retractions and expiratory grunting may be present in varying degrees of severity. The clinical signs and symptoms of TTN may mimic those seen in the early phase of RDS or group B streptococcal pneumonia. The diagnosis of TTN is usually made by excluding other, less benign, causes of respiratory distress (Table 1).

The most common presentation is one in which the respiratory rate is normal for the first hour of life and gradually increases during the next 4 to 6 hours. The rate usually peaks between 6 and 36 hours, then gradually returns to normal by 48 to 72 hours. The maximum rate may reach 120 breaths per minute. Mild hypercarbia, hypoxia, and acidosis may be present at 2 to 6 hours.[12]

Most infants are able to correct their acid-base imbalances through compensation. Tachypnea resulting in hyperventilation causes hypocapnea. Blood gases most frequently show a mild respiratory alkalemia with $PaCO_2$ often less than 30 mmHg. Hypoxemia results from maldistribution of ventilation and ongoing perfusion of nonventilated areas of the lung.

Physical examination may reveal a barrel-shaped chest. Consequently, subcostal retractions may be less prominent. As the respiratory symptoms improve, the chest will resume a more normal size.[13] Retained lung fluid may obstruct the lower airway, resulting in overdistention from a ball-valve effect. Grunting in these infants may be associated with forced expiration due to partial airway obstruction from retained lung fluid rather than being a means of increasing intraalveolar pressure as lung compliance worsens.[12]

Etiology and Pathophysiology

Delayed postnatal reabsorption of normal lung fluid is the most likely explanation for the clinical findings in infants with TTN. *In utero*, the potential airways and air spaces are filled with fluid formed by the fetal lung. This fluid is normally cleared from the chest prior to the first breath by the "thoracic squeeze" that occurs during vaginal delivery. The remainder of the fluid is quickly cleared by the pulmonary veins and lymphatics.

Factors that predispose the infant to wet lung disease include prematurity, cesarean section, breech delivery, hypervolemia, and hypoproteinemia. A premature infant undergoes less thoracic compression than a term infant because of his smaller thorax. The normal thoracic squeeze is absent in infants delivered by cesarean section, resulting in an increased volume of interstitial and alveolar fluid and a decreased thoracic gas volume during the first few hours after birth.[14] Premature infants are hypoproteinemic in comparison with term infants. A lower plasma oncotic pressure may result in delayed resorption of lung fluid. Hypervolemia may increase the capillary and lymphatic hydrostatic pressure. Elevated central pressure may result from placental transfusion and delay clearance of lung fluid through the thoracic duct.

An excess of interstitial fluid in the lung causes air trapping. The resulting hyperinflation is one mechanism that can raise pulmonary vascular resistance. When pulmonary vascular resistance is higher than systemic vascular resistance, the fetal pattern of circulation may occur with shunting through the ductus arteriosus and foramen ovale. Severe hypoxemia results. This manifestation of TTN may be seen more frequently than expected.[15,16]

Radiographic Findings

Because the presenting signs of transient tachypnea are commonly found in other neonatal respiratory diseases, the radiographic pattern becomes the key to diagnosis. The characteristic finding is prominent perihilar streaking and fluid in the interlobar fissures. The prominent perihilar streaking may represent engorgement of the periarterial lymphatics that function in the clearance of alveolar fluid. There may be small collections of liquid, particularly at the costophrenic angles. There is progressive clearing of the lung fluid from the alveoli from peripheral to central and upper to lower lung fields. Within 48 to 72 hours, the chest radiograph is normal.[7]

Hyperaeration of the lungs is evidenced by flattened hemidiaphragms and an increased anterior-posterior diameter of the chest. One factor differentiating infants with RDS from those with transient tachypnea is lung size. The lungs appear small and granular in infants with RDS; in those with TTN, they are usually large and granular (Figure 4).[6]

Treatment

Transient tachypnea of the newborn is a self-limited condition requiring supplemental oxygen and supportive care. Pulse oximetry or transcutaneous monitoring allow non-invasive assessment of oxygenation. The infant should be maintained in a neutral thermal environment.

Fluid and electrolyte requirements should be met with intravenous fluids during the acute phase of the disease. Oral feedings are contraindicated because of rapid respiratory rates. If pneumonia is suspected initially, antibiotics may be administered prophylactically. When hypoxemia is severe and tachypnea persists, persistent pulmonary hypertension may complicate the infant's clinical condition and aggressive medical management may be required to break the cycle of hypoxemia (Figure 8, p. 40).

NEONATAL PNEUMONIA

Pneumonia must be considered in every newborn infant with asphyxia or respiratory distress at birth. Pneumonia is the most common neonatal infection, resulting in significant morbidity and mortality. Nearly 20 percent of all stillborn infants autopsied have a congenitally acquired pulmonary infection.[17] Mortality rates are approximately 20 percent for infants who have perinatally acquired pneumonias; the rate approaches 50 percent for infants who acquire infection in the postnatal period.[18]

Etiology and Pathophysiology

Neonatal pneumonia may occur as a primary infection or a part of generalized sepsis. It is often difficult to distinguish the two. Infectious agents include bacteria, viruses, protozoa, and fungi.

Pneumonia may be acquired *in utero*, during labor or delivery, or postnatally. Examination of the placenta and umbilical cord may provide the first evidence suggesting the presence of congenital pneumonia, which may result from the transplacental passage of organisms such as Cytomegalovirus, Rubella, Varicella, and Enterovirus. Listeria, Tuberculosis, and Syphilis are less common agents.

Ascending infection from the maternal genital tract before or during labor is the more common route of contamination. The major predisposing factor is prolonged rupture of fetal membranes, although bacteria can enter the amniotic fluid through intact membranes. Rupture of the membranes for more than 24 hours, excessive obstetrical manipulation, prolonged labor with intact membranes, maternal urinary tract infection, and maternal fever have all been linked to congenital pneumonia. Fetal tachycardia and loss of beat-to-beat variability in the fetal heart rate pattern during labor may reflect the fetal response to sepsis.

Organisms that normally inhabit the maternal genital tract are responsible for infecting the neonate at risk. Bacterial contamination of the infant always occurs during vaginal delivery. Organisms enter the oropharynx and gastrointestinal tract when the fetus continually swallows contaminated amniotic fluid. Aspiration of contaminated secretions present in the oropharynx may follow a complicated labor and delivery. Chlamydia, *Herpes simplex*, and *Candida albicans* can infect the fetus during passage through the birth canal; however, manifestations of pneumonia may not appear until days after birth.

Pneumonia during the postnatal period may also result from nosocomial infection. The neonate may acquire pathogenic organisms by droplets spread from hospital personnel, other infected infants, or the parents. Unwashed hands, contaminated blood products, infected human milk, and open skin lesions are common modes of transmitting various pathogens to the susceptible neonate. Viral pneumonia caused by respiratory syncytial virus and adenovirus may occur in epidemic proportions in the intensive care unit. The most common nosocomial fungal infection is caused by *Candida albicans*. Widespread use of broad-spectrum antibiotics and central lines place the very low-birthweight infant at high risk for pulmonary candidiasis.

Immaturity of the lungs and immune system makes the neonate more susceptible to pulmonary infection. An immature ciliary apparatus leads to suboptimal removal of inflammatory debris, mucus, and pathogens. In addition, the neonatal lung has an insufficient number of pulmonary macrophages for intrapulmonary bacterial clearance.[19] That newborn infants have deficiencies in the neutrophil inflammatory system is suggested by several clinical observations: frequency of neutropenia during serious infection, high bacterial attack rate, high mortality rate, and lack of significant pulmonary neutrophil accumulation observed at postmortem examination in neonates with pneumonia.[20]

Infants who require admission to intensive care units are at higher risk for colonization of the upper respiratory tract with pathogenic organisms than those who are not admitted. Factors predisposing the NICU patient to pneumonia include liberal use of antibiotics, overcrowding and understaffing, invasive procedures such as endotracheal intubation and suctioning, contaminated respiratory support equipment, and frequent invasion of the protective skin barrier for blood sampling and parenteral fluid administration. The specific organisms that colonize the respiratory tracts of NICU infants are influenced by the choice of antibiotics routinely used and the resident flora of the nursery.

Clinical Presentation

Clinical signs characteristic of neonatal sepsis are nonspecific. Some infants with pneumonia demonstrate no pulmonary symptoms. More often, the presentation will include subtle neurologic signs. The key to early diagnosis is a high index of suspicion. Temperature instability, lethargy, poor peripheral perfusion, apnea, tachycardia, and tachypnea are common early signs. The presence of tachypnea, cyanosis, grunting, retractions, and nasal flaring will focus attention on the pulmonary system. These clinical signs indicative of possible pneumonia are also present in other causes of respiratory distress (Table 1).

More specific clinical signs, such as characteristic skin lesions, may be found in association with congenital pneumonia caused by candida, *Herpes simplex*, or syphilis organisms. Hepatosplenomegaly and jaundice suggest a congenital viral infection. Symptoms of intrapartum infection may be delayed for hours following aspiration of infected amniotic fluid because of the incubation period before the onset of infection. In preterm infants, it is often difficult initially to distinguish between pneumonia and respiratory distress syndrome. Some at-risk infants may have pneumonia in combination with RDS or TTN.

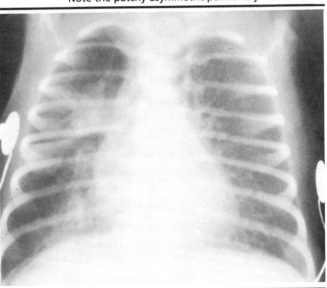

FIGURE 5 ▲ AP view of the chest in infant with pneumonia. Note the patchy asymmetric pulmonary infiltrates.

Diagnostic Workup

The chest film is the most reliable examination for detecting pneumonia; however, appropriate bacterial and viral cultures are needed to identify the specific organism causing the pneumonitis. Rapid viral screening tests allow earlier initiation of appropriate therapy.

Latex agglutination assay of body fluids detects specific antigens and aids in rapid diagnosis of early neonatal sepsis and pneumonia. It is used most frequently in neonates to detect antigen of group B streptococci. Urine latex assay is almost invariably positive initially or within 12 hours of clinical presentation in infants with group B streptococcal bacteremia.[21] Blood cultures, which are usually positive in infants with congenital pneumonia, should be obtained on all infants with suspected pneumonia.[22]

The best indirect indication of congenital infection and pneumonia is the presence of bacteria on a Gram's stain of tracheal aspirates obtained during the first 8 hours of life.[23] A culture of tracheal secretions obtained through a newly inserted endotracheal tube or by tracheal aspiration through a catheter under direct laryngoscopy during the first 12 hours of life has proved useful in diagnosing neonatal bacterial pneumonia.[18] Because of rapid coloniza-

tion, results of tracheal cultures obtained later may be difficult to interpret. The most definitive method of diagnosis is culture and Gram's stain of pleural fluid, but the procedural risks may result in increased morbidity and outweigh any benefits.

The peripheral neutrophil count is valuable in identifying infants with congenital pneumonia or septicemia. Neutropenia in the presence of respiratory distress in the first 72 hours of life suggests bacterial disease. Additionally, an increase in the ratio of immature to total neutrophils on the leukocyte differential is frequently observed during neonatal sepsis.[24]

Radiographic Findings

Chest x-ray examinations are required to support the diagnosis of pneumonia and to distinguish it from other causes of respiratory distress. In some cases, no abnormalities will be found if the studies are performed soon after the onset of symptoms, but radiologic diagnosis should be possible within 24 to 72 hours.

Patchy opacifications become more impressive during subsequent days. In some infants, an area of radiopacification is present but may be attributed to atelectasis. Bilateral homogenous consolidation is a common finding when the pneumonia has been acquired *in utero*.

A wide spectrum of findings is commonly seen following aspiration of infected amniotic fluid: Mild cases may be evidenced by patchy, bilateral bronchopneumonic infiltrates; severe cases may show diffuse bilateral alveolar infiltrate in the lungs with moderate hyperaeration.[7] Although it is difficult to distinguish RDS and group B beta streptococcus pneumonia radiologically, the presence of pleural effusions suggests pneumonia. Serial chest films are useful in following the course of the disease and the effectiveness of treatment (Figure 5).

Treatment

Antibiotic therapy should be instituted immediately following appropriate diagnostic studies and before identifying a pathogenic organism. The initial choice of therapy is broad-spectrum parenteral antibiotics. Therapeutic agents such as ampicillin and gentamicin or cefotaxime will provide coverage for the majority of pathogens found in the maternal genital flora. Many nosocomial infections are caused by organisms that have developed resistance to commonly used antibiotics. Once the pathogen has been identified and sensitivity patterns obtained, therapy can be altered to provide the most effective agent. A combination of antibiotics may be used for synergistic effect. The length of antibiotic therapy should be guided by the response of the infant and the identity of the pathogen. The average duration of therapy is 10–14 days but may be longer in severe cases.

Viral pathogens may respond to a limited number of drugs. Ribavirin therapy may be instituted following the diagnosis of respiratory syncytial virus (RSV). When *Herpes simplex* infection is suspected, acyclovir or vidarabine should be used.

In addition to antimicrobial therapy, the neonate with pneumonia requires careful monitoring of oxygenation and acid-base status.

Supplemental oxygen and ventilatory assistance are often necessary. Volume expanders, blood products, and buffers may be needed for the infant with cardiovascular collapse from septic shock. Exchange transfusion, granulocyte transfusion, and administration of intravenous gamma globulin have been utilized in cases of overwhelming sepsis when conventional therapy has failed.[25] Extracorporeal membrane oxygenation has also been used in attempts to improve survival rates in neonates with little chance of survival.[11]

MECONIUM ASPIRATION SYNDROME

The passage of meconium by the fetus *in utero* is estimated to occur in 8 to 29 percent of all deliveries.[26] However, this occurrence is seen primarily in fetuses born at term or post-term or among those who are small for gestational age. It commonly happens in breech deliveries and is often ignored.

When meconium-stained amniotic fluid is detected, careful and continuous monitoring of fetal well-being is required during labor. The passage of meconium into the amniotic fluid is considered a sign of fetal distress when accompanied by fetal heart rate abnormalities.[27] Increased stillbirth and neonatal mortality rates have been associated with meconium staining. The perinatal mortality when meconium is present without other signs of fetal distress ranges from 5 to 9 percent.[28]

Etiology and Pathophysiology

Meconium is first seen during the fifth month of gestation. It is free of bacteria and contains residuals of gastrointestinal secretions.[26] The pathophysiologic stimuli that trigger the fetal passage of meconium are not clearly understood.

The following theories have been proposed to explain the relationship between fetal hypoxia and the passage of meconium *in utero*:
▶ fetal gut ischemia resulting from decreased perfusion during the "diving reflex"

FIGURE 6 ▲ Pathophysiology of meconium aspiration syndrome

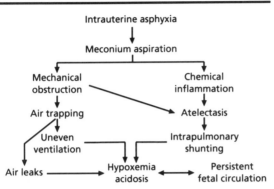

From: Fanaroff AA, and Martin RJ, eds.; Neonatal-Peri-natal Medicine: Diseases of the Fetus and Infant, 4th ed., St. Louis, 1987, CV Mosby, p. 604. Reprinted with permission.

▶ hyperperistalsis following an episode of intestinal ischemia

▶ vagal stimulation elicited by umbilical cord compression, resulting in increased peristalsis and anal sphincter dilation[26]

Meconium passage *in utero* is considered by some to be a normal physiologic function of the term and postterm fetus, indicating fetal maturity.[27] It is rarely observed in fetuses of less than 37 weeks gestation.

Fetal breathing movements occur in the healthy fetus at a rate of 30–70 times per minute. Normally, fluid from the airways moves out into the amniotic fluid with fetal respiratory movements. During an episode of fetal asphyxia, these movements cease and apnea occurs. As the asphyxial episode continues, apnea is replaced by deep gasping. Amniotic fluid containing particulate material may be inhaled into the trachea and large bronchi, and the infant may demonstrate airway obstruction at birth. After the onset of air breathing, meconium migrates rapidly to the distal airways.

The amount of meconium passed into the amniotic fluid will affect the appearance and viscosity of the fluid. As a result, the amniotic fluid may have a light green tinge or have the consistency and appearance of thick pea soup.

Yellow or "old" meconium indicates prolonged fetal hypoxia and is an omnious sign.[29]

Mechanical obstruction of the airways results in a ball-valve phenomenon. With complete obstruction of the smaller airways, atelectasis of alveoli distal to the obstruction occurs. Partial airway obstruction results in areas of overexpansion as air passes around the obstruction to inflate the alveoli. As the airway collapses around the obstruction during expiration, residual air becomes trapped distally. Pneumothorax occurs when the overdistended alveoli rupture and air leaks out into the pleural space. Pneumomediastinum results when extra-alveolar air moves through interstitial tissue to the mediastinum.

The chemical composition of meconium causes local toxic effects. Bile salts, pancreatic enzymes, desquamated intestinal epithelium, and biliverdin in meconium initiate a chemical pneumonitis that further compromises pulmonary function (Figure 6).[30]

Clinical Presentation

Typically, an infant with meconium aspiration syndrome (MAS) has a history of fetal distress and meconium-stained amniotic fluid. The classic postmature infant will show signs of weight loss with little subcutaneous fat remaining. The umbilical cord may be thin with minimal Wharton's jelly. The nails, umbilical cord, and skin may be meconium stained. Respiratory distress may develop immediately after birth. Tracheal occlusion by a meconium plug causes severe gasping respirations, marked retractions, and poor air exchange.

Respiratory distress at birth may be mild, moderate, or severe. The severity of meconium aspiration syndrome is related to the amount of aspirated meconium. In mild cases, hypoxemia is present but easily corrected with minimal oxygen therapy; tachypnea is present but usually resolves within 72 hours. A low $PaCO_2$ and normal pH may be seen. Infants with moderate disease will gradually worsen during the first 24 hours.

FIGURE 7 ▲ AP view of the chest in infant with meconium aspiration syndrome. There are areas of patchy asymmetrical alveolar consolidation and volume loss in addition to areas of overexpansion due to obstruction (ball-valve effect). The lung fields are hyperexpanded.

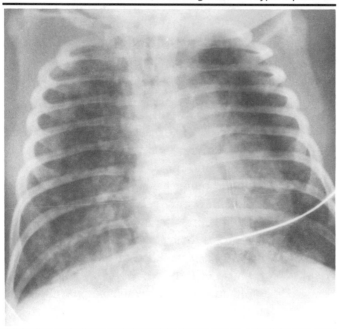

Severely affected infants have neurologic and respiratory depression at birth resulting from the hypoxic insult precipitating the passage of meconium. They develop respiratory distress with cyanosis, nasal flaring, grunting, retracting, and tachypnea. The chest appears overinflated. Rales and rhonchi are common. Diminished breath sounds or heart tones may indicate a pulmonary air leak. Arterial blood gases typically show hypoxemia and acidosis. These infants will have combined respiratory and metabolic acidosis secondary to respiratory failure and asphyxia. Because of large intrapulmonary shunts and persistence of fetal circulation patterns, hypoxemia is often profound despite administration of 100 percent oxygen.

Radiographic Findings

The classic radiographic picture of meconium aspiration syndrome includes coarse, patchy, irregular pulmonary infiltrates. Areas of irregu-

lar aeration are common, with some appearing atelectatic and others appearing emphysematous. Hyperaeration of the chest with flattening of the diaphragm is frequently seen. Pneumothorax and pneumomediastinum are common.[7] Chemical pneumonitis may be apparent after 48 hours.[6] Massive aspiration is characterized by a "snowstorm" appearance. The extent of clinical and radiographic findings will depend upon the amount of meconium aspirated into the lungs (Figure 7).

Treatment

Prevention is the key to managing the infant at risk for meconium aspiration. Several studies have demonstrated decreased mortality and morbidity when meconium is removed from the mouth, pharynx, and trachea before the onset of breathing.[31-33] This requires an obstetrical and pediatric team approach. The obstetrician should begin the resuscitation by suctioning the nose and pharynx with a DeLee catheter or wall suction apparatus immediately after the head is delivered. The infant should then be handed to a designated member of the resuscitation team who is skilled in intubating the trachea under direct laryngoscopy.

When meconium is present below the vocal cords, direct suctioning of the trachea should be accomplished before the infant makes inspiratory efforts. Suctioning should always precede positive pressure ventilation. The urgent need for oxygenation and ventilation in these infants should not be ignored.

Some investigators have questioned the need for routine tracheal suctioning at birth of meconium-stained infants who are delivered vaginally and have a 1-minute Apgar score of more than 8. In a prospective study, meconium-stained but vigorous infants who made their first inspiratory effort before being handed to the pediatrician did not benefit from immediate tracheal suction.[34] Furthermore, case reports have demonstrated that aggressive airway management during and immediately after birth does not always prevent aspiration of meconium.[35]

Nursery Management

Supportive respiratory therapy is required for infants who develop meconium aspiration syndrome. The infant should be monitored continuously for tachypnea. Frequent assessment of blood gases is essential. The need for oxygen and assisted ventilation will be dictated by arterial blood gas values. Continuous monitoring of oxygenation by pulse oximetry or transcutaneous oxygen pressure will alert the nurse to early deterioration. Vigorous pulmonary toilet with percussion, vibration, and suctioning should be performed frequently in the first few hours to remove any residual meconium. Chest x-rays should be obtained to confirm the diagnosis of meconium aspiration and to rule out pulmonary air leaks.

Broad-spectrum antibiotic therapy is indicated when sepsis is suspected. Appropriate cultures should be obtained before starting therapy. There is no objective evidence to suggest that prophylactic antibiotic therapy improves the outcome in meconium aspiration syndrome. Prophylactic use of antibiotics is a common practice in infants with this disease because it is difficult to distinguish it from superimposed bacterial pneumonia on the chest x-ray. The use of steriod therapy to minimize airway inflammation caused by the presence of meconium is controversial.[36]

The infant should be carefully monitored for signs of seizure activity reflecting anoxic cerebral injury. Anticonvulsant therapy may be required. Metabolic derangements such as hypoglycemia and hypocalcemia require appropriate therapy and monitoring. Fluid balance is critical in these infants because cerebral edema and inappropriate secretion of antidiuretic hormone often occur following an asphyxial insult.

Fluid restriction may be initiated early in the course of the disease. Careful monitoring of urine output is essential in the postasphyxial stage. Hematuria, oliguria, and anuria may indicate anoxic renal damage.

Ventilatory assistance is indicated when adequate oxygenation cannot be achieved or maintained in a high concentration of oxygen. Respiratory failure commonly occurs in severe cases of meconium aspiration and may necessitate prolonged assisted ventilation. Once the infant requires assisted ventilation, morbidity and mortality increase. Sedatives and neuromuscular blocking agents may be added to the therapeutic regime when the infant's own ventilatory efforts interfere with the effectiveness of mechanical ventilation.

Recovery from meconium aspiration syndrome usually occurs within three to seven days in infants who do not require assisted ventilation. Those requiring assisted ventilation are usually ventilator-dependent for three to seven days. Although the infant may be weaned successfully from assisted ventilation, tachypnea may persist for weeks. Pulmonary air leaks, persistent pulmonary hypertension, and pulmonary barotrauma often complicate the course of the disease. Prolonged ventilator therapy may occur when MAS progresses to bronchopulmonary dysplasia with resulting oxygen dependency. More long-term deficits are usually seen as a sequela of asphyxia.

The major cause of death in infants with meconium aspiration syndrome is respiratory failure.[37] In some cases, the infant cannot be adequately oxygenated and ventilated with conventional respiratory support. Extracorporeal membrane oxygenation has been used in many of these infants to improve survival.[38]

PERSISTENT PULMONARY HYPERTENSION OF THE NEWBORN

Persistent pulmonary hypertension of the newborn (PPHN) is a clinical syndrome characterized by cyanosis secondary to shunting of

FIGURE 8 ▲ Cycle of hypoxemia in persistent pulmonary hypertension of the newborn

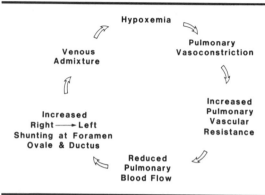

From: Harris TR, Physiologic Principles *in* Goldsmith JP, and Karotkin EH, eds., Assisted Ventilation of the Newborn, 2nd ed., Philadelphia, 1988, W.B. Saunders. Reprinted with permission.

unoxygenated blood through the ductus arteriosus and foramen ovale. Gersony originally described this condition in infants with no parenchymal lung disease or cardiac lesion who developed central cyanosis shortly after birth; he applied the term "persistence of the fetal circulation" (PFC) to them.[39] A variety of other terms has also been used to describe infants with cyanosis and respiratory disease during the first few days of life who have no structural cardiac lesion. These terms include progressive pulmonary hypertension, persistence of fetal cardiopulmonary circulation, pulmonary vascular obstruction, as well as persistence of the fetal circulation and persistent pulmonary hypertension of the newborn.

Because of the variable criteria used to define the syndrome, the true incidence of PPHN is unknown. Although elevated pulmonary vascular resistance is the key pathophysiologic element in the syndrome, there is a wide spectrum of etiologies. Classification according to etiology helps us understand the pathophysiology and manage the condition.

Etiology and Pathophysiology

Pulmonary artery pressure is the product of pulmonary blood flow and pulmonary vascular resistance. The majority of infants with PPHN will have elevated pulmonary vascular resistance; few will have increased pulmonary blood flow as an important component of PPHN. Pulmonary artery pressure may be equal to or greater than systemic arterial pressure in infants with PPHN. Right ventricular and right atrial pressures rise.

When right atrial pressure exceeds left atrial pressure and pulmonary arterial pressure is greater than systemic pressure, blood flow follows the path of least resistance through the foramen ovale and ductus arteriosus. This right-to-left shunt causes hypoxemia due to venous admixture. Hypoxemia increases pulmonary vasoconstriction, and the cycle continues (Figure 8).

Persistent pulmonary hypertension may occur in association with a wide spectrum of neonatal diseases (Table 3). Gersony classified the causes of pulmonary hypertension in terms of cardiopulmonary pathophysiology as follows: (1) pulmonary venous hypertension, (2) functional obstruction of the pulmonary vascular bed, (3) pulmonary vascular constriction, (4) decreased pulmonary vascular bed, and (5) increased pulmonary blood flow.[40]

The time period in which pulmonary vasoconstriction occurs may clarify the pathophysiology of PPHN. Etiologies can be categorized into intrauterine, intrapartum, or postpartum

TABLE 3 ▲ Clinical Conditions Associated with Persistent Pulmonary Hypertension of the Newborn

Pathophysiologic	Anatomical
Utero-placental insufficiency	Diaphragmatic hernia
Perinatal asphyxia	Hypoplastic lungs
Hematologic	**Cardiac**
Polycythemia	Myocardial dysfunction
Hyperviscosity	Congenital heart defects
Metabolic	**Respiratory**
Hypocalcemia	Aspiration syndromes
Hypoglycemia	Infection (GBBS)
Hypothermia	Hyaline membrane disease
	Transient tachypnea of the newborn
Other	
Maternal drugs (aspirin, indomethacin, phenytoin, lithium)	

periods. The terms primary, or idiopathic, and secondary have also been used to describe PPHN. Regardless of the classification used, it is essential to understand that a combination of etiologies may be responsible for PPHN.

Clinical Presentation

Infants presenting with clinical evidence of PPHN are usually greater than 32 weeks gestational age and born following complications of pregnancy, labor, and delivery. The syndrome occurs most commonly in full-term or postterm infants following an intrauterine or intrapartum asphyxial episode. The degree of hypoxemia is usually much greater than the severity of lung disease. Onset of symptoms is usually immediate in infants with congenital diaphragmatic hernia and severe asphyxia. Others may have a more subtle presentation, but most infants at risk will have clinical manifestations before 24 hours. Clinical symptoms may initially be indistinguishable from those of cyanotic congenital heart disease.

There is marked variability in the clinical course. Evidence of respiratory distress may be mild to severe. Signs of heart failure may be present in more adversely affected infants. Central cyanosis may be present despite a high inspired oxygen concentration. Arterial blood gases reveal severe hypoxemia and metabolic acidosis. Arterial PaO_2 values or transcutaneous oxygen values may fluctuate widely when the infant is handled or stressed. The $PaCO_2$ is usually normal but may be mildly elevated. Physical examination reveals varying degrees of respiratory distress and cyanosis.

A single, loud second heart sound or a narrowly split second heart sound with a loud pulmonic component is heard. A long, harsh systolic heart murmur may be heard at the lower left sternal border. This is due to tricuspid insufficiency. Inspection of the chest reveals a hyperactive precordium with a prominent right ventricular impulse that is visible or easily palpable at the lower left sternal border.

The chest may be barrel shaped following aspiration of meconium or the use of high positive inflating pressures with mechanical ventilation. Retractions are present when pulmonary compliance is decreased. Peripheral perfusion is often poor, and pulses are diminished.

Radiographic Findings

There is no classic radiograph for PPHN because the etiologies are varied. The chest radiograph may show normal or decreased pulmonary vascular markings. When the syndrome is complicated by pulmonary disease such as meconium aspiration, pneumonia, and hyaline membrane disease, the radiographic findings will reflect the primary pulmonary disorder. Cardiomegaly is a frequent finding on the initial chest radiograph and may be present without clinically detectable cardiac dysfunction.[41] Pleural effusions, pulmonary venous congestion, and marked cardiomegaly may be seen when there is myocardial dysfunction.

Diagnostic Workup

The diagnosis of PPHN should be suspected in any infant who has hypoxemia that is out of proportion to the severity of lung disease. Parenchymal lung disease is the most common etiology of hypoxemia. However, persistent pulmonary hypertension often complicates the clinical course of infants with primary lung disease.

The most important differential diagnosis to exclude in these infants is cyanotic congenital heart disease. A series of noninvasive bedside tests can be performed using arterial blood gas determinations and ventilation techniques to differentiate between cyanotic heart disease and PPHN. These include the hyperoxia test, preductal and postductal arterial blood sampling, and the hyperoxia-hyperventilation test.[42]

The hyperoxia test is used in term infants to differentiate between the fixed right-to-left shunt in congenital heart disease or PPHN and a ventilation-perfusion mismatch as seen in parenchymal lung disease. The infant is placed

FIGURE 9 ▲ A. Preductal and postductal sampling sites. **B.** Right-to-left shunt across the patent ductus arteriosus. **C.** Right-to-left shunt across the foramen ovale.

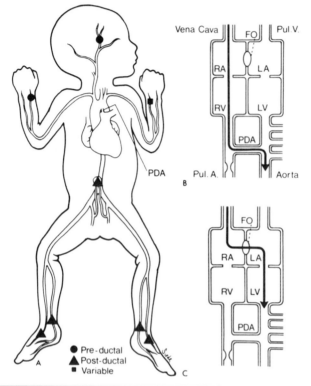

From: Phillips B, Blood Gases: Technical Aspects and Interpretation, *in* Goldsmith JP, and Karotkin EH, eds., Assisted Ventilation of the Newborn, 2nd ed., Philadelphia, 1988, W.B. Saunders, p. 228. Reprinted with permission.

in 100 percent oxygen concentration for five to ten minutes before an arterial or transcutaneous oxygen pressure is determined. If a ventilation-perfusion problem is the cause of the hypoxemia, oxygen will diffuse into the poorly ventilated areas of the lung, and the PaO_2 will usually rise about 100 mmHg. A right-to-left shunt is demonstrated when the PaO_2 remains low in 100 percent oxygen. However, this shunt may be secondary to congenital heart disease or PPHN. Further evaluation is needed to determine if the right-to-left shunt is occurring at the ductal level.

Comparison of arterial oxygenation of blood obtained from preductal and postductal arterial sampling is used to demonstrate the pres-

ence of a right-to-left shunt through the ductus arteriosus. Preductal samples can be obtained from the right radial, right brachial, or either temporal artery; postductal sites most frequently sampled include the umbilical, femoral, and posterior tibial arteries (Figure 9). The left radial artery may represent a mixture of preductal and postductal blood because of the proximity of the left subclavian artery to the ductus.

Preductal and postductal samples must be obtained simultaneously from the quiet infant if they are to be considered reliable. In the hypoxemic infant, a PaO_2 difference greater than 15–20 mmHg indicates significant right-to-left shunting at the ductal level. If the test reveals no difference in PaO_2 between preductal and postductal sites, pulmonary hypertension is not ruled out because shunting may be primarily at the atrial level (Figure 9). Additional testing is needed to differentiate between PPHN and cyanotic heart disease.

The hyperoxia-hyperventilation test is the next step in evaluation. This test is most effectively performed on infants who are intubated. Their oxygen requirements are generally high. An anesthesia bag with an in-line pressure manometer is used to hyperventilate the infant using 100 percent oxygen at rates between 100 and 150 per minute. Inflating pressure is determined by adequacy of chest wall movement.

The clinical response to adequate hyperventilation is assessed by observing color change in the infant or visually examining the umbilical artery catheter blood sample, which will change from dark to bright red, and closely monitoring blood gases by transcutaneous monitors or direct blood gas determinations.

Once hyperoxygenation is achieved, it is important to note the carbon dioxide pressure level at which the change occurred. Hyperventilation has been shown to decrease pulmonary artery pressure and alveolar-arterial oxygen difference.[43] The "critical carbon dioxide pressure" can serve as a useful index for guiding ventilator therapy.[44] The need to use inflating pressures above 35–40 cm H_2O and ventilatory rates above 130 to obtain a critical carbon dioxide pressure of 20 torr or less is a sign of a poor prognosis.[45]

Echocardiography is used to confirm the presence of a structurally normal heart in infants with PPHN. Additionally, it can be utilized to measure the ratio of the systolic time intervals of the right ventricle: The ratio of the right ventricular preejection period (RPEP) to the right ventricular ejection time (RVET) is elevated in infants with pulmonary hypertension.[46]

Contrast echocardiography can be used to demonstrate shunting through the foramen ovale. When myocardial ischemia is present, the electrocardiogram will show ST-segment depression. Invasive diagnostic tests such as cardiac catheterization and pulmonary artery pressure monitoring are rarely needed to make the diagnosis of PPHN.

Treatment

When the fetus has been identified to be at risk for persistent pulmonary hypertension, efforts should be directed toward skilled resuscitation and stabilization. Preventing hypoxemia, acidosis, and hypothermia during the immediate newborn period is essential. The time, site, and delivery route of the fetus with a known risk factor such as congenital diaphragmatic hernia may be scheduled in order to minimize intrapartum and postnatal stress.

The aim of therapy for infants with PPHN is correcting hypoxemia by reversing the right-to-left shunt. This is accomplished by decreasing pulmonary artery pressure or elevating the systemic arterial blood pressure. Treatment includes mechanical ventilation, drug therapy, and supportive care.

Mechanical ventilation. Initially, the fraction of inspired oxygen should be increased until the PaO_2 is greater than 50 mmHg. In most cases, the infant will require an FiO_2 of 0.70 to maintain a PaO_2 of 50 or greater. Mechanical ventilation is most effective when it is begun early. The goal is to reduce the $PaCO_2$ to a level where the PaO_2 rises above 100 mmHg. Each infant has a critical level of $PaCO_2$ at which optimum oxygenation occurs because of decreased pulmonary vascular resistance and a decrease in right-to-left shunt.[44]

Ventilator rates of 120–150 breaths per minute may be required to reach the critical level of carbon dioxide. It may be necessary to hand ventilate the infant if the critical carbon dioxide level is not achieved with the use of a mechanical ventilator. The initial peak inflating pressure is determined by the minimal pressure required to move the chest wall while decreasing the $PaCO_2$ to the critical level. The oxygen concentration should be maintained at a level that will result in the infant maintaining a PaO_2 greater than 120 mmHg.

Weaning should be done cautiously while the pulmonary vasculature is reactive because aggressive changes in FiO_2 may result in pulmonary vasospasm and sudden hypoxemia. Inspired oxygen concentration is decreased cautiously, 1 percent at a time. If the PaO_2 remains greater than 120 mmHg, weaning should be continued. High peak inflating pressure should also be decreased 1 cm each time as long as the critical carbon dioxide pressure and adequate oxygenation are maintained.

The transitional phase of PPHN is the point in the disease process when the hypoxemia is no longer due to pulmonary artery hypertension but to chronic parenchymal lung disease.[47] During the transition phase, the $PaCO_2$ may be allowed to rise by decreasing ventilator settings without causing a sudden decline in the PaO_2. This is usually seen after two or three days. Failure to wean from high pressures and rates during the transition phase can result in severe barotrauma.

Mechanical hyperventilation using high rates and high inspiratory pressure to induce hypocarbia is widely used in treating pulmonary hypertension. There are many unanswered questions regarding risks versus benefits of this therapy. Induced hypocarbia and alkalosis shift the oxygen-hemoglobin dissociation curve farther to the left, which reduces oxygen release at the tissue level. Venous blood return to the heart is impeded, and cardiac output is reduced when extremely high inspiratory pressure and ventilatory rates are used. Hypotension and reduced cardiac output cause a further reduction in oxygenation. Induced hypocarbia can diminish cerebral blood flow and increase cerebrospinal fluid lactate levels.[48]

Another approach in ventilatory treatment of PPHN is to minimize barotrauma while maintaining a PaO_2 between 50 and 70 mmHg. $PaCO_2$ is maintained in the 40–60 mmHg range. The appropriate peak inspiratory pressure is determined by clinical assessment of chest excursion. This conservative approach has been used successfully to manage a group of infants with PPHN and severe respiratory failure.[49]

Drug therapy. A variety of pharmacologic agents has been used in managing PPHN. Sedation may be utilized early in the course of treatment if the infant's spontaneous respiratory effort is out of synchrony with the ventilator. Morphine sulfate is administered to decrease the infant's spontaneous activity and resistance to controlled ventilation. The use of fentanyl as an alternative to morphine for sedation of mechanically ventilated neonates is gaining popularity.[50,51]

Skeletal muscle paralysis may be pharmacologically induced with agents such as pancuronium bromide (Pavulon) when sedation fails to produce a desired improvement in oxygenation and ventilation. Meticulous nursing care and continuous assessment of all bodily functions are required when neuromuscular blocking agents are used.

Vasodilator therapy has been utilized in attempts to reverse the direction of shunting by decreasing pulmonary vascular resistance. To date, no available drug selectively dilates the pulmonary vessels in infants with PPHN. The most widely used drug at present is tolazoline (Priscoline), but serious complications such as hypotension, hemorrhage, and renal dysfunction have been reported following its use.[52] The systemic vasodilator effects of tolazoline often predominate over its pulmonary vascular effects and result in increased right-to-left shunt.[52] Additionally, prostagladins have been employed experimentally in infants with high pulmonary vascular resistance. Success with pharmacologic therapy for infants with PPHN has been varied and unpredictable (Chapter 5).

Volume expanders and pressor agents may be required to maintain normal blood pressure. When vascular volume has been restored and hypotension still exists, dopamine may be utilized to increase myocardial contractility and cardiac output. Dobutamine is sometimes used in combination therapy as a coinfusion with dopamine (Chapter 5).

Supportive care. Protocols for minimal stimulation are utilized in many neonatal centers for infants with PPHN. The infant may be secluded in a quiet, darkened room with restricted caretakers and visitors. Sedation and skeletal muscle paralysis are used to facilitate ventilation. Sensitivity to noise and handling during the acute stage of the disease is manifested by sudden and prolonged periods of hypoxia.

Pulse oximetry or transcutaneous oxygen monitors may be utilized simultaneously at preductal and postductal sites. Continuous arterial blood pressure monitoring is imperative. In term infants, the mean arterial pressure should be maintained above 50 mmHg. Maintaining systolic pressures between 60 and 80 mmHg reduces the systemic and pulmonary pressure gradient, resulting in a decreased right-to-left shunt.[45] Vasopressor therapy is usually required.

Fluid balance must be maintained to ensure adequate intravascular volume and blood pressure. Central venous pressure monitoring may aid in determining adequacy of fluid replacement. General nursing care measures to ensure maintenance of skin integrity are essential because these infants may not tolerate frequent position changes.

Despite ventilatory, pharmacologic, and supportive therapies, many infants do not survive. Others have been saved with ECMO therapy.[53] But whatever the treatment, the outcome will vary according to etiology.

REFERENCES

1. Raj JU: Hyaline membrane disease, *in* Emmanouilides GC, and Baylen G, eds., Neonatal Cardiopulmonary Distress, Chicago, 1988, Yearbook Medical Publishers, pp. 54–55.
2. Collaborative Group on Antenatal Steroid Therapy: Effect of antenatal dexamethasone administration on the prevention of respiratory distress syndrome, American Journal of Obstetrics and Gynecology 141, 1981, pp. 276–286.
3. Jobe A: Respiratory distress syndrome: Pathophysiologic basis for new therapeutic efforts, *in* Emmanouilides GC, and Baylen G, eds., Neonatal Cardiopulmonary Distress, Chicago, 1988, Yearbook Medical Publishers, p. 317.
4. Avery ME, and Taeusch HW: Hyaline membrane disease, *in* Schaeffer's Diseases of the Newborn, 5th ed., Philadelphia, 1984, W.B. Saunders, pp. 133–147.
5. Cotton RB: Relationship of PDA to respiratory distress in preterm infants, *in* Stern L, ed., Clinics in Perinatology 14(3), Philadelphia, 1987, W.B. Saunders, pp. 621–633.
6. Swischuk LE: Imaging of the Newborn, Infant and Young Child, 3rd ed., Baltimore, 1989, Williams and Wilkens, pp. 35, 52, 56.
7. Wesenberg RL: The Newborn Chest, Hagerstown, 1973, Harper & Row, pp. 45–46, 62, 74–83, 119–124.
8. Papageorgiou A, et al.: Reduction of mortality, morbidity, and respiratory distress syndrome in infants weighing less than 1000 grams by treatment with betamethasone and ritodrine, Pediatrics 83, 1989, pp. 493–497.
9. Shapiro D: Surfactant replacement therapy *in* Nelson N, ed., Current Therapy in Neonatal-Perinatal Medicine-2, B.C. Decker, Philadelphia, 1990, pp. 477–480.
10. Bancalari E, and Goldberg R: High-frequency ventilation in the neonate, *in* Stern L, ed., The Respiratory System in the Newborn, Clinics in Perinatology 14(3), 1987, pp. 581–597.
11. Short BL, Miller MK, and Anderson KD: Extracorporeal membrane oxygenation in the management of respiratory failure in the newborn, *in* Stern L, ed., Clinics in Perinatology 14(3), 1987, pp. 737–749.
12. Sundell H, et al.: Studies on infants with type II respiratory distress syndrome, Journal of Pediatrics 78(5), 1971, pp. 754–764.
13. Auld P: Respiratory distress syndromes of the newborn, *in* Scarpelli EM, ed., Pulmonary Diseases of the Fetus, Newborn and Child, Philadelphia, 1978, Lea and Febiger, pp. 502–503.
14. Milner AD, Saunders RA, and Hopkin IE: Effect of delivery by cesarean section on lung mechanics and lung volume in the human neonate, Archives of Disease in Childhood 53, 1978, pp. 545–548.
15. Bucciarelli RL, et al.: Persistence of fetal cardiopulmonary circulation: One manifestation of TTN, Pediatrics 58(2), 1976, pp. 192–197.
16. Bonita BW: Transient pulmonary vascular lability: A form of mild pulmonary hypertension of the newborn not requiring mechanical ventilation, Journal of Perinatology 8(1), 1987, pp. 19–23.
17. Merritt TA: Respiratory distress, *in* Zia M, Clark T, and Merritt TA, eds., Assessment of the Newborn, Boston, 1984, Little, Brown, p. 168.
18. Dennehy PH: Respiratory infections in the newborn, *in* Stern L, ed., The Respiratory System in the Newborn, Clinics in Perinatology 14(3), Philadelphia, 1987, W.B. Saunders, p. 667.
19. Reid L: Influence of the pattern of structural growth of lung on susceptibility to specific infectious diseases in infants and children, Pediatric Research 11, 1977, pp. 210–215.
20. Christensen RD, Thibeault DW, and Hall RT: Neonatal bacterial and fungal pneumonia, *in* Thibeault DW, and Gregory GC, eds., Neonatal Pulmonary Care, 2nd ed., Norwalk, Connecticut, 1986, Appleton-Century-Crofts, p. 580.
21. Friedman CA, Wender DF, and Fawson JE: Rapid diagnosis of Group B streptococcal infection utilizing a commercially available latex agglutination assay, Pediatrics 73, 1984, p. 27.
22. Sherman MP, Chance KH, and Goetzman BW: Gram's stain of tracheal secretions predict neonatal bacteremia, American Journal of Diseases in Children 138, 1984, pp. 848–850.
23. Sherman MP, et al.: Tracheal aspiration and its clinical correlates in the diagnosis of congenital pneumonia, Pediatrics 65(2), 1980, pp. 258–263.
24. Manroe BL, et al.: The neonatal blood count in health and disease, I: Reference values for neutrophilic cells, Journal of Pediatrics 95(1), 1979, pp. 89–98.
25. Wasserman RL: Unconventional therapies for neonatal sepsis, Pediatric Infectious Diseases 2, 1983, pp. 421–423.
26. Bacsik RD: Meconium aspiration syndrome, *in* Symposium on the Newborn, Pediatric Clinics of North America 24(3), Philadelphia, 1977, W.B. Saunders, pp. 464–468.
27. Fenton AN, and Steer CM: Fetal distress, American Journal of Obstetrics and Gynecology 83, 1962, pp. 352–362.
28. Miller FC, et al.: Significance of meconium during labor, American Journal of Obstetrics and Gynecology 122, 1975, p. 573.
29. Desmond MM, et al.: Meconium staining of the amniotic fluid: A marker of fetal hypoxia, Obstetrics and Gynecology 9, 1957, pp. 91–103.

30. Tyler DC, Murphy J, and Cheney FW: Mechanical and chemical damage to lung tissue caused by meconium aspiration, Pediatrics 62(4), 1978, pp. 454–459.

31. Carson BS, et al.: Combined obstetric and pediatric approach to prevent meconium aspiration syndrome, American Journal of Obstetrics and Gynecology 126, 1976, p. 712.

32. Ting P, and Brady JP: Tracheal suction in meconium aspiration, American Journal of Obstetrics and Gynecology 122, 1975, p. 767.

33. Gregory GA, et al.: Meconium aspiration in infants— A prospective study, Journal of Pediatrics 85(6), 1974, pp. 848–852.

34. Linder N, et al.: Need for endotracheal intubation and suction in meconium-stained neonates, Journal of Pediatrics 112(4), 1988, pp. 613–615.

35. Davis RO, et al.: Fatal meconium aspiration syndrome occurring despite airway management considered appropriate, American Journal of Obstetrics and Gynecology 151, 1985, pp. 731–736.

36. Brady JP, and Goldman SL: Management of meconium aspiration syndrome, *in* Thibeault D, and Gregory G, eds., Neonatal Pulmonary Care, 2nd ed., Norwalk, Connecticut, 1986, Appleton-Century-Crofts, p. 497.

37. Vidyasagar D, et al.: Assisted ventilation in infants with meconium aspiration syndrome, Pediatrics 56(2), 1975, pp. 208–213.

38. Heiss K, and Bartlett R: Extracorporeal membrane oxygenation: An experimental protocol becomes a clinical service, Advances in Pediatrics 36, 1989, pp. 117–136.

39. Gersony WM, Duc GV, and Sinclair JC: "PFC" syndrome (persistence of the fetal circulation), Circulation 40, supplement 3, 1969, p. 87.

40. Gersony WM: Neonatal pulmonary hypertension: Pathophysiology, classification, and etiology, *in* Philips JB, ed., Symposium on Neonatal Pulmonary Hypertension, Clinics in Perinatology 11(3), 1984, p. 517.

41. Henry GW: Noninvasive assessment of cardiac function and pulmonary hypertension in persistent pulmonary hypertension of the newborn, *in* Philips JB ed., Symposium on Neonatal Pulmonary Hypertension, Clinics in Perinatology 11(3), 1984, p. 633.

42. Fox WW, and Duara S: Persistent pulmonary hypertension of the neonate: Diagnosis and clinical management, Journal of Pediatrics 103, 1983, p. 505.

43. Peckham GJ, and Fox WW: Physiologic factors affecting pulmonary pressure in infants with persistent pulmonary hypertension, Journal of Pediatrics 93(6), 1978, pp. 1005–1010.

44. Fox WW: Arterial blood gas evaluation and mechanical ventilation in the management of persistent pulmonary hypertension of the neonate, 83rd Ross Conference on Pediatric Research: Cardiovascular Sequelae of Asphyxia in the Newborn, 1981, p. 102.

45. Duara S, and Fox WW: Persistent pulmonary hypertension of the neonate, *in* Thibeault DW, and Gregory G, eds., Neonatal Pulmonary Care, 2nd ed., Norwalk, Connecticut, 1986, Appleton-Century-Crofts, p. 479.

46. Riggs T, et al.: Neonatal circulatory changes: An echocardiographic study, Pediatrics 59, 1977, p. 338.

47. Sosulski R, and Fox WW: Hyperventilation therapy for persistent pulmonary hypertension of the neonate and occurrence of a transition phase, Pediatric Research 16, 1982, p. 309A.

48. Plum F, and Posner J: Blood and cerebrospinal fluid lactate during hyperventilation, American Journal of Physiology 212, 1967, pp. 864–870.

49. Wung J, et al.: Management of infants with severe respiratory failure and persistence of the fetal circulation, without hyperventilation, Pediatrics 76(4), 1985, pp. 488–494.

50. Bell SG, and Ellis LS: Use of fentanyl for sedation of mechanically ventilated infants, Neonatal Network 6(2), 1987, pp. 27–31.

51. Maguire D, and Maloney P: A comparison of fentanyl and morphine use in neonates, Neonatal Network 7(1), 1988, pp. 27–32.

52. Roberts RJ: Drug Therapy in Infants, Philadelphia, 1984, W.B. Saunders, pp. 191–192.

53. O'Rourke P, et al.: Extracorporeal membrane oxygenation and conventional medical therapy in neonates with persistent pulmonary hypertension of the newborn: A prospective randomized study, Pediatrics 84, 1989, pp. 957–963.

3 Nursing Assessment and Care for the Neonate in Acute Respiratory Distress

Kathleen Koszarek, RNC, MSN
Ochsner Foundation Hospital
New Orleans, Louisiana

No other health professional spends as many hours at the patient's bedside as the nurse. This intense, lengthy contact allows the nurse to become totally familiar with an infant's status and promotes an awareness of the subtle cues that warn of a change in the infant's clinical condition. The impact of nursing care on decreasing neonatal morbidity and mortality should never be underestimated.

This chapter discusses respiratory care for the neonate from delivery to admission and routine care with special attention to clinical assessment, interpretation of blood gases and radiograph findings, and parenteral support.

INFANTS AT RISK

Responsibility for the neonate precedes admission to the NICU. Appropriate measures for resuscitation and an orderly admission must be in place prior to the birth. Essential to this preparation is an awareness of the maternal-fetal factors that place the neonate at risk. Thorough knowledge of the perinatal history allows the clinician to identify risk factors for the neonate and to begin prophylactic measures. Pulmonary immaturity must be anticipated in preterm infants; asphyxia is seen more often in term infants with congenital anomalies or those experiencing fetal distress. Table 1 lists high-risk antepartum and intrapartum conditions associated with acute respiratory distress of the neonate at delivery.

An institution that provides perinatal health services must have an adequately staffed and equipped resuscitation room. If acute respiratory distress is anticipated, personnel must be available to receive the infant from the moment of delivery. When resuscitative measures are required, an orderly approach must be employed to optimize results (Figure 1).[1]

The Apgar score has become a standard for initial clinical assessment throughout the country (Table 2).[2] Despite the simplicity of this standard, improper and biased scoring occurs, and effort must be made by the observer to use the scale as objectively as possible.[3] Further examination of the infant should be done in the delivery room to identify any abnormalities requiring immediate treatment. A brief examination routine can provide valuable information regarding the infant's status (Table 3).

Anticipation of problems extends to the nursery as well. The prepared environment should include a heat source for temperature stabilization, cardiopulmonary monitoring equipment, oxygen and suction apparatus, manual resuscitator with appropriately sized face masks, emergency drugs, intubation supplies, and

TABLE 1 ▲ Neonatal Risk Factors for Respiratory Distress at Delivery

Antepartum Factors	Intrapartum Factors
Maternal diabetes	Elective or emergency cesarean section
Pregnancy-induced hypertension	Abnormal presentation
Chronic hypertension	Premature labor
Previous Rh sensitization	Rupture of membranes more than 24 hours prior to delivery
Previous stillbirth	
Bleeding in the second or third trimester	Foul-smelling amniotic fluid
Maternal infection	Precipitous labor
Hydramnios	Prolonged labor (greater than 24 hours)
Oligohydramnios	Prolonged second stage of labor (greater than 2 hours)
Postterm gestation	Nonreassuring fetal heart rate patterns
Multiple gestation	Use of general anesthesia
Size-dates discrepancy	Uterine tetany
Drug therapy:	Narcotics administered to mother within 4 hours of delivery
Reserpine, lithium carbonate, magnesium, adrenergic-blocking drugs	Meconium-stained amniotic fluid
Maternal drug abuse	Prolapsed cord
	Abruptio placenta
	Placenta previa

From: Bloom R, and Cropley C: Textbook of Neonatal Resuscitation, American Heart Association/American Academy of Pediatrics, Dallas, 1987, American Heart Association, p. 1-16. Reprinted with permission.

FIGURE 1 ▲ Overview of resuscitation in the delivery room

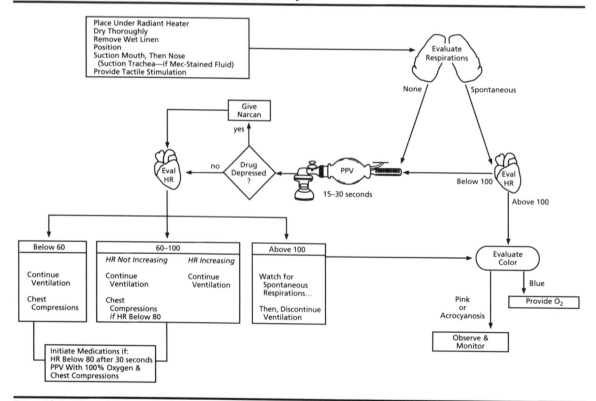

From: Bloom R, and Cropley C: Textbook of Neonatal Resuscitation, American Heart Association, p. 0-5. Reprinted with permission.

TABLE 2 ▲ Apgar Scoring System

Sign	Score		
	0	1	2
Heart rate	Absent	Slow (<100)	>100 beats/minute
Respirations	Absent	Hypoventilation, weak cry	Good, strong cry
Muscle tone	Limp	Some flexion	Active motion
Reflex irritability	No response	Grimace	Cough or sneeze
Color	Blue or pale	Body pink, extremities blue	Completely pink

From: Apgar V, et al.: Evaluation of the newborn infant—Second report, JAMA 168:1985, 1958, copyright 1958, American Medical Association. Reprinted with permission.

blood pressure monitoring equipment. Constant attention to the patient's respiratory status must be maintained during the admission procedure. Medical and nursing procedures carried out on any infant in acute distress should be coordinated and modified to minimize stress that could lead to further compromise.

ADMISSION AND TRANSITION

Immediate assessment should include auscultation of cardiac and breath sounds as well as vital signs including heart rate, respiratory rate, blood pressure, and temperature. The serum blood sugar and hematocrit should be measured by the time the infant is 1 hour of age. Weight can be estimated if the infant is too compromised to tolerate this stressful procedure. If the infant is to be weighed, the utmost care must be taken to assure adequate ventilation and oxygenation during the process. Monitoring equipment (cardio-respiratory, temperature, and oxygen saturation or transcutaneous oxygen/carbon dioxide) should be applied as quickly as feasible.

Common sense can be used to determine those procedures that should and can be delayed. Although measurements and gestational age assessment provide vital information, they should not be carried out to the detriment of the patient. Table 4 provides a list of admitting procedures that should be done within a reasonable time frame, patient status permitting.

The first 6 hours of life are a period of transition for the newborn. Some infants may exhibit acute distress at delivery; others may develop signs and symptoms of ineffective adaptation to extrauterine life during the first hours. Not every infant who exhibits difficulty during transition will require extraordinary supportive measures, but careful assessment and monitoring will ensure that supportive measures are in place when needed to prevent further compromise. An awareness of "expected" behavior and clinical presentation can help the nurse identify those infants who are not successfully adapting to extrauterine life.

Normal recovery from the birth process has been outlined by Desmond and coworkers, who described a characteristic series of changes in vital signs and physical behavior during the first hours of life (Figure 2). A normal transition period can be divided into two major periods of reactivity:

TABLE 3 ▲ Delivery Room Inspection

General: Inspect for asymmetry of growth and major birth defects or birth marks, checking trunk front and back as well as extremities and spine. Note head shape, fontanels, and suture lines. Check genitalia for normalcy.
Neurologic: Note posture, activity, responsiveness.
Respiratory: Auscultate breath sounds, assessing air entry and equality. Inspect movement of the thorax and rate of respirations.
Cardiac: Note underlying skin color, and calculate capillary refill time to assess perfusion. Ausculate cardiac sounds, noting rate, rhythm, and presence or absence of murmur. Note point of maximal impulse. Palpate brachial and femoral pulses.
Abdomen: Palpate for abdominal mass.

TABLE 4 ▲ Admission Procedures

Weigh, measure length and head circumference.
Obtain vital signs: temperature, heart rate, respiratory rate, blood pressure, serum glucose, hematocrit.
Apply and calibrate monitoring equipment, including setting of alarm limits.
Implement priority orders, including medication and diagnostic studies.
Obtain perinatal history; perform physical examination and gestational age assessment.

FIGURE 2 ▲ Newborn adaptations following birth

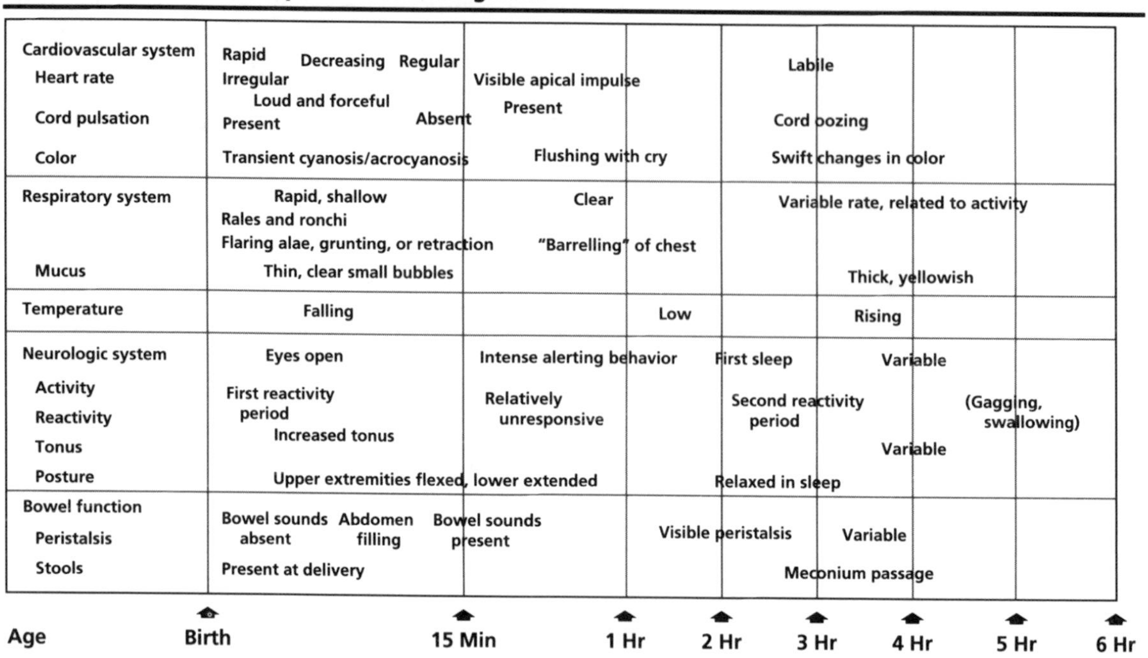

	Birth	15 Min	1 Hr	2 Hr	3 Hr	4 Hr	5 Hr	6 Hr
Cardiovascular system Heart rate	Rapid Decreasing Regular Irregular	Visible apical impulse			Labile			
Cord pulsation	Loud and forceful Present Absent	Present			Cord oozing			
Color	Transient cyanosis/acrocyanosis	Flushing with cry			Swift changes in color			
Respiratory system	Rapid, shallow Rales and ronchi Flaring alae, grunting, or retraction	Clear "Barrelling" of chest			Variable rate, related to activity			
Mucus	Thin, clear small bubbles				Thick, yellowish			
Temperature	Falling		Low		Rising			
Neurologic system Activity	Eyes open	Intense alerting behavior	First sleep		Variable			
Reactivity	First reactivity period	Relatively unresponsive		Second reactivity period			(Gagging, swallowing)	
Tonus	Increased tonus					Variable		
Posture	Upper extremities flexed, lower extended		Relaxed in sleep					
Bowel function Peristalsis	Bowel sounds Abdomen Bowel sounds absent filling present		Visible peristalsis	Variable				
Stools	Present at delivery				Meconium passage			

From: Desmond MM, et al.: The clinical behavior of the newly born: I, The term baby, Journal of Pediatrics 62, 1963, p. 307. Reprinted with permission.

1. During the first 60 minutes of life, the infant is alert with eyes open and displays intensive activity and increased muscle tone. This is followed by an unresponsive interval occurring between 1 and 4 hours of age and lasting 2 to 4 hours.
2. The infant then exhibits variable levels of responsiveness and a tendency toward increased muscle tone.[4]

The immature infant will exhibit a prolonged period of unresponsiveness following the initial reactive period, with the second period of reactivity beginning at a later age. Drugs given prenatally alter the time sequence, and infants requiring resuscitation exhibit a general neurologic decline following the first reactivity period.[4,5]

THERMOREGULATION

Excessive cooling or heating is detrimental to the neonate. Heat balance in the newborn is a result of internal heat production and heat supplied by external sources measured against heat loss.

A neonate has three basic methods of heat production, although they are not all fully developed or totally efficient. The infant may produce heat by shivering, voluntary muscle activity, or the metabolic production of heat. Shivering will produce heat through muscle activity, but the immature nervous system limits this reaction in the term infant and it is not available to the preterm infant. The infant may generate heat through voluntary muscle activity such as crying or moving, and heat loss is reduced by changing position to limit the exposed skin surface. This response is again limited in preterm or compromised infants, especially those who are sedated or physically restrained. Although a term newborn may become restless and increase muscular activity with cold stress, a premature infant is likely to show little response or to become hypotonic.

The main method of heat production is chemical (nonshivering) thermogenesis. This requires an increase in the metabolic rate and increased oxygen consumption. Stimulation of

TABLE 5 ▲ Standard of Care*

Medical Diagnostic Category: Newborns and other neonates with conditions originating in the perinatal period
Medical Diagnosis: All
Nursing Diagnosis: Ineffective thermoregulation

Defining Characteristics	Expected Outcome	Nursing Interventions
• Abnormal body temperature (above or below 36.5–37.2°C) • Respiratory changes: increased oxygen needs, apnea, grunting, nasal flaring • Hypoglycemia/hyperglycemia • Metabolic acidosis • Color change: pallor, mottling, acrocyanosis • Change in activity (lethargy, agitation) • Poor feeding/gastric residuals • Poor weight gain • Specific for hyperthermia: flushed skin tachycardia tachypnea seizures elevated BUN (blood urea nitrogen)	• Infant free of the signs or symptoms of altered thermoregulation as evidenced by normal axillary temperature • Vital signs within normal limits for patient • Oxygen saturations ≥88% • Blood gases within indicated parameters • No evidence of respiratory distress • Serum electrolyte and fluid balance within normal limits • Acceptable perfusion (capillary refill ≤2 seconds) • Absence of lethargy or agitation • Growth within normal parameters as evidenced by Babson growth chart • Normal feeding pattern	• Maintain in stable thermal environment • Place in radiant warmer or double-walled incubator as indicated; Set skin probe at 36.5° C • Utilize equipment alarms and skin probes • Monitor skin probe values • Consult neutral thermal environment chart to estimate initial ambient temperature for incubator (Table 6) • Utilize heated water pad as needed; set at desired body temperature • Assess and document: Temperature q 15–30 minutes until stable, then q 2–4 hours as indicated Signs of alteration in thermoregulation (as per "Defining Characteristics") Skin temperature, ambient temperature, and heater output; relate findings to axillary temperatures • To prevent heat loss: Cover with heat shield or, if in radiant warmer and intubated, use plastic film wrap Prewarm linen and equipment on which infant will be placed Use radiant overhead warmer for procedures Keep neonate dry; change wet linen promptly Weigh or bathe only if infant's temperature is stable Keep infant away from outside windows and air drafts Use porthole sleeves on incubator Dress medically stable infants in incubators with hats, gowns, and booties • Begin weaning to room environment by bundling and discontinuing skin probe control

*Table sources are references 7–15.

thermal receptors in the skin, especially those located in the trigeminal area of the face, will result in an increase in the metabolic rate. The central regulating mechanism for thermoregulation is situated in the hypothalamus. This control center can be impaired by various drugs and by conditions such as intracranial hemorrhage, cerebral malformation, and severe birth asphyxia.[6]

Brown fat, which is stored prenatally in the interscapular, paraspinal, and perirenal areas, is used initially as the fuel source. In response to cold stress, norepinephrine and thyroid hormones are released, resulting in metabolism of the brown fat. Brown fat is broken down into fatty acids and glycerol, and the metabolism of these fatty acids results in metabolic acids. Under conditions of stress, epinephrine is also released, activating the utilization of glycogen stores. Glycolysis may be inhibited, however, in the presence of lipolysis, which occurs during the utilization of brown fat.

Prolonged stress, central nervous system damage, sedation, shock, hypoxia, sepsis, drug narcosis, and nutritional depletion will limit heat production.[6] The term infant's heat production

TABLE 6 ▲ Neutral Thermal Environmental Temperatures (in °C)

Weight (gm)	Age:	0–6 hours	12–24 hours	36–48 hours
Less than 1,200		35.0	34.0	34.0
1,200–1,500		34.1	33.8	33.5
1,501–2,500		33.4	32.8	32.5
More than 2,500 (and 36 weeks gestation)		32.9	32.4	31.9

Modified with permission from: Frigoletto FD, Little GA, eds., Guidelines for Perinatal Care, 2nd ed., Elk Grove Village, Illinois: American Academy of Pediatrics and American College of Obstetricians and Gynecologists, 1988, p. 277. Data from Scopes JW, Ahmed I: Minimal rates of oxygen consumption in sick and premature infants, Archives of Disease in Childhood 41, 1966, pp. 407–416; Scopes JW, Ahmed I: Range of critical temperatures in sick and premature newborn babies, Archives of Disease in Childhood, 1966, pp. 417–419.

abilities can be quickly exhausted, and brown fat, once metabolized, is not replaced. Premature infants have limited ability to increase their metabolic rate, minimal brown fat and glycogen stores, and, if they have lung disease, impaired oxygenation—all of which put them at increased risk for hypothermia.

Thermoregulation is further complicated by the neonate's susceptibility to heat loss. The large body surface when compared to total body mass accelerates heat loss. Heat reaches the body surfaces by direct conduction through body tissue or via the circulation. The insulation layer of subcutaneous fat as well as the skin is thin, especially in the preterm infant, thereby allowing greater heat and evaporative water loss.[16,17]

Vasoconstriction of peripheral vessels will keep internal heat, generated by normal metabolic processes, from being lost to the external environment. However, this mechanism is compromised during periods of vasodilatation associated with phases of shock, and in the presence of certain autonomic drugs which produce vasodilatation. Preterm infants have limited subcutaneous tissue to serve as an insulation layer, an extremely thin epidermal skin layer, and impaired ability to limit skin blood flow.[6]

Heat is lost through four mechanisms:[16]

▶ **Conduction** refers to heat transfer through solids, liquids, or gases; it is dependent on physical contact between surfaces of different temperatures.

▶ **Convection** refers to heat transfer via gas involving a mixing of cooler and warmer air, facilitated by air movement.

▶ **Evaporation** refers to the heat taken from a surface that is required to change a given amount of liquid into a gas.

▶ **Radiation** refers to transmission of heat by electromagnetic waves from the surface of one mass to another; it requires no direct contact.

These principles can be applied to many practical aspects of nursing care (Table 5).

Ideally, infants should be maintained in environmental temperatures and conditions that permit maintenance of normal core temperature in a resting state when oxygen consumption and metabolic rate are minimal. This has been called the infant's neutral thermal environment (NTE), the components of which are environmental air temperature, radiant surfaces, ambient air flow, and relative humidity. Although environmental air temperature is usually easily controlled, factors such as temperature of radiant surfaces, air flow, and humidity are more difficult to assess and control. Because thermal needs vary with weight and gestational age, the proper NTE for individual infants must be estimated accordingly (Table 6).

Thermal instability, whether hypothermia or hyperthermia, places the infant at risk for further complications, and diligent nursing care may markedly decrease the incidence of these complications. The cold-stressed infant, if capable, will increase his metabolic rate to produce heat, thereby increasing caloric consumption. Poor weight gain and hypoglycemia are a consequence of this caloric consumption. The increased metabolic rate requires oxygen as fuel, and increased oxygen consumption may produce hypoxia and a resultant metabolic acidosis. Secondary effects of cold stress include

FIGURE 3 ▲ Neonatal morbidity by birthweight and gestational age

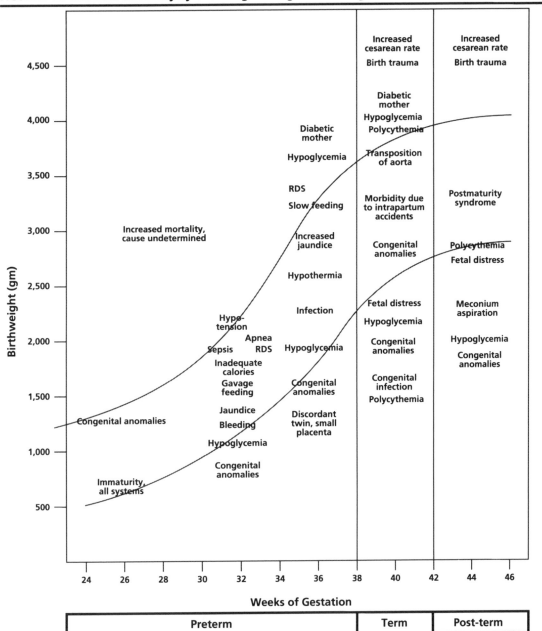

Modfied from: Lubchenco LO: The High Risk Infant, Philadelphia, 1976, W.B. Saunders. Reprinted with permission.

metabolic acidosis as a consequence of vaso-constriction and fat metabolism. Pulmonary vasoconstriction can occur, leading to further hypoxia, acidosis, and increasing severity of respiratory distress.

Although hypothermia is more common,

hyperthermia may also occur very readily in the neonate. Hyperthermia is usually iatrogenic, but it may also indicate sepsis or dehydration. Blood flow to the skin is increased by the over-heated baby's attempt to release heat. This can result in hypotension and increased insensible

FIGURE 4 ▲ Finnstrom's gestational age assessment criteria

Criteria	Score 1	2	3	4	Total
Breast size, transverse diameter	Less than 5 mm	5 to 10 mm	More than 10 mm		
Nipple formation by inspection	Barely visible, no areola	Nipple well defined, areola not raised	Nipple well defined, edge of areola raised above the skin		
Skin opacity by inspection of abdomen	Numerous veins, tributaries and venules seen clearly	Veins and tributaries seen	Few large vessels seen	Few large vessels indistinctly or no vessels seen	
Scalp hair by inspection	Fine, wooly or fuzzy; strands indistinct	Coarse and silky; each hair appears as a single strand			
Ear cartilage by palpation	No cartilage in antitragus	Cartilage in antitragus	Cartilage in antihelix	Cartilage formation complete in helix	
Finger nails by inspection and palpation	Nails do not reach fingertips	Nails reach fingertips	Nails reach or pass fingertips, edge distinct and relatively firm		
Planter skin creases by inspection of broader creases	No skin creases present	Anterior transverse creases only	Occasional creases in anterior two-thirds	Whole sole covered with creases	

Gestational age (physical exam)_____   **Total Score**_____

Appropriateness of growth SGA/AGA/LGA

Adapted from: Finnstrom O: Studies on maturity in newborn infants, IX: Further observation on the use of external characteristics in estimating gestational age, Acta Paediatrica Scandinavica 66, 1977, pp. 601–604.

water loss. Hyperthermia causes increased oxygen consumption and places the infant at risk for apnea, dehydration, and seizures.

Although term newborns have functioning sweat glands to assist with heat dissipation, infants of less than 32 weeks gestation have virtually no ability to sweat. Those between 32 and 37 weeks have limited ability, usually confined to the head and face. The functional ability of the sweat glands improves rapidly with chronological age and matures rapidly during the first 4 postnatal weeks.[6]

GESTATIONAL AGE ASSESSMENT

The American Academy of Pediatrics recommended in 1967 that newborns be classified by birthweight, gestational age, and intrauterine growth to identify existing or potential problems (Figure 3). Weight alone is an inadequate predictor of gestational age.

Clinical assessment tools have been developed

FIGURE 4A ▲ Transforming maturity score to gestational age (days)

Maturity score (7 criteria)	Gestational age in days
7	191
8	198
9	204
10	211
11	217
12	224
13	230
14	237
15	243
16	250
17	256
18	263
19	269
20	276
21	282
22	289
23	295

From: Finnstrom O: Studies on maturity in newborn infants, IX: Further observation on the use of external characteristics in estimating gestational age, Acta Paediatrica Scandinavica 66, 1977, p. 602. Reprinted with permission.

TABLE 7 ▲ History and Physical

History

Maternal:
   Age, gravida, para, abortions, living children
   Blood type, serology (date and results)
   Complications of pregnancy

Labor and Delivery:
   Labor spontaneous or induced; complications of labor, fetal monitoring
   Rupture of membranes—hours prior to delivery, character of fluid
   Medications given
   Fetal presentation; delivery—vaginal or cesarean section (indication); use of forceps
   Apgars 1, 5, 10 minutes (if indicated); specify lost points
   Resuscitation measures required

Family:
   Mother/father—married, single, co-habitating, apart, father in contact
   Environment—living arrangements, telephone

Physical Examination

Vital signs:	Temperature (axillary)	Hematocrit
	Pulse	Blood glucose
	Respirations	BP (central or peripheral, 4 limb)
General:	Resting posture, activity, gross abnormality or overt distress, color	
Skin:	Condition, texture, lanugo, vernix; note meconium staining, jaundice, hemangioma, nevi, rash, excoriation, petechiae, bruises	
Head:	General shape; note molding, caput, cephalhematoma, craniotabes; sutures, fontanels (anterior and posterior), hair texture	
Eyes:	Size or shape of eye, clarity of lens, reactivity of pupils; note edema or discharge	
Nose:	Shape, patency; note drainage, nasal flaring	
Ears:	Cartilaginous development, position of ear lobe, shape of auricle	
Mouth:	Palate, tongue (size), lips and mucous membranes (color)	
Neck:	Trachea position, movement, note masses	
Chest:	Clavicles, symmetry, diameter breast buds; note retractions, abnormal rate or respiratory pattern	
Lungs:	Breath sounds, equality, character; note grunt, crackles, rales, rhonchi, wheezes	
Cardiovascular:	Point of maximal impulse, heart rhythm and rate, murmur (quality, radiation, location of intensity); peripheral pulses—femoral, brachial, radial (equality); peripheral perfusion (capillary refill time in seconds)	
Abdomen:	Shape, muscle tone, number of umbilical vessels, size of liver; note any masses palpated	
Genitourinary:	*Female:* note discharges, abnormalities in voiding *Male:* urethral meatus patency and position, testicular descent and scrotal development (rugae); note hernia, hydrocele, abnormalities in voiding	
Anus:	Patency, stools	
Extremities:	Symmetry, range of motion; number, shape, length of digits; length of nails; palmer creases	
Spine:	Alignment; note sacral dimple, scoliosis, myelomeningocele	
Neurologic:	Tone, responsiveness, cry (character, intensity, frequency); behavior (alertness, irritability); reflexes (suck, grasp); note tremors, paralysis (facial, brachial, lower extremities)	

to help the clinician estimate gestational age. In 1970 Dubowitz published an assessment tool incorporating both neuromuscular and physical criteria. Neuromuscular criteria are usually less biased by intrauterine growth retardation and birthweight, though they may be affected by central nervous system insult or trauma. Use of physical criteria may result in overestimation of maturity in the presence of IUGR, but physical criteria are less biased by neuromuscular abnormalities.[18] A shortened version of the Dubowitz tool was developed by Ballard and associates, who eliminated the more stressful maneuvers of the neuromuscular examination.[19]

Both tools have limited application to the extremely preterm infant.[20,21] Ballard is presently collecting data to validate an expanded assessment tool that could be used with premature infants as young as 20 weeks gestation.[22] Numerous other shortened versions of gestational assessment tools are available, but the criteria defined by Finnstrom (Figures 4 and 4A) may be the most useful for assessing critically ill infants who cannot tolerate the manipulation required for neuromuscular assessment.[23,24]

Gestational age assessment should be performed as soon as feasible because early, accurate identification of infants at risk is essential. Even a properly done gestational age examination will provide estimates that vary up to two weeks (plus or minus) from the actual gestation. Despite this limitation, gestational age assessment remains a valuable tool. This assessment is usually not as urgent when the mother has received early and continuous prenatal care. Ultrasound dating, especially when done in the first or second trimester, can provide very accurate dating.

CLINICAL ASSESSMENT

Particular attention should be paid to the infant's clinical presentation. The presenting clinical signs indicate the etiology of the respiratory distress; sequential monitoring traces the progression of the respiratory disease. An orderly approach to physical examination provides a consistent, complete assessment. Any critically ill infant should be monitored with a transcutaneous ($TcPO_2$) instrument or pulse oximetry (SpO_2).

Assessment interventions must be tempered by an understanding of infant tolerance for such stressful procedures. Some clinicians prefer to group their care procedures; others space them, assuming that the rest periods decrease stress. The superiority of either method is unclear, but it is certain that the infant should be allowed to recover from any procedure, as evidenced by normalization of $TcPO_2$, SpO_2, or heart rate and color, before further stressful procedures are implemented.

The initial assessment procedures in the nurs-

ery are essential to gain a baseline of information. Because this is often the patient's first complete physical examination, each nursing unit should have an established format for this procedure (for an example, see Table 7). The nursing admission note should be exact, including name, age, sex, admitting diagnosis, mode of admission, and any pertinent findings from the examinations. Any significant perinatal history should also be included. All the data will be used to prepare a nursing care plan for the neonate.

CLINICAL ASSESSMENT OF RESPIRATORY STATUS

Clinical assessment of the infant's respiratory status begins with basic observation. Color is judged by looking at generalized color as well as that of the oral mucous membranes. Cyanosis is a blue discoloration of the skin, nail beds, and mucous membranes. Because fetal hemoglobin is easily saturated with oxygen, clinical cyanosis does not occur until severe hypoxia is present.

The presence of oral or nasal secretions should be noted. Chest movement, including depth of respirations, symmetry, and synchrony, is evaluated. The rate of respiration is counted for a full minute. Tachypnea is the most frequent indicator of respiratory disease, although an infant in severe respiratory failure may exhibit slow, gasping respiration or experience episodes of apnea.

Because the infant's cartilage is soft, airway resistance or lung disease produces visible retractions. Retractions can occur intercostally (between the ribs) or subcostally (immediately below the rib cage). Sternal as well as suprasternal and subxiphoid retractions may be present. Severe lung or airway resistance can also produce see-saw respirations, characterized by a collapsing chest and a rising abdomen on inspiration. Nasal flaring during inspiration is the result of widening of the nasal alae in an attempt to decrease upper airway resistance.

Auscultation is performed to determine air

TABLE 8 ▲ Silverman Retraction Score

Stage 0	Stage 1	Stage 2
Upper chest and abdomen rise synchronously	Lag or minimal sinking of upper chest as abdomen rises	"See-saw" sinking of upper chest with rising abdomen
No intercostal sinking on inspiration	Just visible sinking of intercostal spaces on inspiration	Marked sinking of intercostal spaces on inspiration
No xiphoid retraction	Just visible xiphoid retraction	Marked xiphoid retraction
No nasal flaring	Nasal flaring minimal	Marked nasal flaring
No expiratory grunt	Expiratory grunt heard with stethoscope only	Expiratory grunt heard with naked ear

Modified from: Silverman WA, and Andersen DH: A controlled clinical trial of effects of water mist on obstructive respiratory signs, death rate and necropsy findings among premature infants, Pediatrics 17(1), 1956, pp. 1–10.

movement and the quality of breath sounds. Grunting, a sound produced when air is exhaled against a partially closed glottis, may be audible without the aid of a stethoscope. This maneuver delays expiration and increases gaseous exchange by increasing end-expiratory pressure and lung volume.

Auscultation of the chest should progress in an orderly manner, with the examiner comparing and contrasting each side of the chest for equality of breath sounds. Because sound is easily transmitted through the small chest of the newborn, the clinician must be able to identify subtle differences. The presence of crackles (fine or coarse), wheezes, grunting, or other extraneous sounds should be assessed and documented.

A scale has been developed to provide an objective means of assessing the progression or improvement of respiratory distress (Table 8). This scale is especially useful in helping the novice perform a complete evaluation. As she gains experience in caring for the critically ill neonate, the nurse will be able to recognize patterns of clinical signs and symptoms associated with specific disease states. For example, a round barrel chest is seen with volume trapping disorders such as transient tachypnea of the newborn and meconium aspiration syndrome; retractions and hypoexpansion are present with restrictive disease such as hyaline membrane disease. (Chapter 2 discusses pathophysiology and clinical presentation more specifically.)

Although nursing care will depend on the infant's clinical diagnosis, each unit is responsible for developing a standard of care for the infant experiencing respiratory distress. Table 9 provides an example of such a standard. The individual patient's care plan can be used for communicating information unique to that patient that falls outside the established standards of care.

Interpretation of Blood Gases

An adjunct to clinical assessment of respiratory disease is chemical assessment via blood gases. The medical plan of care for the patient includes the frequency of blood gas determinations, and it is every nurse's responsibility to be cognizant of each blood gas sample drawn on her patient. To assist in the interpretation of the blood gas values, the nurse also needs to be aware of the patient's status before the sample is obtained. Assessment of any abnormalities identified and institution of appropriate treatment is often the responsibility of the staff nurse or respiratory therapist, working within the parameters established by the physician. Although the etiology of abnormalities can be complex and multifactorial, the nurse must have a basic knowledge of acid-base disorders in order to interpret blood gases.

There are four major components to the arterial blood gas: pH, $PaCO_2$, bicarbonate (HCO_3^-) or base excess, and PaO_2. The pH scale is a mathematical expression of the acid-base balance of a solution. The number of hydrogen ions in a solution determines the acidity of that solution. An acid solution can donate hydrogen ions; a base solution can accept hydrogen ions. Blood pH is determined by the balance between acids, which results from the byproducts of metabolism, and the body's buffer

TABLE 9 ▲ Standard of Care*

Medical Diagnostic Category: Newborns and other neonates with conditions originating in the perinatal period

Medical Diagnosis: Respiratory distress syndrome, transient tachypnea of the newborn, meconium aspiration syndrome, pneumonia, congenital diaphragmatic hernia, persistent pulmonary hypertension of the newborn, pulmonary insufficiency of prematurity

Collaborative Medical/Nursing Problem	Expected Outcome	Nursing Interventions
Respiratory insufficiency	Normal blood gases maintained	• Administer and monitor ventilation parameters
Fluid and electrolyte balance/ nutrition	Normal fluid and electrolyte balance maintained	• Administer muscle relaxants and sedation
Infection	Infection treated appropriately	• Administer parenteral and enteral fluids
		• Monitor electrolyte values
		• Weigh and measure growth parameters as required
		• Administer antibiotics
		• Monitor culture reports and complete blood cell count (CBC) results

Nursing Diagnosis
Impaired gas exchange

Defining Characteristics	Expected Outcome	Nursing Interventions
Respiratory distress: grunting, flaring, retractions, apnea, tachypnea	Infant will maintain adequate gas exchange during acute phase as evidenced by:	• Assess blood gases:
Abnormal breath sounds: crackles, wheeze, decreased, absent, unequal	Blood gases within stated parameters	Assess ventilation and oxygenation (PaCO$_2$/PaO$_2$) and acid-base balance (pH/PaCO$_2$/HCO$_3^-$)
Cyanosis, pallor	Adequate and appropriate breath sounds	Follow serially to detect deterioration: acidosis, hypoxia, hypercapnea
Tachycardia, bradycardia	Lack of cyanosis	Notify MD if deterioration occurs
Abnormal blood gases, transcutaneous carbon dioxide, oxygen, or oxygen saturation	Oxygen saturation ≥88%	• Assess and document q 2 hours:
	Vital signs within normal parameters	Breath sounds
		Vital signs
		Ventilatory/oxygen parameters and alarm limits
		Signs of impaired gas exchange secondary to extubation, pulmonary air leak, ventilator malfunction
		• Assess response to muscle relaxants:
		Duration of effect
		Change in cardiovascular or pulmonary status
		Need for continuation of paralysis
		• Minimize handling to prevent hypoxia, use readings from pulse oximeter to modify care
		• Explain treatment rationale to infant's family

Nursing Diagnosis
Ineffective Airway Clearance

Defining Characteristics	Expected Outcome	Nursing Interventions
Presence of endotracheal tube, nasal prongs, nasal pharyngeal tube	Infant will be able to clear airway adequately as evidenced by:	• Follow two-person suctioning procedure for endotracheal tube; individualize to prevent hypoxia
Excessive amounts of mucus	Clear and equal breath sounds	• Suction nares prn when utilizing nasal prongs or nasal pharyngeal tube
Atelectasis on chest film	Lack of respiratory difficulty	• Reposition q 2 hours as tolerated
		• Place small roll under neck to promote maintenance of airway
		• Report absent or unequal breath sounds, tenacious secretions, or clinical deterioration

*Table sources are references 7,25,26.

systems. If the carbon dioxide, for example, is not excreted effectively by the lungs, it combines with water to form carbonic acid, which leads to an excess of hydrogen ions and the development of acidemia.

Blood buffers are used to neutralize acid in order to maintain the acid-base balance. Of the three major buffers in the blood—hemoglobin, serum protein, and bicarbonate—the bicarbonate system is predominant. Bicarbonate will combine with hydrogen ions to form carbon dioxide and water, thereby buffering the acids and balancing the pH. If the carbon dioxide cannot be excreted via the lungs, the hydrogen ions can return to solution, and an acidemia will again develop:[27–29]

$$H^+ + HCO_3^- \rightleftharpoons H_2CO_3 \rightleftharpoons H_2O + CO_2$$

The lungs are primarily responsible for the carbon dioxide level ($PaCO_2$); the kidneys control plasma bicarbonate (HCO_3^-). A value of 7.4 is the normal biologic blood pH. In the clinical setting, values between 7.35 and 7.45 are considered normal for adults: A value less than 7.35 indicates acidemia, and one greater than 7.45 indicates alkalemia. Because of their immaturity and their attempts to adapt to extrauterine life, normal newborns and preterm infants have serum pH values that vary from those of adults (Table 10).

The pH is a product of the *ratio* of the respiratory component, measured as carbon dioxide, and the metabolic component, measured as bicarbonate. A normal blood pH of 7.4 is the result of a bicarbonate to carbon dioxide ratio of 20:1. Because it is not the absolute value but the ratio of CO_2 to HCO_3^- that controls the pH, abnormalities can be compensated for by proportional increases or decreases in carbon dioxide or bicarbonate.

Carbon dioxide will add hydrogen ions, thereby acting as an acid. Bicarbonate will accept ions, acting as a base. As the $PaCO_2$ rises (more acid) or the HCO_3^- falls (less base),

TABLE 10 ▲ **Acceptable Neonatal Arterial Blood Gas Values**

	<28 weeks gestation	28–40 weeks gestation
pH	>7.28	>7.30
$PaCO_2$	40–50	40–50
PaO_2	45–65	50–70

From: Phillips B, McQuitty J, and Durand D: Blood gases: Technical aspects and interpretation, *in* Goldsmith J, and Karokin E, eds., Assisted Ventilation in the Neonate, 1988, W.B. Saunders, p. 226. Reprinted with permission.

the pH will become more acidotic. As the carbon dioxide falls (less acid) or the HCO_3^- rises (more base), the pH will become more alkalotic. Because the level of $PaCO_2$ is directly related to respiratory status, pH abnormalities resulting from abnormal $PaCO_2$ are considered respiratory in origin.

Bicarbonate is part of the body's buffer system, and any abnormalities in HCO_3^- are considered metabolic in origin. Base excess (BE) reflects the concentration of buffer, principally bicarbonate, and expresses numerically the metabolic status. Positive values express an excess of base or a deficit of acid; negative values express a deficit of base or an excess of acid. When the base excess is negative, it is sometimes referred to as the base deficit.

The body attempts to maintain a normal pH in two ways:

1. By correcting or altering the component responsible for the abnormality. For example, if an increased level of carbon dioxide in the blood is causing respiratory acidosis, the body will attempt to increase excretion of carbon dioxide by the lungs and bring the causative factor, increased CO_2, back to normal levels.

2. By compensating through alterations in the component that is not primarily responsible for the abnormality. Carbon dioxide and/or bicarbonate will be excreted or retained in order to counteract or balance the abnormal values. For example, if a high $PaCO_2$ is causing respiratory acidosis, the body will attempt to excrete more acid and conserve HCO_3^- to compensate, although compensation by

TABLE 11 ▲ Examples of Arterial Blood Gas Levels for Different Conditions

Normal parameters

	pH	7.35
	$PaCO_2$	42
	BE (base excess)	−2
	HCO_3^-	23
	PaO_2	60

Respiratory acidosis

	pH	7.22
	$PaCO_2$	55
	BE	−4
	HCO_3^-	21
	PaO_2	58

Respiratory alkalosis

	pH	7.49
	$PaCO_2$	30
	BE	0
	HCO_3^-	22
	PaO_2	65

Metabolic acidosis

	pH	7.18
	$PaCO_2$	40
	BE	−10
	HCO_3^-	16
	PaO_2	55

Metabolic alkalosis

	pH	7.60
	$PaCO_2$	45
	BE	+8
	HCO_3^-	32
	PaO_2	70

renal function is a slow mechanism and may take several days. If the $PaCO_2$ (acid) is low, the body will rid itself of bicarbonate (base). The inverse is also seen. High HCO_3^- will be compensated by a high $PaCO_2$; a low HCO_3^- will be compensated by a low $PaCO_2$. Thus, subsequent abnormal values of carbon dioxide or bicarbonate may result from the compensation mechanism of the body attempting to bring the ratio of HCO_3^- to CO_2 back to 20:1. Critically ill neonates may be limited in their ability to compensate for problems. Respiratory disease limits the body's ability to effectively lower $PaCO_2$, and the neonatal kidney may be ineffective in conserving bicarbonate.

Interpreting of blood gas data should follow a logical pattern. Initially evaluate the pH to determine if an acidemia or alkalemia is present. Then evaluate the respiratory parameter ($PaCO_2$) and the metabolic parameter (HCO_3^-) to determine if the acidemia or alkalemia is respiratory or metabolic in origin. Examples are given in Table 11. The clinical picture can become quite complex because abnormalities can exist in both systems simultaneously. A review of the infant's clinical status, previous blood gas values, and treatment measures will help determine whether this is an ongoing compensation mechanism or two somewhat independent abnormalities. Figure 5 lists common clinical etiologies of acid-base disturbances.[28,29]

Blood gas levels also allow assessment of oxygenation, measured as PaO_2 or as oxyhemoglobin saturation (SaO_2). The PaO_2 value is measured directly from the blood sample while the SaO_2 is usually calculated.

Ninety-eight percent of total blood oxygen content is bound to hemoglobin in the red cells. Oxygenation depends on the transfer of oxygen across the alveolar-capillary interface to be bound with hemoglobin. Hemoglobin's ability to pick up oxygen and release it at the tissue level is affected by several factors, which are: pH, $PaCO_2$, temperature, 2, 3-diphosphoglycerate (2, 3-DPG), and hemoglobin type. A by-product of glucose metabolism, 2, 3-DPG accumulates in the presence of sustained tissue hypoxia. Additionally, fetal hemoglobin differs from adult hemoglobin in its oxygen affinity because fetal hemoglobin is less sensitive to the effects of 2, 3-DPG. The relationship between SaO_2 and PaO_2 is not linear; it is expressed in the oxygen-hemoglobin dissociation curve (Figure 6).[30,31]

Alkalosis, hypocapnia, hypothermia, decreased concentrations of 2, 3-DPG, and the presence of fetal hemoglobin change the binding characteristics of hemoglobin, increasing its affinity for oxygen. This causes decreased oxygen

FIGURE 5 ▲ Acid-base disturbances

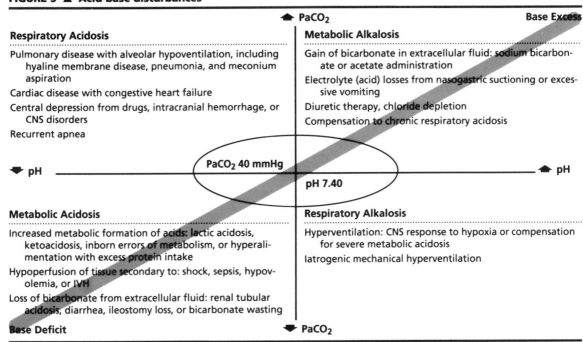

Respiratory Acidosis

Pulmonary disease with alveolar hypoventilation, including hyaline membrane disease, pneumonia, and meconium aspiration

Cardiac disease with congestive heart failure

Central depression from drugs, intracranial hemorrhage, or CNS disorders

Recurrent apnea

Metabolic Alkalosis

Gain of bicarbonate in extracellular fluid: sodium bicarbonate or acetate administration

Electrolyte (acid) losses from nasogastric suctioning or excessive vomiting

Diuretic therapy, chloride depletion

Compensation to chronic respiratory acidosis

PaCO₂ 40 mmHg
pH 7.40

Metabolic Acidosis

Increased metabolic formation of acids: lactic acidosis, ketoacidosis, inborn errors of metabolism, or hyperalimentation with excess protein intake

Hypoperfusion of tissue secondary to: shock, sepsis, hypovolemia, or IVH

Loss of bicarbonate from extracellular fluid: renal tubular acidosis, diarrhea, ileostomy loss, or bicarbonate wasting

Respiratory Alkalosis

Hyperventilation: CNS response to hypoxia or compensation for severe metabolic acidosis

Iatrogenic mechanical hyperventilation

release at the tissue level, potentially leading to tissue hypoxia. Increased affinity, depicted to the left of the normal oxygen-hemoglobin dissociation curve, is called a "shift to the left."

Acidosis, hypercapnia, hyperthermia, adult hemoglobin and increases in 2, 3-DPG diminish hemoglobin's affinity for oxygen, thus impairing oxygen pickup at the alveolar-capillary level. This decreased ability to saturate or load hemoglobin with oxygen at the alveolar-capillary level is usually not a factor clinically unless there is an extreme shift of the curve or impaired saturation already exists due to pulmonary or cardiac disease. Oxygen is released more readily at the tissue level under these conditions. This decreased affinity, depicted to the right of the normal oxygen-hemoglobin dissociation curve, is called a "shift to the right." The extent to which the curve shifts depends on the condition causing the shift and its severity.[29,32,33]

The shape of the curve is of clinical significance. The initial portion of the curve is steep, reflecting somewhat proportional changes in SaO_2 and PaO_2. Oxygen saturations less than

FIGURE 6 ▲ Oxygen dissociation curves of fetal and adult hemoglobins*

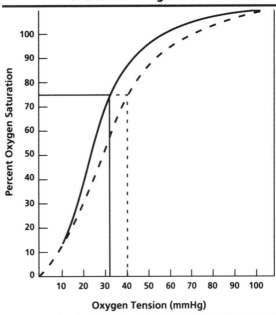

*Hemoglobin saturation at 75 percent is the level at which cyanosis appears. The corresponding PaO_2 can be estimated on the graph for both fetal (——) and adult (– – –) hemoglobin.

Adapted from Klaus M, and Meyer BP: Oxygen therapy for the newborn, Pediatric Clinics of North America 13, 1966, p. 731; From: Coen RW, and Koffler H: Primary Care of the Newborn, 1987, Little, Brown, p. 73. Reprinted with permission.

80 percent usually represent a PaO_2 inadequate for tissue oxygenation. The upper portion of the curve is flat, indicating that small changes in saturation may result in large changes in PaO_2. This limits the ability to estimate PaO_2 from saturations greater than 92 percent.

Monitoring a critically ill infant with a pulse oximeter will provide continuous information on his status by determining the pulse oxygen saturation (SpO_2). Intermittent assessment of the arterial blood gases will yield specific information on PaO_2.

Interpretation of Chest X-ray Films

Radiographic examination is a medical standard of care for the neonate with respiratory distress. The frequency of such examinations is at the discretion of the physician, but in an emergency the nurse is often the first health care worker available to view the film. On transport, it is usually the primary transport nurse's responsibility to interpret the available films.

The NICU staff nurse should also have the ability to recognize acute or dramatic changes in the infant's x-ray film and to convey this information to the physician who is not immediately available to view the films. The best way for nurses to develop this skill is through consistent exposure to the diagnostic interpretation of such films. If the unit has radiographic rounds, the staff nurse should make every effort to attend.

Proper technique includes columination or coning of the x-ray field, which provides a better quality film as well as diminishing radiation scatter. The cassette must be in proper position under the neonate with appropriate coning to expose only those structures that are to be evaluated. Nursing responsibility includes placing a small lead shield over the infant's reproductive organs to further limit radiation exposure.

Proper interpretation of the x-ray film requires a systematic approach, beginning with evaluation of the quality of the film. Exposure, seen as density and contrast, must be noted. Overpenetration will result in a dark film, with the infant's lungs appearing hyperlucent or overaerated. Underpenetration will produce a "white" film, giving the false impression of atelectasis or hypoexpansion.

Density and contrast can be evaluated by looking at the appearance of air in the stomach, which is usually partially filled with air, providing a baseline for comparison. The technician documents on each film the settings used when obtaining it. Use of consistent settings with appropriate modification of the technique is the best means of obtaining quality films.

Film interpretation continues with a survey of the infant's positioning. Rotation, if any, should be identified. The ribs should appear of equal length on either side of the vertebral column, and the clavicles should appear symmetric. A rotated film will skew the appearance of the lung field and prevent the evaluation of a mediastinal shift. One side may appear falsely atelectatic, and the heart may obscure the left lung field.

If the area to be exposed is not perpendicular to the beam from the x-ray tube, an oblique view will be obtained. Such a film will slant all structures and misrepresent positioning of the indwelling tubes and lines. With proper angulation, the clavicles will be at a 90° angle to the vertebral bodies. Errors can be avoided by proper positioning of the infant, who should be held flat and prevented from rolling to one side or the other. If the infant is to be held during the procedure, the staff member must wear a lead apron, and her hand coned out of the field.

Motion during the film could make assessment of the lung fields inaccurate. Evidence of motion is best detected by looking for the blurring of normally distinct structures such as electrocardiograph lead wires.

Next the film should be evaluated for extraneous objects that may prevent interpretation or lead to a false conclusion. Radiopaque objects will appear clearly on the film and are thus easily identified. If possible, these should be removed from the field prior to the x-ray study to prevent obstruction of body structures. Electrocardiograph leads, thermo-skin probes, and transcutaneous sensors will block the viewing of structures and should be moved, if feasible. For an anterior-posterior chest film, it is best to place electrocardiograph leads in the axillary line and skin sensors on the shoulder or abdomen.

Nonradiopaque objects will not appear clearly on the film but will leave shadows that may be difficult to differentiate from pathologic findings in the chest. Warming mattresses produce a wafflelike appearance that prevents any realistic interpretation of the film. Bunched linen or plastic tubings lying under or over the infant will produce lines. Incubator tops often have a small hole for inserting tubes. If film is shot through the plexiglass incubator top, a small, circular bleb may appear on the film. A skin fold may be falsely interpreted as a pneumothorax; this is best identified on the film by tracking the skin fold line outside the thoracic cavity.

Finally, a systematic clinical examination of the film can be made.

1. Heart size, position, and shape should be evaluated. The cardiac silhouette of the newborn is large, especially during the first 24 hours of life. Cardiac size is estimated by determining the cardiothoracic (CT) ratio. The longest horizontal diameter of the heart is divided by the greater internal diameter of the chest. The heart will normally measure half the distance of the thorax, with a CT ratio of 0.5, although the CT ratio of normal newborns may be slightly larger. This measurement, used to determine cardiomegaly, is further limited in the neonate because a large shadow from the thymus, a film obtained during expiration, or areas of atelectasis will create a generous cardiac silhouette that may exceed this ratio.[34]

Cardiomegaly is seen with volume overload, and an extremely small silhouette will be seen in infants who are hypovolemic, dehydrated, or whose high intrathoracic pressure is causing decreased venous return. Initially, the apex of the heart is elevated secondary to the right ventricular hypertrophy associated with fetal circulation. As the left ventricle predominates in extrauterine life, the cardiac apex will descend caudally. The configuration is affected by the size of the thymus, but abnormal shapes still can be seen with various congenital heart diseases. A globular shape is seen with hypoplastic left heart disease or coarctation of the aorta, an egg shape is seen with transposition of the great vessels, and a boot shape is seen with tetralogy of Fallot.

2. The lung fields should be surveyed. Pulmonary expansion can be determined by locating the level of the diaphragm. During inspiration, the dome of the hemidiaphragm will usually move to the level of the eighth rib or below. The diaphragm will be higher if the lungs are severely hypoventilated or if the film was taken during the expiratory phase. Overinflated lungs appear hyperlucent, with their normally domed diaphragms flattened.

3. The aeration of the lungs should be determined. Are they clear (dark) or opaque (white)? Is there evidence of granularity, seen as coarseness or a "ground glass" appearance? Are there areas of streaking, haziness, or consolidation? Lung tissue should extend fully to the pleura.

Hyperlucent (extremely clear) areas over the entire lung or at its margins may indicate a pneumothorax (free air in the thoracic cavity surrounding the lung). A decubitus film, made by placing the unaffected side down and using an anteroposterior position, will more clearly define a pneumothorax because the free air will layer to the upmost area. Free air in the mediastinal area, called a pneumomediastinum, will often outline the thymus, producing a sail or butterfly appearance. A pneumopericardium, free

TABLE 12 ▲ Disorders Indicated by Abnormal Roentgenographic Patterns

Granular: hyaline membrane disease (HMD), transient respiratory distress of the newborn, neonatal pneumonitis (especially group B-streptococcal)

Bubbly: HMD with overdistended terminal airways (associated with mechanical ventilation), pulmonary interstitial emphysema, bronchopulmonary dysplasia, Wilson-Mikity syndrome

Opaque: absent or greatly reduced functional residual volume, pulmonary hemorrhage, bilateral chylothorax or hydrothorax

Vascular Congestion: transient respiratory distress of the newborn, congenital heart disease (CHD) >12 hours of age, myocardial dysfunction with congestive heart failure

Infiltrate: pulmonary infections (viral/bacterial), meconium aspiration, amniotic fluid aspiration, segmental atelectasis, pulmonary hemorrhage, vascular congestion secondary to cardiac disease, transient respiratory distress of the newborn, early Wilson-Mikity syndrome

Hazy: underaeration, pulmonary edema, resolving phase of HMD, bilateral diaphragmatic paralysis

Overaerated, Clear: hyperventilation, CHD with decreased pulmonary vascularity, central obstructing lesions (vascular ring or mediastinal mass)

Unequal Aeration: secondary to mucus plugging or improper placement of endotracheal tube, unilateral pulmonary hypoplasia, congenital lobar emphysema

Hyperlucent: pulmonary air leak

Adapted from: Swischuk L: Radiology of pulmonary insufficiency, *in* Thibeault D, and Gregory G, eds., Neonatal Pulmonary Care, Norwalk, Connecticut, 1986, Appleton, Century, Crofts, pp. 235–279.

air around the heart, will be seen as a complete halo encircling the heart.

Table 12 lists the classical radiographic findings associated with the major neonatal respiratory pathology. Because many of the abnormalities have similar radiographic findings, a knowledge of the patient's history and clinical presentation is essential. Developing a basic competence in x-ray interpretation and familiarity with associated respiratory pathophysiology will be of invaluable assistance to the nurse in providing appropriate patient care, which includes the ability to knowledgably communicate patient status to the physician.

ROUTINE CARE

After the admission of the infant, a routine should be established in regard to frequency of assessment. Table 13 provides an example of routine nursing orders for the critically ill patient. Premature infants often tolerate handling poorly, so the relative importance of all interventions versus the potential disturbance must be evaluated.

Monitoring the vital signs does not necessarily mean that the baby must be disturbed. Heart rate, blood pressure, and skin temperature can usually be obtained from monitoring equipment. At least once each shift the monitored vital signs should be verified by counting pulse and respirations for one minute, and direct blood pressure reading should be correlated with an indirect (cuff pressure) reading method.

The nurse is responsible for verifying the proper functioning of all monitoring equipment, setting appropriate alarm limits for the patient, and analyzing the information gathered for significant changes. The nurse should review and interpret changes in vital signs, evaluate temperature fluctuations and thermal environment, calculate urine output (cc/kg/hour), and compare fluid intake with output. Normal parameters for vital signs are as follows:

Temperature (axillary): 36.5–37.2° C

Heart rate (apical): 120–140 beats/minute (term),
140–160 beats/minute (preterm)

Respiratory rate: 30–60 breaths/minute

Blood pressure (systolic): 50–70 mmHg, increases by 4 days of age to 60–90 mmHg

Blood pressure (diastolic): 25–45 mmHg, slight rise by 4 days of age

The nurse should also review hematocrit, serum glucose, urine checks, stool checks, acid-

TABLE 13 ▲ Nursing Care Guidelines for Critically Ill Infants

Vital Signs

1. Take temperature (axillary), pulse, and respirations:
   • q 1 hour or more frequently on critical unstable infants
   • q 2 hours on all mechanically ventilated, CPAP, or oxyhood patients
   • q 3 hours on stable infants
2. Record blood pressure q 1 hour on all infants with arterial lines (lines must be recalibrated every 12 hours and should be correlated with an indirect, peripheral BP measurement.)
3. Take peripheral blood pressure (documenting extremity used):
   • q 4 hours on all acute care neonates without arterial lines
   • q 12 hours on all infants

Obtain Specimen for

1. Hematocrit (label as central or peripheral):
   • on admission and q 8 hours on all unstable infants
   • daily on stable NICU patients
   • 4 hours after a transfusion
2. Blood glucose:
   • on admission and q 1–2 hours until stable (60–150 mgm%)
   • q 4–8 hours on NPO patients
   • q 8 hours while patient on IV fluids
3. Urine specific gravity and combstix:
   • q 8–12 hours on all patients receiving parenteral fluids

Intake and Output

1. Compute q 8–12 hours
2. Calculate urine output (cc/kg/day) q 4–8 hours if urine output low or excessively high
3. Record all fluid intake, including medication, flush, and blood products
4. Record all output, including urine, blood, stool, gastric output, and drainage

are relatively small, extreme care is needed in the preparation and administration of medications. Complicating this problem are the patient's possible fluid restriction and dependence on a continuous infusion of glucose. Drugs infused over several minutes or hours must be mixed with glucose solutions when compatible to provide optimal calories.

The literature is rich with information about drug doses, routes, and intervals but often lacks the necessary information about administration rates and drug compatibilities. Table 14 is a protocol sheet for drug information that should be available on every drug administered. *Drug Administration in the NICU: A Handbook for Nurses* is a valuable guide containing this pertinent drug information.[35]

base status, and recent laboratory studies and check for outstanding laboratory test results. Each NICU should have a listing of normal laboratory values specific for its hospital's laboratory available to the nursing staff. These values, properly interpreted, along with sound nursing judgment of overall status, can provide an accurate picture of the neonate's condition.

Fluid Requirements

Infants in respiratory distress are usually managed initially with intravenous fluids. Umbilical catheters and percutaneously inserted intravenous catheters are used. Central venous lines may be utilized if prolonged parenteral fluids are required. Nursing personnel are responsible for ongoing assessment of these flu-

Administration of Medication

A major nursing responsibility is the prompt and accurate administration of medication. Dosages of drugs given to the neonate are based on body weight, and each nurse must be capable of calculating such doses. Because doses and volumes

TABLE 14 ▲ Protocol for Essential Drug Information

Name: Generic name with trade name in parentheses (indexed by both names)

Indication/Action: Class, indication/action of drug

Dose/Route/Interval: Dose (single dose, not by total daily dose), route, and interval of administration

Preparation: Type of fluid for reconstitution and for dilution; preferred fluids first with alternative fluids in parentheses (See drug label for the reconstitution instruction.)

Administration Rate: Desired rate of administration

Comments: Drug levels, side effects, antidotes, incompatibilities, tips on administration, other comments

References: References referred to by number, followed by page numbers in parentheses (references listed in back of the handbook)

TABLE 15 ▲ Estimated Fluid Requirement for Full-Term Infants' Daily Fluid Requirements

To Replace Fluid from:	cc/kg/day
Insensible water loss	15–20
Renal water loss	60–90
Stool water loss*	10
Growth*	10–15
Water of oxidation	−15
Total	80–120

*On day 1 of life, these values should be zero, rising to the stated numbers by day 3.

From: Wassner SJ: *in* Nelson N, ed., Current Therapy in Neonatal-Perinatal Medicine 2, Toronto, 1990, B.C. Decker, p. 153. Reprinted with permission.

ids to assure both the accuracy of infusion rates and the patency of the line. Intravenous infiltrates or catheter accidents are major iatrogenic complications.

Fluid requirements vary with gestational and chronological age. Fluid is required to replace water retained for growth and water lost in urine, stool, and other body drainage such as gastrointestinal or wound drainage as well as fluid lost from the respiratory tract and skin (insensible water loss) (Table 15). Insensible water loss is especially significant in the neonate

TABLE 16 ▲ Factors Influencing Insensible Water Loss*

Increasing

1. Radiant warmers (50–100%)
2. Phototherapy (30–50%)
3. Increased body temperature
4. Increased environmental temperature
5. Increased respiratory rate
6. Decreased ambient humidity
7. Motor activity and crying
8. Low birthweight
9. Decreased gestational age
10. Skin breakdown or injury
11. Congenital skin defects

Decreasing

1. Endotracheal intubation on mechanical ventilation
2. High ambient humidity
3. Heat shield, plastic-wrap blanket, double-walled incubator
4. Malnutrition
5. Decreased activity

*Table sources are references 36–38.

because it increases proportionally as birthweight and gestational age decrease and may be 60 to 70 ml/kg/day in an infant with a birthweight under 1 kilogram.[36] Table 16 lists factors that can increase or decrease insensible water loss in the neonate.

During the first week of life, physiologic extracellular dehydration normally causes a 5–20 percent weight loss. A higher fraction of weight loss is experienced by smaller, more preterm infants because of their proportionately larger extracellular water and greater tissue catabolism.[37]

Fluid requirements increase with postnatal age and the introduction of enteral feedings. Fecal water losses are greater, and urine output increases in response to the increased renal solute load. Oxidation of metabolic fuels (carbohydrates, fats, and protein) results in a gain in fluid, but this is offset by the deposit of water in tissue associated with growth. Clinical assessment of hydration includes evaluation of vital signs, skin turgor, mucous membranes, anterior fontanel, body weight, and urine output.

Nutritional Requirements

The neonate has high nutritional requirements to support growth, and the ill newborn's needs are even greater. Enteral feedings are the ideal method of providing calorie needs in a balanced diet. Unfortunately, the critically ill neonate may not be a candidate for enteral feedings for several days or weeks.

Parenteral nutrition is begun with glucose infusions, usually 5 or 10 percent dextrose in water, depending on the infant's tolerance of the glucose load. The glucose intake is increased during the first week of life, with a usual goal of 11–12 mg/kg/minute. A minimum of 50–60 calories/kg/day is needed for maintenance, and additional calories are required for growth. Glucose intolerance, as evidenced by blood glucose levels greater than 150 mg/dl and/or glucosuria, can be precipitated by stress, thermal instability, sepsis, acidosis, or respiratory failure.

TABLE 17 ▲ Neonatal Enteral Feedings*

	Advantages	Disadvantages
Gastric (bolus)	Utilizes stomach capacity and digestive capabilities Potential for greater absorption More physiologic than continuous Tube easier to place and less likely to perforate	Potential compromise in neonates with severe respiratory distress, delayed gastric emptying, esophageal chalasia, or during the use of nasal CPAP Bradycardia with tube placement
Gastric (continuous)	May be better tolerated in very low-birthweight infants, infants with bowel disease, or infants with severe cardiopulmonary disease	Higher risk of contamination of formula with bacterial growth Fat concentration of human milk changes during delivery
Transpyloric (continuous)	Useful in infants with delayed gastric emptying or gastroesophageal reflux and aspiration Used in infants on ventilatory support, such as nasal CPAP	As per continuous gastric feedings Greater risk of bowel perforation Increased radiation exposure because of more frequent x-ray exams for placement May experience decreased absorption of potassium and fat

*Table sources are references 39, 41–44.

Protein, provided as parenteral amino acids, can be started by one or two days of age if the infant is receiving at least maintenance calories as carbohydrate (glucose). The infant is started on 0.5–1 gm/kg/day of protein, which is gradually increased over a week's time to 2–2.5 gm/kg/day if renal and liver function is adequate. Electrolytes, vitamins, minerals, and trace elements must also be provided as part of the peripheral alimentation.

Fat, given as intralipid, can also be started by one or two days of age. The infant receives 0.5–1 gm/kg/day, which is usually increased over several days to 3 gm, although preterm infants may tolerate only 2 gm/kg/day. Visible lipemia or a serum triglyceride of more than 200 mg/dl requires a decrease in intralipids. Lipids contain high calories in minimal fluid volumes, thereby providing an excellent source of calories. Up to 50 percent of the neonate's calories can be given as fat.[39,40]

Enteral feedings should be started as soon as feasible. They remain the best source of nutrition for the neonate, especially for the low-birthweight infant who is particularly vulnerable to malnutrition. Even infants requiring mechanical ventilation should be considered candidates for early enteral feedings. Determination of the formula, volume, and route of feeding is based on the infant's gestational age, weight, and clinical status (Table 17). The time when suck, swallow, and respirations are coordinated varies, but generally infants can successfully nipple by 32–34 weeks gestation if they are alert and vigorous.

A previously ill neonate or a preterm infant usually must be started on gavage feedings in small volumes gradually increased over several day's time. Each nursery should have personnel capable of properly placing a gavage tube and correctly administering the feeding to the neonate.[45] Infants who use pacifiers during feedings have been found to nipple feed earlier, gain weight better, and be discharged earlier.[46,47]

The infant's clinical status should be assessed with each feeding or every 2–3 hours if feedings are continuous. Abdominal distention, regurgitation, absence of bowel sounds, bile-stained aspirates, and large feeding residuals are indications of feeding intolerance.

Most infant formulas contain 20 calories per ounce. This is considered the caloric content of breast milk as well, although the actual caloric content can vary greatly. Utilization of breast milk requires special care measures by the mother and the nursery staff to prevent contamination. Use of breast milk in continuous

TABLE 18 ▲ Standard of Care*

Medical Diagnostic Category: Newborns and other neonates with conditions originating in the perinatal period
Medical Diagnosis: All
Nursing Diagnosis: Potential for impaired skin integrity

Defining Characteristics	Expected Outcome	Nursing Interventions

Developmental factors: less than 2 weeks postnatal age, premature
Altered tissue perfusion
Altered nutritional status
Altered skin turgor
External factors
  Excretions and secretions
  Physical immobility
  Humidity (excessive or decreased)
  Iatrogenic factors:
  • *Mechanical*—epidermal stripping from removal of adhesives, restraints, pressure points
  • *Chemical* burns—external burns from topical agents such as alcohol or betadine; internal burns from intravenous infiltrates
  • *Thermal* burns from heating units or transcutaneous probes
	Skin integrity maintained
	Skin moist or slightly dry, flaky
		• Assess skin and document integrity, color, perfusion, turgor, temperature, edema each shift and prn
		• Notify physician of significant findings requiring medical intervention
		• Minimize use of adhesives
		• Utilize pectin barriers and kara base electrodes; change as indicated by infant's skin integrity
		• Remove adhesives with patience and water-soaked cotton balls
		• Utilize pressure gauze dressings for stasis of bleeding
		• Allow transparent dressings to peel off naturally
		• Avoid hot packs or heat retaining plastic
		• Avoid use of emollients and agents with preservatives and dyes
		• Using sterile water, remove excess betadine on skin after procedures and before dressing wounds
		• Rotate sites for temperature probes q 24 hours
		• Prevent pressure points by turning q 2 hours and prn and utilizing egg-crate foam or water mattress
		• Avoid pressure points or constriction of blood flow (from dressings, tubing, probes, clothes)
		• Bathe the acutely ill infant only in diaper area or soiled skin as tolerated; bathe convalescent infants with soap only once or twice per week
		• Utilize the less alkaline soaps such as Lowila, Aveeno, Basis, Neutrogena, Purpost, Oilatum
		• Treat excessively dry skin with a nonperfumed emollient, such as HEB cream base

*Table sources are references 7,48–50.

feedings is associated with high bacterial growth and loss of fat content.[41,51]

Steady growth can normally be achieved when the infant is receiving 100–120 calories/kg/day. If the infant cannot tolerate the high fluid volumes necessary to achieve this goal, a modified formula of increased caloric density (24 calories/ounce) can be utilized.[39] Formulas that provide the additional calories, vitamins, and minerals required by the premature infant are also available.

Skin Care

Skin integrity relates directly to neonatal well-being, and skin care has been recognized as a vital nursing care function for the newborn. Skin maturity and integrity have a major impact on thermoregulation, insensible water loss, and susceptibility to infection.

The skin is composed of the epidermis and the dermis. The outer layer of the epidermis is known as the stratum corneum (horny layer). Composed of several layers of flattened and dehydrated cells, it is tough, fairly impermeable, and constitutes a barrier against bacteria while decreasing water and heat loss. The dermo-epidermal junction is a specialized attachment between the epidermis and the papillary or outer layer of the dermis. The dermis lies beneath the epidermis, formed of connective tissue containing lymphatics, nerves and nerve endings, blood vessels, sebaceous and sweat glands, and elastic fibers. Underlying this is subcutaneous tissue first seen around 14 weeks gestation but not significant in quantity until near term.

When an infant is born prematurely, the stratum corneum is underdeveloped, and the dermo-epidermal junction is weak, which results in a markedly increased permeability of the skin—especially in infants less than 32 weeks gestation and 2 weeks chronological age. Premature infants also display functional immaturity of eccrine sweat glands, altered vasomotor tone, and a deficit in the shivering reflex. Consequently, the infant is at increased risk for temperature instability, high insensible water loss, and skin injury.[52,53]

Normally, the stratum corneum acts as a diffusion barrier, aided by skin surface lipids formed from epidermal cells and sebaceous glands. The premature's skin is quite susceptible to percutaneous absorption of substances due to an underdeveloped stratum corneum and a thin layer of keratinocytes. Factors influencing absorption are temperature, hydration, perfusion, surface lipids, chronological and gestational age, skin condition, and the chemical and vehicle used. An acidic skin pH develops during the first four days after delivery, providing an acid mantle that has a bacteriocidal quality. Bathing alters the status of the skin, and care must be exercised to promote the acid mantle that provides protection.[48]

Skin care needs of the sick infant include preventing physical injury (stripping of the epidermis, thermal burns, pressure necrosis), preventing chemical injury (chemical infiltrates, chemical burns), minimizing insensible water loss, minimizing risk of infection, and avoiding excessive transdermal absorption of topical agents. Table 18 provides a standard of care, listing nursing interventions designed to protect the integrity of the neonate's skin.

CARE OF THE PARENTS

Care for parents begins with a respect for their rights as parents and an understanding that they are individuals in a crisis situation. A crisis develops when an individual's coping skills are inadequate to deal with a problem or threat. It is important to remember that it is the parents and not the health team members who define the magnitude or significance of the crisis. Reaction to the crisis causes a temporary disruption of the normal psychological equilibrium, resulting in tension and discomfort. Feelings of guilt, anxiety, fear, shame, and helplessness may occur. As a result of this effective upset, the cognitive process may be impaired, resulting in confusion and disorganized behavior.[54,55]

Because parents usually anticipate a normal birth and a healthy infant, a crisis develops when this does not occur. Parents, specifically the mother, prepare during pregnancy for the perfect child. The premature infant may be perceived by the parents as defective. The birth of a premature or critically ill infant may also be viewed by the mother as failure on her part to produce a normal or complete child. The guilt feelings arising from such perceptions often discourage or prohibit a closeness between the parent and the child as well as between the parents themselves. Guilt coupled with the threatening situation further interferes with the parents' ability to understand and deal with the problem.[56] The following techniques may assist the nurse when she must communicate bad news or diagnostic information to parents:[57]

1. Maintain eye contact; use touch and space appropriately.
2. Use the client's name.
3. Begin with a tone-setting statement.
4. Give a brief description of the problem in layman's terms.
5. Follow with the correct medical term(s), verbal and written.
6. End with a continuity statement, explaining what will happen next.

Parents of a premature infant have also been denied the time to psychologically prepare for the birth of their child. The last weeks of a pregnancy are spent physically and mentally preparing for the birth. With a preterm delivery, the parent's state of unpreparedness combined with what may be a life-threatening situation for both the mother and the infant lead to extremely high levels of stress. The birth experience and the delivered infant are not what the parents had wanted or expected. Perceptual distortions are often out of proportion to the severity of the situation. Parents are hampered by both physical and mental barriers in their attempt to become acquainted with and form emotional ties to their child. Going home without the baby also reinforces their feelings of disappointment and failure.[58]

According to the findings of Kaplan and Mason, parents of premature infants have four developmental tasks following the birth of their child: (1) expressing grief, in anticipation of the loss of the infant, (2) acknowledging maternal failure to produce a term or healthy infant, (3) resuming the process of relating to the infant when the infant begins to recover, and (4) understanding the special needs of their infant.[59] To provide appropriate support, the nurse needs to recognize the stage at which the individual parent is functioning.

Throughout the hospitalization, the parents' needs should be identified along with those of their infant. The family's strengths should be identified and capitalized upon to help them through a difficult time. The family's weaknesses, which are sometimes easy to see and other times hidden, will eventually impact the parents' ability to deal with their infant's problems.

The initial phase of crisis is usually marked by a period of physical, functional, and emotional disorganization. Parents feel they cannot take on the parental role because they do not have a child to care for. The hospital staff assumes the care of their child, and feelings of inadequacy and disorganization intensify. Parents may mimic the physician or nurse in an attempt to define their role as parent. When they cannot perform at the same level, further feelings of inadequacy develop.

Denial may be used as a coping mechanism to control the disorganization precipitated by the crisis. Withdrawal may be a form of denial as well as a part of the anticipatory grief for the potential loss of their child. Anger and resentment are also seen during this phase. The anger may be directed at themselves or displaced to others, including family, friends, or health care workers.[60]

Caplan has described three coping patterns used by mothers in dealing successfully with this type of crisis situation: (1) The mother masters the situation by cognitive understanding of the cause and consequence of the prematurity. (2) The mother copes emotionally, verbalizing her feelings and sharing them with others. (3) The mother actively seeks help from others.[61] The nurse can attempt to identify the successful coping strategies employed by parents and assist them in their attempt to deal with the situation.

Once the parents work through their grief and sense of failure, they can begin a phase of emotional adaptation and enter a more positive relationship with their child. They begin to focus on their infant as an individual and must resume the task of interacting with the infant that began during the pregnancy.

The parents are getting acquainted with their child during their first weeks together. The acquaintance process has been described as consisting of three main components. Participants in the process (1) acquire information about each other, (2) assess one another's attitudes, and (3) continue to collect data to change or reinforce existing impressions and develop further impressions about each other.[62]

The term infant can communicate in various ways, focusing on the human face and listening attentively to a human voice. The child will latch onto the mother by grasping, sucking, or rooting, and the mother interprets these behaviors as methods of seeking contact. Signals such as crying, smiling, babbling, and arm gestures from the infant are identified by the parent as personal communications.[63]

Infant cues play a major part in the acquaintance process. Research by Robson and Moss has shown that for many mothers, the first positive maternal feelings toward their infants were associated with the baby's responses to them.[64] The mother uses the infant's behavior to judge or assess his attitude toward her. Fathers also attempt to assess their infant's attitudes early in the acquaintance process by interpreting his behaviors. Success in gaining information and assessing infant attitudes may influence the positive development of subsequent parent-infant relationships, resulting in attachment formation.[65]

Unfortunately, the premature or critically ill newborn does not respond in the typical manner. During the acute phase of illness, these infants may be hypotonic or motionless. As they recover, they may be irritable, inconsolable, or easily exhausted. Parents may perceive the premature infant's immature reflexes as abnor-

FIGURE 7 ▲ Example of weekly update note sent home to parents

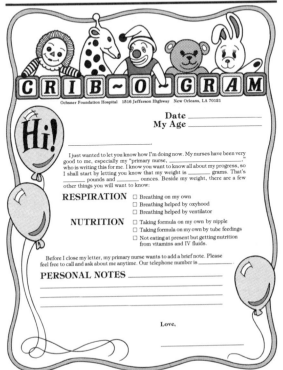

From: Primary Nursing Care Manual, Ochsner Foundation Hospital. Reprinted with permission.

TABLE 19 ▲ Guidelines for Effective Parent Teaching

1. Use "everyday" terms.
2. Utilize two or more modes of communication.
3. Recognize parents' limitations.
4. Make comparisons.
5. Repeat information.
6. Progress from simple to difficult.
7. Summarize information.
8. Check for understanding.
9. Encourage questions.
10. Allow ventilation of feelings.

Adapted from: Sumrall BC: Personal communication.

mal.[66] Such behaviors, as well as those exhibited by a frankly neurologically abnormal infant, can hinder parent-infant interaction, and parents must come to terms with the infant's abilities and limitations.

As parents of critically ill and premature infants are making their emotional adaptation and attachment to their infant, they should be encouraged to assume caretaking responsibilities. Table 19 lists a few basic principles that the nurse can employ to help the parent learn caretaking skills. Mastering these skills reinforces the role of the parent and diminishes feelings of inadequacy. Reluctance to assume this role may be an indication that the individual is still grieving the anticipated loss of the child, and forcing him or her to assume responsibilities prematurely may reinforce feelings of disorganization. At this time parents start to recognize their child's special needs. How is this infant like other "normal" infants, and how does he differ? As parents recognize the uniqueness of their infant and develop an understanding of that child's needs, they are accepting and integrating him into their family. These tasks may be only partially completed at discharge, but if a positive relationship is to be established, they eventually must be accomplished.

The individuality of each parent, infant, and situation must be recognized. Table 20 provides a care plan to help the NICU parent through this crisis.

TABLE 20 ▲ Parental Support Care Plan

Medical Diagnostic Category: Newborns and other neonates with conditions originating in the perinatal period
Medical Diagnosis: All
Nursing Diagnosis: Knowledge deficit, parental/family

Defining Characteristics	Expected Outcome	Nursing Interventions
Parents verbalize their lack of knowledge Parents relate incorrect information to other family members or to the health care team	Parents will be able to verbalize their understanding of infant's present condition, planned treatment, and likely progress	• Prepare parents for their first contact with infant when possible • Provide tours of the NICU to parents who have been indentified by the obstetrician as high risk for delivering a preterm or ill infant • Explain what equipment is being used and why • Encourage parents to ask questions frequently • Coordinate information and explanations within the health care team so that information given to the parents is consistent • Carefully plan timing and content of information to avoid information overload • Periodically reclarify with parents their understanding of infant's status • Provide significant information to both parents to avoid confusion • Provide written literature when appropriate
Inability to meet own basic needs	Parents get appropriate meals and rest	• Assist family in recognizing their own health care needs • Collaborate with social services in finding alternate housing, such as boarding home or hotel, or assistance with meals when appropriate • Encourage the parent's utilization of their family support system
Inability to express fears and concerns	Parents will verbalize feelings about infant's illness and hospitalization	• Provide supportive climate in which parents may feel comfortable sharing their concerns • Allow parents to fully express their feelings; do not minimize or repudiate their stated concerns
Failure to understand rationale for prescribed treatment regimen	Parents will verbalize an understanding of infant's condition, treatment, and progress after initial shock and/or denial	• Interpret hospital environment and events for parents • Offer brief explanation of infant's condition and treatment • Refer pertinent questions to physician. Reinforce or clarify explanations
Inappropriate anger toward staff	Parents will collaborate with health team members regarding decisions about infant	• Recognize parents' ethnic/cultural background and identify customs or attitudes that will affect their interaction with health care personnel • Utilize primary nursing to provide a consistent caretaker who can develop a trusting relationship with parents • Allow for ventilation of anger with a nondefensive response from staff • Offer additional support avenues, such as social workers, pastoral care, or parent support group • Arrange interdisciplinary family conferences for difficult or complex patients/family
Unwillingness to participate in infant care	Parents will demonstrate attachment behaviors toward infant	• Provide an open visiting policy • Identify special characteristics of infant to assist parents in seeing their baby as a unique individual
	Parents will participate in infant's care	• Involve parents in decisions about infant's care, offering choices whenever possible • Encourage participation in basic care; be aware that parents can easily be intimidated by the expertise of the hospital staff • Provide privacy at the bedside • Encourage the bringing of clothes, small toys, or religious articles such as medals • Encourage picture taking • If parents cannot visit, maintain contact by arranging times to call parents to provide updates and send weekly information letters (Figure 7)

SUMMARY

Nursing care of the infant in acute respiratory distress is all encompassing. Responsibilities begin with direct patient care and extend to the family of the infant. Although the focus of patient care activities will be directed by the patient's diagnosis, the nurse must provide total assessment and care. Each intervention with the neonate has a purpose and will impact the patient's status. The nurse must continue to scrutinize each aspect of the neonate's care and recognize that nursing activities are creating the environment in which the infant lives. The neonate's well being is truly in the hands of his nurse.

REFERENCES

1. Bloom R, and Cropley C: Textbook of Neonatal Resuscitation, American Heart Association/American Academy of Pediatrics, Dallas, 1987, American Heart Association.

2. American Academy of Pediatrics/American College of Obstetricians and Gynecologists: Guidelines for Perinatal Care, 2nd ed., Elk Grove Village, Illinois, 1988, American Academy of Pediatrics.

3. Clark DA, and Hakanson DO: The inaccuracy of Apgar scoring, Journal of Perinatology 8(3), 1988, pp. 203–205.

4. Desmond M, Rudolph A, and Phitaksphraiwan P: The transitional care nursery, Pediatric Clinics of North America 13(3), 1966, pp. 651–668.

5. Brazelton TB: Psychophysiologic reactions in the neonate, Journal of Pediatrics 58(4), 1961, pp. 513–518.

6. Hey E, and Scopes JW: Thermoregulation in the newborn, in Avery G, ed., Neonatology: Pathophysiology and Management of the Newborn, 3rd ed., Philadelphia, 1987, J.B. Lippincott, pp. 201–211.

7. Axton SE: Nursing Diagnosis Pocket Guide: Neonatal and Pediatric Care Plans, Baltimore, 1986, Williams & Wilkins.

8. Baumgart S, et al.: Effect of heat shielding on convective and evaporative losses and on radiant heat transfer in the premature infant, Journal of Pediatrics 99(6), 1981, pp. 948–956.

9. Greer PS: Head coverings for newborns under radiant warmers, Journal of Obstetric, Gynecologic, and Neonatal Nursing 17(4), 1988, pp. 265–271.

10. Hull D: Thermal control in very immature infants, British Medical Bulletin 44(4), 1988, pp. 971–983.

11. Kaplan M, and Eidelman A: Improved prognosis in severely hypothermic newborn infants treated by rapid rewarming, Journal of Pediatrics 105(3), 1984, pp. 470–474.

12. Malin SW, and Baumgart S: Optimal thermal management for low birth weight infants nursed under high-powered radiant warmers, Pediatrics 79(1), 1987, pp. 47–54.

13. Marks KH, et al.: Thermal head wrap for infants, Journal of Pediatrics 107(6), 1985, pp. 956–959.

14. Moen JE, et al.: Rectal temperatures in preterm infants under radiant warmers, Journal of Obstetric, Gynecologic, and Neonatal Nursing 16(5), 1987, pp. 348–352.

15. Yeh TF, et al.: Oxygen consumption and insensible water loss in premature infants in single- versus double-walled incubators, Journal of Pediatrics 97(6), 1980, pp. 967–971.

16. Baumgart S: Physiology and physics of heat exchange in the premature newborn nursed under a radiant warmer, Journal of the California Perinatal Association 4(2), 1984, pp. 15–18.

17. Topper WH, and Stewart TP: Thermal support for the very-low-birth-weight: Role of supplemental conductive heat, Journal of Pediatrics 105(5), 1984, pp. 810–814.

18. Dubowitz L, Dubowitz V, and Goldberg C: Clinical assessment of gestational age in the newborn infant, Journal of Pediatrics 77(1), 1970, pp. 1–10.

19. Ballard JL, Novak KK, and Driver M: A simplified score for assessment of fetal maturation of newly born infants, Journal of Pediatrics 95(5), 1979, pp. 769–774.

20. Spinnato JA, et al.: Inaccuracy of Dubowitz gestational age in low birth weight infants, Obstetrics and Gynecology 63(4), 1984, pp. 491–495.

21. White PL, Fomufod AK, and Rao MS: Comparative accuracy of recent abbreviated methods of gestational age determination, Clinical Pediatrics 19(5), 1980, pp. 319–321.

22. Gunderson L: Infant development, in Gunderson L, and Kenner C, eds., Care of the 24–25 Week Gestational Age Infant, Petaluma, California, 1990, Neonatal Network, pp. 1–22.

23. Finnstrom O: Studies on maturity in newborn infants, IX: Further observation on the use of external characteristics in estimating gestational age, Acta Paediatrica Scandinavica 66, 1977, pp. 601–604.

24. Constantine NA, et al.: Use of physical and neurologic observations in assessment of gestational age in low birth weight infants, Journal of Pediatrics 110(6), 1987, pp. 921–928.

25. Sconyers S, Ogden B, and Goldberg H: The effect of body position on the respiratory rate of infants with tachypnea, Journal of Perinatology 7(2), 1987, pp. 118–121.

26. Nugent J: Acute respiratory care of the newborn, Journal of Obstetric, Gynecologic and Neonatal Nursing (supplement), May/June 1983, pp. 31–44.

27. Brouthton J: Understanding blood gases, Ohio Medical Products Medical Article Reprint Library #456, August 1971.

28. Effros RM: Acid-base balance, in Murray J, and Nadel J, eds., Textbook of Respiratory Medicine, Philadelphia, 1988, W.B. Saunders, pp. 129–148.

29. Hodgkin J: Blood gas analysis and acid-base physiology, in Burton G, Gee G, and Hodgkin J, eds., Respiratory Care: A Guide to Clinical Practice, Philadelphia, 1977, J.B. Lippincott, pp. 234–257.

30. Coen R, and Koffler H: Primary Care of the Newborn, Boston, 1987, Little, Brown.

31. Klaus M, and Meyer BP: Oxygen therapy for the newborn, Pediatric Clinics of North America 13, 1966, p. 731.

32. Phillips B, McQuitty J, and Durand D: Blood gases: Technical aspects and interpretation, in Goldsmith J, and Karotkin E, eds., Assisted Ventilation of the Neonate, Philadelphia, 1988, W.B. Saunders, pp. 213–232.

33. Blanchette V, and Zipursky A: Neonatal hematology, *in* Avery G, ed., Neonatology: Pathophysiology and Management of the Newborn, 3rd ed., Philadelphia, 1987, J.B. Lippincott, pp. 638–686.

34. Park M: Pediatric Cardiology for Practitioners, 2nd ed., Chicago, 1988, Yearbook Medical Publishers.

35. Pawlak RP, and Herfert LA: Drug Administration in the NICU: A Handbook for Nurses, 2nd ed., Petaluma, California, 1990, Neonatal Network.

36. Wassner S: Fluid therapy, *in* Nelson N, ed., Current Therapy in Neonatal-Perinatal Medicine-2, Toronto, 1990, B.C. Decker.

37. Bell EF, and Oh W: Fluid and electrolyte management, *in* Avery G, ed., Neonatology: Pathophysiology and Management of the Newborn, 3rd ed., Philadelphia, 1987, J.B. Lippincott, pp. 775–794.

38. Costarin A, and Baumgart S: Modern fluid and electrolyte management of the critically ill premature infant, Pediatric Clinics of North America 33(1), 1986, pp. 153–178.

39. American Academy of Pediatrics/Committee on Nutrition: Nutritional needs of low-birth-weight infants, Pediatrics 75(5), 1985, pp. 976–986.

40. Rubaltelli FF, Carnielli V, and Orzali A: Parenteral nutrition of the newborn, *in* Stern L, ed., Feeding the Sick Infant, Nestle Nutrition Workshop Series, vol. 11, New York, 1987, Nestec Ltd, Vevey/Raven Press, pp. 241–255.

41. Greer F, McCormick A, and Loker J: Changes in fat concentration of human milk during delivery by intermittent bolus and continuous mechanical pump infusion, Journal of Pediatrics 105(5), 1984, pp. 745–749.

42. Parker P, Stroup S, and Greene H: A controlled comparison of continuous versus intermittent feeding in the treatment of infants with intestinal disease, Journal of Pediatrics 99(3), 1981, pp. 360–364.

43. Pereira GR, and Lemons JA: Controlled study of transpyloric and intermittent gavage feeding in the small preterm infant, Pediatrics 67(1), 1981, pp. 68–71.

44. Vidyasagar D, et al.: Nutritional problems in neonatal intensive care units, *in* Stern L, ed., Feeding the Sick Infant, Nestle Nutrition Workshop Series, vol. 11, New York, 1987, Nestec Ltd, Vevey/Raven Press, pp. 153–175.

45. Weibley TT, et al.: Gavage tube insertion in the premature infant, Maternal Child Nursing 12, January/February 1987, pp. 24–27.

46. Bernbaum JC, et al.: Nonnutritive sucking during gavage feeding enhances growth and maturation in premature infants, Pediatrics 71(1), 1983, pp. 41–45.

47. Goldson E: Nonnutritive sucking in the sick infant, Journal of Perinatology 8(1), 1986, pp. 30–34.

48. Rutter N: Percutaneous drug absorption in the newborn: Hazards and uses, Clinics in Perinatology 14(4), 1987, pp. 911–930.

49. Lund C, et al.: Evaluation of a pectin-based barrier under tape to protect neonatal skin, Journal of Obstetric, Gynecologic and Neonatal Nursing 15(1), 1986, pp. 39–44.

50. NAACOG: Neonatal Skin, OGN Nursing Practice Resource, vol. 12, March 1985.

51. Lemons P, Miller K, Eitzen H, Strodtbeck F, and Lemons J: Bacterial growth in human milk during continuous feeding, American Journal of Perinatology 1(1), 1983, pp. 76–80.

52. Rutter N: The immature skin, British Medical Bulletin 44(4), 1988, pp. 957–970.

53. Solomon LM, and Esterly NB: Neonatal Dermatology, Major Problems in Clinical Pediatrics, vol. 11, Philadelphia, 1973, W.B. Saunders, pp. 1–22.

54. Aquilera D, and Messick J: Crisis Intervention: Theory and Methodology, St. Louis, 1978, C.V. Mosby.

55. Lam C: Crisis intervention in respiratory distress, Journal of the California Perinatal Association 2(2), 1982, pp. 104–107.

56. Kennell J, and Klaus M: Caring for the parents of premature or sick infants, *in* Klaus M, and Kennel J, eds., Parent-Infant Bonding, 2nd ed., St. Louis, 1982, C.V. Mosby, pp. 151–226.

57. Sumrall BC: Personal communication.

58. Mercer R: Nursing Care for Parents at Risk, New Jersey, 1977, C.B. Slack.

59. Kaplan D, and Mason E: Maternal reactions to premature birth viewed as an acute emotional disorder, American Journal of Orthopsychiatry 30, 1960, pp. 359–552.

60. Sammons W, and Lewis J: Premature Babies—A Different Beginning, St. Louis, 1985, C.V. Mosby.

61. Caplan G: Patterns of parental response to the crisis of premature birth, Psychiatry 23, 1960, pp. 365–367.

62. Newcomb T: The Acquaintance Process, New York, 1961, Holt, Rhinehart and Winston.

63. Brazelton TB, Koslowski B, and Main M: The origins of reciprocity: The early mother-infant interaction, *in* Lewis M, and Rosenblum L, eds., The Effect of the Infant on Its Caregiver, New York, 1974, Wiley.

64. Robson K, and Moss H: Patterns and determinants of maternal attachment, Journal of Pediatrics 77(6), 1970, pp. 976–985.

65. Gay JT: A conceptual framework of bonding, Journal of Obstetric, Gynecologic, and Neonatal Nursing 10, 1981, pp. 440–444.

66. Johnson SH, and Grubbs J: The premature infant's reflex behaviors: Effect on the maternal-child relationship, Journal of Obstetric, Gynecologic and Neonatal Nursing 4(3), 1975, pp. 15–20.

4 Nursing Procedures

Barbara S. Turner, RN, DNSc, FAAN
Madigan Army Medical Center
Tacoma, Washington

Most infants admitted to newborn intensive care units are there due to compromise or complications of their respiratory systems. Caring for the critically ill infant requires refined observational and assessment skills combined with a knowledge of the physiologic processes underlying the infant's admission to the unit.

This chapter reviews respiratory system assessment and discusses various nursing interventions used in treating infants with respiratory problems. Possible solutions and interventions to common nursing problems are outlined. Both the nurse who is new to neonatal nursing and the more experienced nurse will find help with some of the most frequent and challenging aspects of caring for the newborn with respiratory compromise.

RESPIRATORY ASSESSMENT

A nurse completes a physical examination on each infant admitted to the NICU. This examination is updated as needed during the current and following shifts and is an invaluable tool for assessing the impact of nursing interventions on the respiratory status of the infant. The initial physical assessment provides the basis for gauging changes that occur over time and enables the nurse to relate those changes to the earlier status of the infant. Because this initial evaluation will be referred to frequently by other caretakers, it is imperative that it be completed immediately after a nurse assumes care of an infant.

A respiratory assessment begins with observation of the infant at rest. The respiratory rate is counted for a full minute, the chest is observed for symmetry of movement and retractions, and the nares are watched for signs of flaring. The nurse also listens to the infant for grunting, stridor, wheezing, or crying. The infant's color is assessed; signs of cyanosis must be evaluated as to their origin. Central cyanosis is evidenced by cyanotic gums and mucous membranes; peripheral cyanosis is usually confined to the hands and feet.

The chest is then auscultated along the anterior, posterior, and mid-axillary line. Sounds from each side of the chest are compared for equality of breath sounds and presence or absence of rales, rhonchi, and other abnormal sounds. Rales are fine rustling noises that result from air passing fluid in the alveoli. Rhonchi are deeper, coarser, snoring sounds that result

The opinions or assertions are the private views of the author and are not to be interpreted as reflecting Department of the Army or Department of Defense policies.

from air passing plugs of mucus or debris in the bronchi.

Problem: How do I assess an infant who is breathing at a rate of 80 breaths per minute and has nasal flaring and audible grunting?

This infant is exhibiting the classic signs of respiratory distress. Rapid respirations occur when the infant is unable to meet his oxygenation demands with a normal respiratory rate and thus must increase the respiratory rate in an effort to meet these needs. The normal respiratory rate for newborn infants is 40 to 60 breaths per minute.

Nasal flaring is the infant's attempt to bring additional air into the lungs. When the infant's nares flare with inspiration, the airway is enlarged and as a result resistance is decreased.

Expiratory grunting occurs when the infant exhales against a partially closed glottis. This maintains end-expiratory pressure in the lungs by increasing transpulmonary pressure. When the alveoli are partially expanded, as they normally are, further expansion consumes relatively little additional energy; when the alveoli are collapsed, it is more difficult to expand them with each breath.

By maintaining positive end-expiratory pressure in the lung, the infant overcomes the breath-to-breath problems of inflating the alveoli. It is much the same as inflating a balloon: Initial expansion is difficult, but once the balloon has begun to inflate, it is easier to inflate the remainder.

Problem: What causes an infant's chest to appear depressed with each breath?

This is a classic sign of respiratory distress in the premature infant. This phenomena, known as retraction, occurs when the lungs are non-compliant (or stiff) and the chest wall is compliant. In the adult, the lungs are compliant, and the chest wall is not as compliant. Therefore, with each inspiration, the lungs expand while the chest wall resists movement. In the premature infant the stiff lungs resist movement while the compliant chest wall moves readily with the respiratory cycle, making the chest appear to be depressed with each breath.

INTUBATION

Intubation is the insertion of an endotracheal tube or artificial airway into the trachea for the purpose of supporting ventilation and oxygenation. Endotracheal tubes are generally of two types:

1. Cole tubes have a narrow distal opening and a wide proximal opening. The area that narrows is the shoulder of the endotracheal tube, which rests on the larynx and prevents the tube from slipping farther into the trachea, thus preventing a right main stem bronchus (RMSB) intubation.[1]

2. Murphy tubes are of the same diameter throughout. Both types of tubes have a single end hole.

Some of the newer types of endotracheal tubes have side-hole opening(s) in addition to the end-hole opening. A variety of endotracheal tubes is commercially available, including nonkinking tubes and tubes with side ports for monitoring mean airway pressure or administering transtracheal medication.

Neonatal endotracheal tubes are uncuffed to prevent excessive pressure against the tracheal wall and to allow the largest endotracheal tube to be inserted. Cuffed tubes, because of the extension of the cuff, require relatively more room than uncuffed tubes. A cuffed endotracheal tube can be inflated, thereby exerting pressure that restricts tube movement.

Because neonatal endotracheal tubes are uncuffed, they move within the trachea. The respiratory cycle of the ventilator can account for up to 2 cm of tube movement; movement of the infant's head can result in 1 cm or more of tube movement.[2] Flexion of the infant's head moves the endotracheal tube toward the carina and beyond into a main stem bronchus. Extension of the head moves the tip of the tube toward the glottis away from carina.[3] Nasotracheal tubes have been reported to

FIGURE 1 ▲ Example of a bedside card listing endotracheal tube size and endotracheal suctioning information

FIGURE 1 ▲ Example of a bedside card listing endotracheal tube size and endotracheal suctioning information

Baby:	Jones
Weight:	2,200 gm
GA:	34 weeks
ET tube size:	3.5
Inserted:	8 cm at the lips
Suction catheter size:	6½ Fr
Suction depth:	12 cm

result in more intratracheal movement than orotracheal tubes.[4]

Nurses are responsible for assessing the integrity of the airway as well as determining when the endotracheal tube is incorrectly positioned. If the tube is positioned too low, it may be in one bronchus, resulting in only one lung or segment of a lung being ventilated.

A correctly placed endotracheal tube, as shown on x-ray examination, is positioned below the clavicle and above the carina. Because the term newborn's trachea is approximately 4 cm in length, the endotracheal tube should be positioned 1–2 cm below the vocal cords and approximately 2–3 cm above the carina.[5] Endotracheal tube placement can also be determined by sonography.[6] When the tip of the endotracheal tube is visualized 1 cm above the aortic arch, the tube is correctly positioned.

Once the tube is determined to be in the correct position, it is secured by tape or other methods. The depth of insertion should be noted and posted on the infant's incubator or radiant warmer. For endotracheal tubes that have centimeter markings, the marking located at the infant's lips is the depth that is recorded. For those tubes that do not have depth markings, the lettering on the tube can be used as a marker. Figure 1 is an example of a bedside card used to document the depth of insertion.

Recording the depth of insertion helps nurses determine if the tube has moved from the correct position. Because excessive secretions, tape, or other securing mechanisms become loose, and movement of the infant's head and neck result in endotracheal tube movement, assessing endotracheal tube position is an ongoing process.

The "1–2–3, 7–8–9" rule can generally be used for determining tube depth for orotracheal intubation. An infant weighing 1 kg would have the endotracheal tube placed at a depth of approximately 7 cm, a 2 kg infant would have the endotracheal tube inserted to an 8 cm depth, and a 3 kg infant would have it inserted to 9 cm. For nasotracheal intubation, 1 cm is added to the 7–8–9 rule to compensate for the increased distance that nasotracheal intubation requires. This additional depth changes the 1–2–3, 7–8–9 rule to 1–2–3, 8–9–10.

Intubation is not a benign procedure and should be carried out with care. In the premature infant, intubation has been associated with cardiac rhythm changes, apnea, increased blood pressure, and decreased heart rate and transcutaneous oxygen tension.[7] Other complications of intubation are noted in Table 1. Thermal support, adequate ventilation, oxygenation, and physiologic monitoring as well as necessary equipment and supplies should be in place before intubation is begun.

Care of the Neonate with an Endotracheal Tube

The inadvertent or accidental displacement of an endotracheal tube out of the trachea is an emergency that occurs in an estimated in 2–40

TABLE 1 ▲ Complications Associated with Intubation

Complication	Reason
Palatal grooves[8–10]	Pressure of tube on palate
Nasal erosion and stricture[11–13]	Pressure of nasal tube on nares
Defective dentition[14–15]	Pressure of tube on gums
Subglottic stenosis[16–17]	Irritation from tube
Esophageal perforation[18–20]	Insertion trauma
Aspiration[21]	No cuff on the tube
Bacterial colonization[1,22]	Presence of ET tube
Tracheal granuloma[23]	Irritation from tip of ET tube

percent of all intubated neonates.[24] Nurses are responsible for assessing and maintaining the endotracheal tube in the correct position.

Assessing the position of the endotracheal tube takes only a few minutes and is noninvasive; it is therefore imperative that this be done frequently enough to assure that effective ventilation is not impeded by an incorrectly positioned tube. The tip of the endotracheal tube should be situated approximately 1.5 cm below the glottis. Radiographically, this corresponds to the tip lying at T 2–4.

Problem: How can I determine whether the endotracheal tube is in the correct position?

Several methods can be used to determine the relative position of the endotracheal tube:

1. Auscultation of the chest. Auscultation of the infant's chest will provide clues to the relative position of the endotracheal tube. The nurse should routinely auscultate the chest along the mid-axillary line, comparing the right and left breath sounds. Endotracheal tubes that are positioned too low may enter the right main stem bronchus instead of the left because of the degree of angulation of each bronchus from the trachea. It was believed previously that in the infant the angulation of each bronchus from the trachea was 55° and that with growth and development it gradually assumed the adult angulation of 25° for the right bronchus and 45° for the left bronchus.[25] It is now known that the angulation of each bronchus from the trachea in newborns and infants is approximately equal to that of the adult.[26,27]

With an RMSB intubation, there will be ipsilateral hyperinflation of the right lung and contralateral collapse of the left lung because only the right side of the chest will be ventilated. However, breath sounds may not always be decreased on the left because some of the breath sounds from the right may be referred to the left side of the chest.

An infant with a left-sided pneumothorax presents with many of the same clinical signs as one with an RMSB intubation. The electrocardiogram (ECG) complex is often used to distinguish between the two conditions. With a pneumothorax the R-S voltage may be decreased because the extrapulmonary air does not transmit electrical activity as well as fluid.

The treatment for an RMSB intubation is to pull the endotracheal tube back until bilateral breath sounds are heard. The distance the tube is pulled back can be measured from a recent radiograph, if one is available. If the cause of the decreased breath sounds is a pneumothorax rather than a misplaced endotracheal tube, pulling the tube back may result in accidental extubation. So if a pneumothorax has not been ruled out and there is no radiographic confirmation of a misplaced endotracheal tube, the tube should *not* be pulled back.

2. Observation of chest movement. With accidental extubation or intubation of the RMSB, chest movement may not be observable or may be unequal. In a RMSB intubation, the inflated lung will cause the chest to rise higher on the right side than the left.

3. Auscultation of the chest and abdomen. Breath sounds should be heard better in the chest than in the abdomen. Breath sounds clearly heard in the abdomen accompanied by distention of the abdomen may indicate that the endotracheal tube has slipped out of the trachea and into the esophagus. If this occurs, the endotracheal tube is removed, and the infant is reintubated. An oral gastric tube is placed for decompression of the abdomen.

4. Observation of the endotracheal tube for fogging or condensation upon exhalation. The endotracheal tube will fog or show evidence of condensation when the infant exhales if the tube is placed in the trachea. Condensation upon exhalation will not be found in endotracheal tubes positioned in the oral pharynx or in the esophagus. If it is difficult

to see the fogging in the endotracheal tube during ventilation and if the infant has some spontaneous respirations, the ventilator can be momentarily disconnected while the flat end of the laryngoscope is placed near the end of the endotracheal tube. Fogging of the laryngoscope should be evident.

Problem: How can the endotracheal tube be secured in position?

Endotracheal tubes can be secured using a variety of methods, including adhesive tape, "pink tape," suture and tape, locking mechanisms, Velcro, umbilical clamps, logan bows, and cloth ties. Descriptions of step-by-step methods of securing endotracheal tubes in position can be found in the literature.[28,29] Securing the tube requires two persons: one to hold the tube in the correct position while simultaneously ventilating the infant, another to anchor the tube. For those methods of securing endotracheal tubes that require adhesive tape, "tagging" the end of the tape by folding it over on itself to create a "flag" or "tag" facilitates tape removal and repositioning of the endotracheal tube.

Problem: What causes movement of the endotracheal tube once it is in place?

It is not uncommon to find that the endotracheal tube will be positioned too high on one radiograph and in perfect position on the next without any caregiver intervention. Every uncuffed endotracheal tube has a certain amount of "play" or tube movement. Flexion or extension of the head and neck, body position, and position and tension of the ventilator tubing may affect endotracheal tube position. For radiographic interpretation it is most convenient if the infant is positioned on the x-ray plate with his head in a neutral position to help radiologists, neonatologists, and nurses assess tube position.

Another cause of endotracheal tube movement is what is loosely called the "sliding tube syndrome" in which the infant's oral secretions loosen the securing tape or devices used to hold

---

TABLE 2 ▲ Indicators of Possible Extubation

1. Audible crying
2. Absent breath sounds
3. Visible struggling or extreme agitation
4. Absence of condensation in the endotracheal tube on exhalation
5. Increased abdominal distention
6. Cyanosis
7. Bradycardia
8. Hypoxemia

---

the tube in place. This allows for increased tube movement with movement of the infant's head or the ventilator tubing. There may be sufficient tube movement to allow the infant to become extubated. In these instances the tube must be resecured in the correct position, which requires either removing or reinforcing the old securing.

Accidental extubation requires immediate recognition and intervention. Because any infant may become extubated at any time, each intubated infant should have at his bedside the equipment necessary to reintubate: laryngoscope, appropriate sized blade, endotracheal tubes in a range of sizes, oxygen, and equipment needed to provide bag and mask ventilation.

Posting the correct endotracheal tube size and depth of insertion in a prominent location at the bedside facilitates reintubation. The bag and mask at the bedside should be tested at the beginning of each shift and set up to deliver the appropriate oxygen concentration and positive end-expiratory pressure (PEEP). Oxygen blenders at the bedside and manometers connected to the manual resuscitation bag allow the nurse to ventilate the infant at appropriate and safe positive inspiratory and end-expiratory pressures.

Problem: How can I determine if the infant is extubated?

Indications of possible extubation are summarized in Table 2. The most definitive sign is an audible cry. Intubated infants have silent cries; the endotracheal tube passes through the vocal cords, precluding their ability to make any sound.

FIGURE 2 ▲ Steps to assess the position of the artificial airway

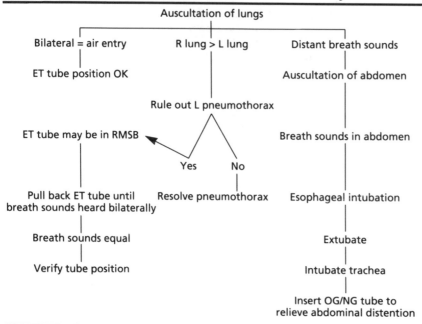

Infants who have progressively increasing abdominal distention and who do not have a nasogastric (NG) or oral gastric (OG) tube in place may be extubated. If the esophagus is intubated, the volume of air will be delivered to the stomach, resulting in abdominal distention. The presence of an NG/OG tube may mask the distention because it will allow excess air to escape from the stomach. The steps used to assess the position of the artificial airway are summarized in Figure 2.

Problem: What causes excessive water collection in the endotracheal tube adapter, and how can I prevent it?

When an infant is correctly intubated, breath sounds can be heard equally well on both sides of the chest. Absent breath sounds may indicate extubation. Breath sounds will not be audible in an extubated infant who is hand or mechanically ventilated; however, breath sounds may be heard bilaterally when the infant initiates a breath because the air is not entering the lungs through the endotracheal tube.

Any infant who is visibly struggling or very agitated should be assessed for potential extubation or blocked endotracheal tube. The endotracheal tube may be blocked with secretions, may be kinked, or may have slipped into the esophagus or oral pharynx.

Failure to see condensation in the endotracheal tube on exhalation suggests extubation. Because exhaled air is fully saturated, there will be condensation in the endotracheal tube on exhalation. Placing the end of the laryngoscope handle near the endotracheal tube adapter will also result in fogging of the laryngoscope on exhalation; however, infants who are apneic or chemically restrained will not have the respiratory effort needed to fog the laryngoscope.

Ventilator tubing circuits have both an inspiratory and an expiratory tubing circuit. Depending upon the type of tubing, the inspiratory and expiratory circuits may be of different colors. By consistently using one color for the inspiratory circuit, the health care team can determine at a glance which tubing is inspiratory and which is expiratory. This is helpful if there is a problem with excessive water accumulation at the site of the endotracheal tube adapter.

When the infant is positioned on his side, the inspiratory tubing should be on the top and the expiratory tubing on the bottom to prevent excessive water buildup in the adapter.

When the fully saturated and warmed gases are propelled toward the infant, they cool, and the water condenses in the tubing as it travels to the infant. This condensation travels by gravity toward the water traps in the ventilator circuit. Excessive "rain out" can also occur at the endotracheal tube adapter site.

FIGURE 3 ▲ Ventilator tubing with in-line thermometer at the proximal airway

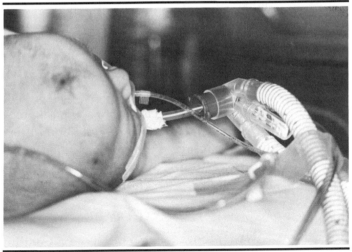

When the inspiratory tube is in the superior position, the excess water drops down into the expiratory circuit and is removed. In contrast, when the inspiratory tube is in the inferior position, the excess water cannot get into the expiratory circuit and thus pools at the end of the inspiratory circuit. Excessive water collected at this point can then run down the endotracheal tube into the infant.

Heated ventilator circuits have been used to combat "rain out." Inspired gas temperatures should be regulated and monitored at the proximal airway site with an in-line thermometer. Safe temperature ranges are 32–34°C. An example of in-line temperature monitoring is shown in Figure 3.

All ventilators have in-line water traps to collect the excess water on both the inspiratory and expiratory circuits. These traps must be drained or emptied to remove any water they collect. Some traps must be removed from the ventilator in order to be drained; these have valves that allow ventilation to continue uninterrupted while the traps are removed.

New Techniques

Two new types of endotracheal tubes that help the health care professional ensure correct tube placement have recently been developed.

Both involve noninvasive methods that can be carried out at the infant's bedside. The first type has an indwelling fiberoptic light that, when connected to a high-intensity light source, illuminates the tip of the endotracheal tube.[30] The light is visible through the skin and thus allows the caretaker to assess tube position as often as necessary without disturbing the infant or subjecting him to excessive radiographs. However, it does not allow the practitioner to differentiate an esophageal from a tracheal intubation.

The fiberoptic filament alters the outer-to-inner diameter ratio of the endotracheal tube. When compared to a conventional endotracheal tube, the inner diameter of the tube with the fiberoptic strand is smaller. Although investigators state that no excess heat was transmitted to the infant's trachea, the temperature at the tip of the light was not reported.[30]

The second type of endotracheal tube has a metallic ring embedded in its wall which does not alter the tube's inner diameter.[31] When a hand-held monitoring device is placed at the infant's suprasternal notch, a green light and audible alarm indicate that the tube is in the correct position. The monitoring device does not discriminate between tracheal and esophageal intubation. This type of noninvasive endotracheal tube position monitor is useful during transport of the critically ill infant when more traditional methods of assessing tube position are not available or are difficult because of ambient noise or vibration.

OXYGEN HOOD

Oxygen hoods or "head boxes" are designed to concentrate the gas mixture around the infant's head. The hoods are plexiglass with openings for the head and neck; some are designed with side access doors and openings for intravenous lines and monitoring cables. Noise that results from the delivery of the gas to the hood can be muffled by placing a foam baffle inside. A thermometer is used to monitor the ambient temperature of the air in the hood. Oxygen delivered via a hood may be all the oxygen support needed by infants who have mild transient tachypnea of the newborn, respiratory distress syndrome, or aspiration syndrome.

The hood size used is based on the size of the infant. A box that is too small may result in pressure areas around the infant's neck or shoulders; one that is too large may allow the infant's head to slip out of the oxygen-enriched environment. Hoods can be used for infants cared for on radiant warmer beds or in incubators. Infants in incubators who require greater than 30 percent oxygen (FiO_2) should have a hood in the incubator to concentrate the oxygen around their face and thus prevent wide fluctuations of FiO_2 when incubator doors or ports are opened.

The percentage of oxygen in the hood is continuously monitored while the infant is inside by an oxygen analyzer placed near the infant's nose. The inspired oxygen percentage is recorded hourly on the infant's flow sheet. Because of drifts in the calibration, the oxygen analyzer should be calibrated at least every eight hours to both high and low FiO_2. The calibration process requires removing the analyzer from the oxygen hood for a few minutes. The probe is placed in room air until the reading has stabilized. If the analyzer does not read 21 percent, it is adjusted to bring the reading to 21 percent. The probe is then exposed to 100 percent oxygen by placing it in a glove along with a source of 100 percent oxygen. If the reading is not 100 percent, the calibrating mechanism is used to bring it to 100 percent. The probe is then re-exposed to room air, and a check is made to ensure that the reading is 21 percent. Linearity of the analyzer can be assessed by placing the probe in a glove containing 50 percent oxygen.

The oxygen/air mixture delivered to the hood should be both warmed and humidified. The temperature probe in the hood is checked with vital signs to ensure that the hood temperature is within the recommended range of 32–35°C.

In order to prevent carbon dioxide accumulation, the gas flow into the hood should be at least 5–7 liters/minute. When there is excessive condensation from the humidified air on the inside of the hood, it can be wiped with a soft cloth so that the infant's head is clearly visible.

NASAL CPAP

Nasal prongs are used to administer continuous positive airway pressure to the neonate. Because infants are predominately nose breathers, the application of continuous distending pressure may help increase end-expiratory pressure. The prongs, made of molded soft plastic and available in sizes to fit the premature as well as the term newborn, fit inside the infant's nares and are attached to the ventilator. Selecting the correct size of prongs is important: If too large, they create trauma to the nares from erosion and pressure; if too small, they may not be as effective in providing sufficient oxygenation and ventilation to the infant.

The disadvantages of using nasal prongs include nasal trauma and the variability of end-expiratory pressure. End-expiratory pressure is lost whenever the infant opens his mouth. Taping the infant's mouth shut, even with a gastric tube in place, is not recommended because of the risk of aspiration.

As with the delivery of any gas to an infant, the air must be both warmed and humidified. Temperature regulation is difficult in the small infant but becomes even more problematic if the inspired gases are not warmed. Unwarmed gases dry out the nasal membranes and create generalized chilling of the infant.

Problem: How do I keep the prongs in position?

The initial positioning of the nasal prongs is not difficult. They can be positioned in the nares using securing devices of Velcro or surgical masks with tie strings.

Maintaining the prongs in the correct position is more difficult. Nasal prongs irritate the nares and result in increased nasal secretions. Patience and creativity are required to maintain proper positioning of the nasal prongs. The goal should be to keep the infant in a quiet awake state, asleep, or at least calm and not struggling. Stroking, creating a quiet environment, and/or playing soft music often help quiet the infant and keep him from fighting the prongs. At times nothing seems to help quiet the infant, and the nurse may find that much time is spent repositioning the prongs.

Frames are available that will hold ventilator tubing in position. Use of these frames with soft linen rolls or intravenous bags positioned on either side of the head will help maintain the infant in position and limit head movement, thus helping to keep the prongs in position.

Care must be taken to change the infant's position frequently to prevent skin breakdown on the head. Use of sheepskin, water mattresses, or foam bedding will help preserve skin integrity. All linen under the infant needs to be free of wrinkles and folds because these can contribute to skin breakdown.

TRANSCUTANEOUS OXYGEN/CARBON DIOXIDE MONITORING

The advent of transcutaneous oxygen and carbon dioxide tension monitoring has heralded a new frontier for nursing management of the infant with respiratory distress. Previously, nurses relied on intermittent arterial or capillary blood samples to determine the degree of hypoxia, hyperoxia, and hypocarbia.

For years nurses have recognized that the values from arterial blood gases were often not in concert with their assessment of the infant's oxygenation status. Infants who have had multiple arterial blood gases drawn often become hypoxemic when their arm is straightened to draw blood; thus timing of the intermittent

samples is important. Nurses who attempt to obtain blood when the child is quiet and appears normoxic find that touching the infant or making the noises associated with gathering and arranging supplies for drawing a blood sample can be enough to upset the infant and as a result change his oxygenation status.

Prior to the advent of transcutaneous monitoring, decisions to change oxygen therapy and mechanical ventilation therapy were based on isolated blood gas values. Because transcutaneous monitoring provides a continuous reflection of the oxygenation status of the infant, health care team members are able to directly observe the infant's responses to different aspects of therapy.

Even parents have become involved in the use of the monitors. They may notice the positive response on the transcutaneous monitor when they touch or speak to their infant. This helps reinforce their importance in his care. Conversely, parents may notice that touch causes the infant to become agitated and upset, thereby decreasing the transcutaneous readings. For these parents counseling by the nurse is of utmost importance to convey the vital role the parents have in their infant's care.

Transcutaneous Oxygen Monitoring

Transcutaneous oxygen monitoring is the measurement of skin oxygen tension rather than arterial oxygen tension. Given an accurate instrument with a specific temperature range under specified conditions, the correlation between skin oxygen tension and arterial oxygen tension is excellent.[32,33] Normally, skin oxygen tension ranges from 1–3 mmHg, and arterial oxygen tension ranges from 60–90 mmHg. Although skin oxygen tension may be elevated in the extremely premature infant, it does not equal arterial oxygen tension.[32]

For skin oxygen tension to approximate arterial oxygen tension, heat must be applied to the skin. Transcutaneous oxygen tension relies on the application of an external heat source to a small area of the skin. The heat produces a hyperemia or increased blood supply to the area. This alters skin oxygen tension by making the skin more permeable to oxygen by altering the lipid layer under the skin and by shifting the oxygen dissociation curve to the right. When the oxygen dissociation curve is shifted to the right, oxygen is not bound as tightly to the hemoglobin molecule and is released more readily at the tissue. These changes alter skin oxygen tension so that it correlates closely with arterial oxygen tension.[32-35] The correlation between skin and arterial oxygen tensions is best when the infant has normal perfusion to the monitoring site, normal body temperature, and normal blood pressure.

For best results it is important that the monitor be calibrated as frequently as recommended in the operating instructions, usually every four hours. With time, transcutaneous oxygen monitors are subject to drifts from their calibration points. Frequent calibration will help improve the correlation between transcutaneous and arterial oxygen tensions. Transcutaneous oxygen monitors have a limited range of accuracy; hypoxia (less than 40 mmHg) and hyperoxia (more than 120 mmHg) may not be accurately reflected by the transcutaneous oxygen tension ($TcPO_2$) monitor.

The heated $TcPO_2$ electrode is applied to any smooth skin surface with a double-sided adhesive ring. Contact liquid enhances the interface of the probe with the skin.

Problem: The reading on the $TcPO_2$ monitor is 159 after I reposition either the baby or the probe. What does this mean?

Readings of 159 on the transcutaneous monitor may reflect the oxygen tension of the ambient room air rather than of the infant (21 percent oxygen multiplied by a barometric pressure of 760 = 159 mmHg ambient oxygen tension). This reading occurs when air is trapped under the probe because it is not in proper contact with the skin. Removing the probe, reapplying the contact liquid and adhesive ring, and

reapplying the probe are required. The reading may be substantially higher if the infant is in an oxygen-enriched environment such as 35 percent FiO_2 (35 percent $FiO_2 \times 760$ mmHg barometric pressure = 266 mmHg).

Problem: During a procedure the infant is lying on the transcutaneous probe for a short time, and the readings do not appear to be accurate. What causes this?

Placing the probe under the infant alters the blood supply to the probe site due to the compression of the tissue between the probe and the infant. Therefore the readings may be inaccurate. Repositioning either the infant or the probe will rectify the problem.

Problem: When the probe is removed, I notice small reddened areas on the skin under the probe. How do I assess this?

Because the transcutaneous monitor requires heat (44–45°C) to increase the blood supply to the skin site, these are local erythematous areas. They will fade, usually within 60 hours, and require no intervention other than not reusing the site until it has healed.[36] The severity of the burns depends on skin sensitivity, probe temperature, and the length of time the probe is left in position. If there are blisters from the monitor, the probe position needs to be changed more frequently (every 2 hours) or the temperature of the probe reduced. Reducing the probe temperature, however, reduces the accuracy of the readings. Skin craters have been reported as a complication of transcutaneous monitoring.[37]

Problem: When drawing arterial blood gases, when do I take the reading from the monitor?

$TcPO_2$ monitoring generally has a 30–40 second delay in responding to changes in arterial oxygenation, therefore the value on the monitor should be recorded approximately 20 seconds after the blood is drawn. Crying, agitation, and handling will cause the values to change.

Problem: Why is it that the longer the monitor is on an infant, the less accurate the reading becomes?

Transcutaneous monitors, like many instruments, are subject to "drifts" from their calibration. With transcutaneous monitors, the drift will increase with time since calibration. To correct and/or control the drift, the monitors should be calibrated every three to four hours while in use. Calibration requires that the probe be removed from the infant for approximately five to ten minutes, depending on the type of monitor used.

Once the monitor has been calibrated and the probe position changed, approximately 15–20 minutes are required for "warm up." The warm-up time period allows the probe and the skin to be heated to the correct temperature so that the alteration in skin oxygen tension can begin. During the calibration and warm-up time, the monitor will not accurately reflect the PaO_2.

Problem: What if the $TcPO_2$ does not accurately reflect the PaO_2 of the infant?

As part of the troubleshooting process, the membrane is routinely checked for air bubbles, wrinkles, and collected debris, which can contribute to inaccurate readings. Readings that do not reflect PaO_2 accurately, despite troubleshooting the equipment and probe, can still be used to follow trends in oxygenation.

If an infant has significant shunting through the ductus, close attention must be given to the site of the transcutaneous monitor and the source of the arterial blood sample. Preductal blood is sampled from the right arm and postductal blood from the lower body. The left arm may contain mixed pre- and postductal blood. Therefore if the $TcPO_2$ probe is on the right chest wall (preductal) and the blood is drawn from the umbilical artery catheter (postductal), there will be poor correlation between $TcPO_2$ and PaO_2 during significant shunting.[38]

In cases of right-to-left shunting, both the $TcPO_2$ probe and the arterial blood should be sampled preductally because the goal is to prevent hypoxia to the lungs, brain, and eyes.[33] Transcutaneous readings are recorded at least every hour and for each arterial blood sample drawn for gas analysis.

Transcutaneous Carbon Dioxide Monitoring

Transcutaneous carbon dioxide ($TcPCO_2$) monitoring may be carried out either separately from or in conjunction with transcutaneous oxygen monitoring. There may be two probes and one monitor, two probes and two monitors, or a single probe and monitor. Although $TcPCO_2$ monitoring is less dependent upon arterialization of the capillary bed, better correlation is obtained with the use of a heated probe.[32,39–42]

As with $TcPO_2$ monitoring, $TcPCO_2$ monitoring requires calibration of the probe and monitor at selected intervals, usually every four hours. The calibration process requires 5–10 percent carbon dioxide gases, which corresponds to 20–60 mmHg $PaCO_2$. Positioning of the probe is similar to that of the $TcPO_2$ probe.[32]

New probes that extend the calibration time are under investigation. Recent reports have indicated that an iridium oxide sensor can both reduce the temperature required for monitoring and increase the duration of monitoring one site without changing probe location and without compromise in accuracy of the monitor.[41]

PULSE OXIMETRY

Transcutaneous pulse oximetry is a method of continuously and noninvasively monitoring the oxygen saturation of the hemoglobin molecule. Unlike $TcPO_2$, which measures skin oxygen tension through the use of a heated probe, oximetry measures oxygen saturation using spectrophotometric principles. Oxygen saturation is measured by placing a probe emitting red spectrum light on one side of a pulsating vessel and a receptor on the opposite side of the vessel.

The oxygen saturation monitor consists of a monitor, a patient probe, and a cable connecting the two. The monitor produces two different wavelengths of red and infrared light

FIGURE 4 ▲ Pulse oximeter probe on an infant's foot

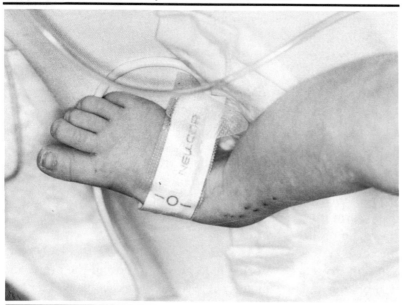

light source does not produce burns, there is no thermal injury to the infant. Oxygen saturation is indicated for use in the extremely small immature infant who may experience serious thermal injury with the $TcPO_2$ monitor. Infants with bronchopulmonary dysplasia (BPD) have been reported as having increased and unpredictable gradients between arterial and transcutaneous oxygen tension. Pulse oximetry has been shown to be a reliable method of measuring oxygen saturation (SpO_2) in these infants when there is greater than 50 percent adult hemoglobin.[43–46]

Problem: Where can the probe be positioned to find an arterial source?

The probe can be positioned on the fingers, toes, hand, foot, or wrist of the neonate (Figure 4). Other sites will depend on the infant's size. Newer probes allow for forehead placement.

Problem: Can ambient light interfere with pulse oximetry readings?

Ambient light containing the red spectrum may interfere with accurate readings from the oxygen saturation monitor. Light from heat lamps and phototherapy lights has been reported to skew readings.[47] The high intensity of light emitted from these sources masks the small changes in light transmission from the probe. The remedy is to shield the probe from the ambient light. Some of the probes designed for use in the newborn population contain a light shield as an integral part.

Problem: How can I determine the accuracy of the monitor?

Most transcutaneous pulse oximeters have a visual representation of the pulse intensity as well as a digital display of the pulse. The

which are transmitted to the patient probe that contains a photodetector. The light and the photodetector are placed opposite each other in such a position that a pulsating arterial bed is between the light and the detector. Light adsorption is measured as the light passes through the tissue. The response time is near instantaneous. The equipment requires no calibration or warm-up time prior to use.

Pulse oximetry requires adequate perfusion of the tissues and near-normal body temperature. The light must be able to detect arterial pulsations in order to differentiate arterial from venous and capillary blood. Advantages of the oxygen saturation monitor include instantaneous detection of changes in oxygen saturation, no required calibration, and digitally displayed output within seconds of probe application.

There are no reported complications associated with the use of the pulse oximeter. The adhesive on the skin probe has the potential to cause some interruption of the infant's skin integrity, but neonatal probes held in place with gentle pressure using an elastic band will circumvent this problem.

Because the probe is not heated and the

TABLE 3 ▲ Comparison of Transcutaneous Oxygen Tension and Pulse Oximetry Monitors

	Transcutaneous Oxygen Tension	Pulse Oximetry
Calibration	8–10 minutes every 4 hours	None (Some pulse oximeters have a pocket tester to test the calibration of the internal mechanics.)
Warm-up time	Approximately 15 minutes after probe application for the skin to reach 43–44° C and capillary bed to "arterialize"	None (displays oxygen saturation level instantly once a pulse is located)
Lag time (time from the change in oxygenation status to its reflection on the monitor)	30–40 seconds	None (instantaneous)
Complications	Thermal injuries resulting in first and second degree burns due to heat generated from probe	Compromised skin integrity under the probe (may go unnoticed because the probe does not need repositioning at set intervals)
Artifacts (factors causing inaccurate readings)	Membrane wrinkles, air between the membrane and skin, pressure on the probe	Movement of extremity with probe, inflated blood pressure cuff proximal to probe, light with red spectrum reaching an unshielded probe

pulse display should be within three beats per minute of the display on the cardiac monitor.[48] Differences greater than this will not reflect accurate oxygen saturation values because the probe is not detecting the arterial pulsations accurately. Some newer monitors have integrated the ECG complex with the oxygen saturation probe.

Problem: What if the readings from the pulse oximeter are inaccurate or do not register?

This can be caused by an incorrectly positioned probe resulting in lack of opposition between the light source and the photodetector or a light source that is partially occluded with debris from the skin or adhesive. These problems can easily be corrected by replacing, repositioning, or cleaning the probe.

Placing the probe distal to a blood pressure cuff will result in inaccurate or no reading when the blood pressure cuff is inflated because the blood supply to the probe site has been interrupted. The monitors are sensitive to motion and will display inaccurate readings when the extremity with the probe is moving.

Soft restraints in the very active infant will preclude this. In infants with severe hypotension, the monitor may not be able to detect and display the heart rate and saturation because of difficulty in detecting a pulsating arterial bed.

Although the monitor requires no calibration, at least one manufacturer has a pocket tester that, when inserted into the monitor in place of the patient probe, emits both a known infrared signal and a pulse signal. This allows the nurse to check the accuracy of the equipment's internal calibration.

Problem: Which infants can be monitored using the oxygen saturation monitor?

The oxygen saturation monitor is reliable, practical, and accurate for use in infants with a wide range of birthweights, postnatal ages, and heart rates.[32,43–50]

Problem: Are there any complications from using the oxygen saturation monitor?

In the newborn population, there are no known complications from oxygen saturation monitoring when the neonatal probes are used as indicated.

Problem: What are the comparative advantages and disadvantages of the transcutaneous oxygen monitor and the oxygen saturation monitor?

A comparison of the two monitoring systems is outlined in Table 3.

Problem: How do the nursing responsibilities compare for infants with transcutaneous as opposed to oxygen saturation monitors?

The nursing care responsibilities for the two types of monitors are compared in Table 4.

TABLE 4 ▲ Nursing Care Responsibilities for Infants with Transcutaneous and Oxygen Saturation Monitors

Transcutaneous Oxygen and Carbon Dioxide Monitors

1. Calibrate the monitor prior to use and every 4 hours thereafter.
2. Change the position of the probe at least every 4 hours, more often if the infant has blistering of the skin.
3. Document the monitor readings at least every hour and with each blood sample taken for gas analysis. Document the current FiO_2 reading.
4. Note the infant's response to nursing procedures based on the monitor readings. Alter the nursing care plan accordingly.
5. Position the probe on a flat, well-perfused area of the infant.
6. Document on the infant's flow sheet when the probe position was changed.
7. Set monitor alarms in accordance with unit policy.

Pulse Oximetry Monitors

1. Calibrate the monitor if applicable for the model and brand.
2. Select the appropriate sized probe, and locate a position for monitoring.
3. Place the probe so that the light source and the photodetector are opposite each other.
4. Set monitor alarms in accordance with unit policy.
5. Document monitor readings and FiO_2 every hour and with each blood sample drawn for gas analysis.
6. Change probe site PRN to avoid skin breakdown.

ENDOTRACHEAL SUCTIONING

Endotracheal suctioning is a nursing procedure that removes accumulated secretions and debris from the tracheobronchial tree of intubated infants. Because the presence of an endotracheal tube does not allow the glottis to close, the infant is unable to cough. This, in conjunction with the inhibition of ciliary activity due to the tube in the trachea, inhibits the infant's ability to move secretions toward the pharynx.

In the newborn the procedure is not without complications (such as hypoxia, bradycardia, atelectasis, tissue trauma, bacteremia, perforation, pneumothorax, and increased intracranial pressure).[51-62] Endotracheal suctioning consists of inserting a sterile catheter into the trachea and applying negative pressure while withdrawing it. In an effort to ameliorate or lessen the complications associated with the procedure, additional components have been added to the procedure, including increasing FiO_2, hyperventilation, maintaining a set catheter-to-endotracheal tube ratio, and regulating the negative pressure used (Table 5).[51,63]

Increasing the amount of inspired oxygen prior to, during, and following suctioning may help decrease the degree of suction-induced hypoxemia. Increasing the FiO_2 10–15 percent above the baseline when suctioning infants as well as close monitoring of $TcPO_2$ or SpO_2 is recommended.

Normal saline solution (0.25 ml–0.5 ml) may be used as an irrigant during endotracheal suctioning. Routine use of saline irrigation is debatable.[63,64] This practice has not been thoroughly investigated and its efficacy established, but rather has been practiced as a matter of tradition. Further research is warranted to verify the necessity of this procedure.

If normal saline is used, the volume should be premeasured to assure delivery of the desired amount and care should be taken to prevent contamination of the solution.[64] The normal saline is administered through the endotracheal tube, and the infant is ventilated two or three times to disperse in saline. The infant is then removed from the ventilator and bagged with a manual resuscitation bag or left on the ven-

TABLE 5 ▲ Components of Endotracheal Suctioning

Oxygen	Increase 10–15 percent over baseline
Pressure	Baseline
Rate	Additional breaths prior to and following suctioning
Irrigant	Normal saline, 0.25–0.50 ml
Catheter size	6 French for ET size 3.0 or less 8 French for ET size 3.5 and 4.0
Negative pressure	75–80 mmHg
Suction duration	5 seconds applied intermittently only during withdrawal of catheter
Suction depth	Length of endotracheal tube or length of endotracheal tube plus one centimeter

tilator and given additional breaths using the manual inspiration mode.

The suction catheter is premeasured according to endotracheal length. The catheter is advanced only the length of the endotracheal tube or the length of the endotracheal tube plus one centimeter.[63] This practice decreases the risk of pneumothorax and tissue trauma. The suction catheter length is posted at the infant's bedside.

The suction catheter is inserted through the endotracheal tube and negative pressure of 75–80 mmHg is applied as the catheter is withdrawn. The infant is placed back on the manual resuscitation bag or the ventilator and given 20–30 seconds of additional ventilation or sufficient ventilation to return the oxygen saturation/transcutaneous monitors to baseline. Pass the catheter only once or twice unless the amount of secretions warrants additional passes. Do not rotate the infant's head.[63] The amount and type of secretions recovered are recorded along with the infant's response to the procedure. After suctioning, the chest is assessed for changes in breath sounds. The secretions recovered from suctioning may vary from thin and watery to thick and viscous. The color may be clear, white, yellow, green, blood tinged, or bloody.

Problem: How much should the FiO_2 be increased during suctioning?

Increasing the FiO_2 from 10 to 20 percent above baseline is the most common practice, but is only a guide. Some infants will require more than a 20 percent increase over baseline; others will need only a 5 percent increase. The purpose of increasing FiO_2 is to decrease both the incidence and severity of suction-induced hypoxemia. The amount of additional oxygen used should be based on the infant's response to past suctioning episodes.

Problem: When withdrawing the suction catheter from the endotracheal tube, should the finger port of the suction catheter be occluded the entire time, or should it be covered intermittently?

In theory, if the finger port is occluded for

the duration of the application of negative pressure, there would be more secretions removed because there is a longer period of time for negative pressure to capture and aspirate the secretions. Continuous negative pressure may cause increased trauma because secretions or tracheal epithelial tissue caught by the negative pressure will be shorn off and removed.

In contrast, using intermittent negative pressure would, in theory, remove fewer secretions, remove less lung gas, and cause less trauma than continuous pressure, because negative pressure is applied to the trachea for a shorter period of time. A concern that has been voiced about intermittent negative pressure is that secretions, once caught at the tip or at the eye-hole openings of the suction catheter, could fall off and drop back down into the trachea when negative pressure is released.

Problem: Is it better to use a manual resuscitation bag or the manual inspiration mode on the ventilator when suctioning?

The purpose of ventilating the infant prior to, during, and following suctioning is to prevent some of the complications associated with endotracheal suctioning by providing the infant with additional oxygen and ventilation.

Both the manual resuscitation bag and the ventilator are used to ventilate the infant while suctioning. There are advantages and disadvantages to each, and the health care practitioner's decision will be based on personal preference as well as unit policy.

Using the manual resuscitation bag during suctioning requires both skill and experience. This method allows the caretaker to control the parameters of ventilation: FiO_2, positive inspiratory pressure (PIP), PEEP, inspiratory time, and rate. If this method is used, an in-line manometer is essential for monitoring the pressures used during ventilation. An extensive review of the existing manual resuscitation bags is available in the literature.[65]

Skill is required to match the controlled waveform of the ventilator breaths. In times of crisis, the caretaker may become anxious and transmit this to the patient by an increased rate and/or pressure. New NICU nurses are often most comfortable giving additional breaths through the ventilator. Experienced NICU nurses may prefer the bag because it gives them an opportunity to "feel" the compliance of the lung.

Using the ventilator to give additional breaths or to ventilate the infant during suctioning allows the caretaker to control the FiO_2 and the rate while the ventilator administers the preestablished PIP and PEEP. Using the ventilator thus prevents inadvertent increases in PIP or PEEP from reaching the infant. Even in inexperienced hands the manual ventilator breaths given in this manner are nearly indistinguishable from controlled ventilator breaths.

Problem: How long after I increase the oxygen on the ventilator do I wait to suction?

Additional oxygen is given to the infant prior to suctioning to help reduce the suction-induced hypoxemia that can occur with endotracheal suctioning. Increasing the oxygen on the ventilator and immediately suctioning the infant does not allow sufficient time for the infant to benefit from the increased oxygen levels; therefore suctioning should be delayed until the infant has a chance to benefit from the hyperoxygenation breaths.

The time needed is based on the "washout time" of the ventilator. This is the time it takes for the increase in oxygen to reach the end of the ventilator's inspiratory circuit. The time will be based on the ventilator; the type, length, and diameter of tubing; the flow rate; and the settings. Some ventilators will reflect the change in oxygen as quickly as 18 seconds; others will require a considerably longer time. The washout time can be measured using a second ventilator, by placing a calibrated oxygen analyzer at the end of the ventilation tubing and measuring the time required for the analyzer to detect the increase in oxygen.

Problem: When I suction the infant, I have to remove him from the ventilator and the ventilatory cycle is lost. Can this be prevented?

In some units modified endotracheal tube adapters are used to help prevent the loss of both oxygenation and ventilation during suctioning. The modified adapters have side-port openings that allow the suction catheter to be inserted while the infant remains on the ventilator, so that only minor disruptions occur in the ventilatory cycle.[66,67] Although this is advantageous, some nurses have observed that it is more difficult to suction the infant using the modified adapters because the opening is small, and it becomes difficult to maintain sterile technique. It is imperative to close the side-port openings following suctioning so that the infant receives the full benefit of the ventilatory cycle.

Problem: With the concern over infections and AIDS, what protection should I use when suctioning?

Health care professionals must be cognizant of the potential danger of contamination from respiratory secretions as well as other body fluids. Current recommendations include wearing goggles and gloves on both hands while suctioning. There have been case reports of cross-transmission of infectious secretions from health care workers not using proper endotracheal suctioning techniques.[68,69]

CHEST PHYSIOTHERAPY

The 1979 Conference on the Scientific Basis of In-Hospital Respiratory Therapy sponsored by the National Heart, Lung, and Blood Institute defined chest physical therapy as "consisting of physical maneuvers such as cough, forced expiration, chest wall percussion and vibration, and postural drainage to improve respiratory function and treat atelectasis and pneumonia."[70]

Cough and forced expiration are not used in newborns as part of chest physical therapy because they are difficult to elicit. In this population, chest physical therapy consists of external chest percussion and/or vibration and postural drainage followed by suctioning.

Chest percussion is generally believed to alter the pressure in the airways of the newborn, which helps dislodge the mucus plugs. Externally administered chest percussion generally ranges from 4–5 Hz. In contrast, vibration is administered at up to 41 Hz and is believed to help propel mucus from the smaller bronchi to the larger airways.

It has been postulated that mucus is cleared by chest percussion or vibration by: improving mucociliary interaction, simulating the ciliary beat frequency, stimulating active substances in the lung, or releasing chemical mediators in the airways.

Percussion, vibration, and positioning are used to move secretions from the periphery of the lungs to the bronchus and up toward the pharynx. Cilia movement is responsible for transporting the secretions from the lower trachea to the pharynx. In the intubated infant the presence of an endotracheal tube inhibits ciliary activity in the area around the end of the endotracheal tube; thus the secretions may pool at the distal end of the tube, where they are removed by suctioning.

There has been considerable interest in the role of chest physiotherapy in the neonatal population. The method of chest physiotherapy may vary, but the procedure generally includes the gentle percussion and/or vibration of the chest and back in a variety of positions to loosen secretions.[71–73]

Before chest physiotherapy is initiated, it should be determined that there is a sufficient volume of secretions to be loosened and moved. Murphy termed this concept the "ketchup bottle effect": "The bottle must contain some ketchup before it can be turned upside down, thumped on the back... and a splash... appears."[74]

Chest physiotherapy is used with newborns who have pneumonia, meconium aspiration, or other conditions resulting in atelectasis and hypercapnea. It is generally believed that there will be an improvement in pulmonary function after chest physiotherapy. Infants with respiratory distress syndrome have few secretions in the early phase of the disease process and probably would derive benefit from chest percussion in the later stages of the disease.

Percussion is given for three to five minutes over the right and left side of the chest and over the back of the infant. Particular emphasis is given to the area of the lung that is atelectatic. Devices used for percussion include face masks, pediatric percussors, nipples, padded medicine cups, a bulb syringe cut in half with padded edges, or the nurse's fingers. The percussion device should deliver a column of air under pressure to the chest wall, ideally at 40 compressions per minute. Percussion is administered every two to eight hours, depending on the infant's condition and ability to tolerate the procedure.

Vibration may be used in conjunction with percussion, or it may be administered separately. A padded electric toothbrush or vibrator can be used. Most infants seem to tolerate vibration better than percussion. Throughout the administration of percussion and vibration the infant should be monitored for signs of distress.

Postural drainage is used to move the loosened secretions to the larger airways so they can be transported toward the pharynx, where they are removed by suctioning. The infant is positioned so that the bronchus supplying the larger airways is in a dependent position during percussion.

In general, infants weighing less than 1,250 gm or with known or suspected intracranial bleeds should not be placed in the head-down position. Infants with abdominal surgery, abdominal wall defects, or umbilical artery catheters should not be placed in the prone position unless the hips and abdomen are supported so that pressure is avoided over the abdomen.[29]

Problem: What position is used to drain which lung segment during postural drainage?

The position of the infant and the corresponding lung segment to be drained are iden-

TABLE 6 ▲ Postural Drainage*

Position	Lung area
Sitting	Upper lobes
Supine	Anterior segment of upper lobe
Side, 30° upright	Posterior segment of upper lobe
Flat, prone	Superior segment of upper lobe
Head down, supine	Anterior basal segment of lower lobe
Head down, side rotated forward	Lateral basal segment
Head down, prone	Posterior basal segment
Head down, left side	Right middle lobe

*Table sources are references 68–70

tified in Table 6. For practical purposes, the infant's condition and tolerance will dictate the amount of time and positions used for postural drainage.

There are conflicting reports in the literature concerning the efficacy of chest physiotherapy.[75–79] The goal is to facilitate the removal of secretions to promote better oxygenation and ventilation; however, the procedure is not without complications such as hypoxia, rib fractures, bruising, and dislodged tubes.[29,80] The advantages of using chest physiotherapy must be weighed against the disadvantages associated with the procedure.

AIR LEAKS AND CHEST TUBES

It has been estimated that 2–10 percent of normal newborns will have a spontaneous pneumothorax.[77] The majority of these infants will be asymptomatic. In the distressed newborn who is subjected to mechanical ventilation, the incidence of air leaks is significantly higher, ranging from 16 to 40 percent, with the highest incidence seen in infants with meconium aspiration syndrome.[81]

Air leaks are caused by alveolar rupture, usually at the base of the alveoli. This can result from a number of factors, including positive pressure ventilation and ball-valve obstruction with distal air trapping. Hand ventilating an infant with a manual resuscitation bag without an in-line manometer to measure inspiratory pressure can result in inadvertent administration of high inspiratory pressure, leading to rupture. Infants who require high inspiratory pressure on the ventilator in order to ventilate the lung adequately are at an increased risk for pneumothorax because the high pressure may only marginally expand some alveoli while overexpanding and rupturing others.

A pneumothorax may also be caused by secretions and debris in the lung causing a ball-valve phenomenon. Air is able to enter the alveoli around the debris but is unable to be exhaled around the debris because the airways narrow during exhalation. This results in air retention in the alveoli during exhalation and the resultant addition of air to the alveoli during the next inhalation causing overdistention and the potential for rupture.

Infants with atelectasis are particularly prone to air leaks because of the presence of both normally expanded and nonexpanded alveoli. The pressure required to ventilate the infants is often sufficient to overexpand the normally expanded alveoli, causing them to rupture. When the alveoli rupture, air escapes into the interstitium and travels along the perivascular spaces to the hilum, where it may rupture into the pleural space, causing a pneumothorax; into the mediastinum, resulting in a pneumomediastinum; or into the pericardium, causing a pneumopericardium.[81]

Recent research has documented that infants with respiratory distress syndrome and pulmonary interstitial emphysema who have one pneumothorax are at 44 percent risk of developing a contralateral pneumothorax.[83]

Signs and Symptoms

The signs and symptoms of a tension pneumothorax in an infant on the ventilator may be overt or subtle, and the condition is often first suspected by the nurse at the bedside. Rapid detection and treatment of a pneumothorax are imperative in the critically ill

FIGURE 5 ▲ Chest tube with bulky dressing covering insertion site

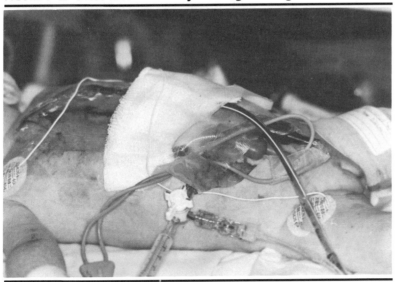

infant. The presence of a pneumothorax causes swings in blood pressure that result in changes in cerebral blood flow. An increase in the cerebral blood flow causes an increased intracranial pressure and may cause rupture of the very fragile vessels of the germinal matrix.

The infant may show a sudden deterioration in color, increasing agitation, hypoxia, and ineffective ventilation. Upon auscultation there may be decreased breath sounds on the affected side and asymmetry of chest movement. The following are some of the more common signs:

1. Increased anterior-posterior chest diameter
2. Decreased breath sounds in one lung upon auscultation
3. Displacement of heart sounds away from the affected side of the chest
4. Distension of the chest on the affected side
5. Duskiness, cyanosis
6. Decrease in the voltage of the QRS complex
7. Increased oxygen and ventilation requirements
8. Bradycardia
9. Generalized cyanosis

The voltage change in the R-S wave on the

ECG complex results from the accumulated air in the extrapleural space not conducting the electrical voltage as well as fluid. This causes a decrease in the R-S wave that can be seen on the bedside monitor.

The diagnosis of a pneumothorax is made from a chest x-ray, but transillumination of the chest may be helpful as an initial noninvasive step. When transillumination is used, ambient room lights should be reduced to facilitate interpretation. A fiberoptic light is placed on one side of the infant's chest and then on the other. The circle of light on the chest wall is compared for size—the right side versus the left. The side with the increased diameter of light is suspected of having a pneumothorax. When possible, a chest x-ray should follow to confirm the diagnosis before treatment is instituted.

The treatment of choice for excess air in the pleural space is removal of the air using needle aspiration or indwelling chest tubes. Needle aspiration is a single procedure in which a scalp vein needle (23–25 gauge), attached to a stopcock and syringe, is inserted through the chest wall to remove excess air. Air is evacuated by the syringe and then vented to the room by turning the stopcock. Because of its potential complications, this procedure is performed by a physician or by a nurse certified to perform needle aspiration.

A chest tube is placed for the continual removal of fluid or air from the pleural space (Figure 5). Using sterile procedures, the chest tube is inserted through a small skin incision, then threaded over the rib and into the pleural space. The tip is placed anteriorly for air removal (air rises) and posteriorly for fluid removal (fluid falls). The tube is held in posi-

FIGURE 6 ▲ Anterior chest tube with purse string suture

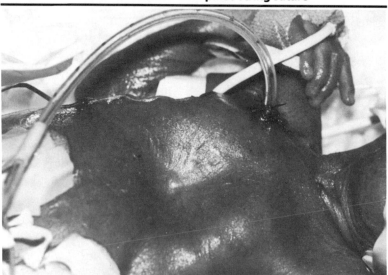

tion with purse string sutures (Figure 6), bulky dressing (Figure 5), and/or tape (Figure 7). The tube may be connected to a Heimlich valve or to underwater sealed vacuum using a one- or two-bottle system or a commercially available chest tube drainage set (Figures 8 and 9). If a one-bottle system is used, the negative pressure must be able to be regulated to prevent trauma to the infant. The negative pressure (10 cm H_2O) connected to the drainage set may be continual or intermittent. The drainage col-

lection system used must be able to be secured to prevent accidental breakage of the bottles or other mishaps.

Problem: How do I prevent tension on the chest tube at the insertion site?

The chest tube is secured to the bed with pins or hemostats to prevent tension on the insertion site.

Problem: What precautions can I take against inadvertent disconnection of the chest tube connections with ensuing respiratory compromise?

All chest tube connections are securely taped with adhesive tape. Rubber protected clamps are kept at the bedside for clamping the tubing should it become disconnected. The bottles are kept below the level of the patient at all times.

Problem: How can I quantify the drainage of fluid from the chest tube?

In general, chest tubes placed after surgery will have greater fluid drainage than those placed to relieve a tension pneumothorax. Fluid output can be quantified by marking the fluid level in the container using a tape strip at the beginning of the shift and again at four to eight hours. If there is a significant fluid output, the drainage is measured more frequently. If small collection bottles (90 ml) are used, it may be necessary to replace or empty the bottle if it becomes more than half filled. The fluid accumulated is measured and documented on the infant's flow sheet.

The negative pressure setting is based on the initial fluid level in the bottle and the diameter of the chest tube; addi-

FIGURE 7 ▲ Chest tubes secured with purse string sutures and tape

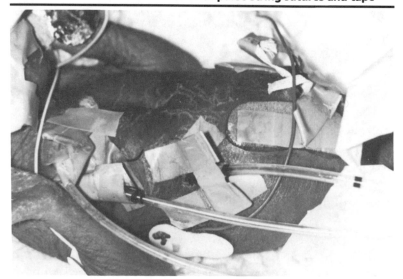

FIGURE 8 ▲ A one-bottle chest tube drainage system

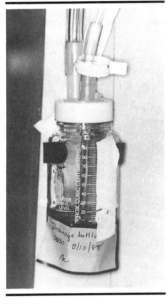

FIGURE 9 ▲ A commercially available chest tube drainage set

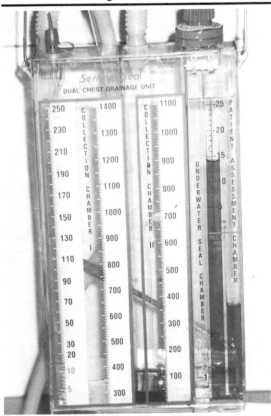

tional fluid alters the negative pressure, as does the addition of another chest tube or changing a chest tube for one of a different diameter.

The assessment of chest tube drainage also includes an evaluation of the degree of bubbling or fluctuation of the fluid in the bottle or tubing. Bubbling or fluctuation of fluid in the chest tubing indicates that the tube is patent and removing air/fluid. Although the position of the tube is evaluated from x-rays, one indicator that the tube may be outside the chest wall is active continual bubbling. This may also indicate an air leak in the collection tubing.

No bubbling or fluctuations may indicate either that the air leak is resolved or that the tube is no longer patent. Chest tubes that are not patent are removed and replaced with new ones.

If the bubbling or fluctuation of the fluid has stopped for 24 hours, the tube is clamped and a chest film obtained to rule out reaccumulation of air, which would indicate that the air leak has not resolved. Many hospitals do not clamp chest tubes prior to removal if the infant remains on positive pressure ventilation.

The chest tube is removed under aseptic conditions, and an occlusive dressing is applied using Vaseline or a similar substance to prevent air from entering through the incision site. A chest film is taken after the tube has been removed to rule out air accumulation.

Problem: What is the relationship of pneumothorax to the incidence of intraventricular hemorrhage?

The relationship of pneumothorax to intraventricular hemorrhage has been reported by several investigators.[84] One study using puppies found that the rate of removal of the air in reducing the pneumothorax was related to cerebral blood velocity.[85] Rapid removal of the air resulted in increased arterial blood pressure and cerebral blood velocity; slow evacuation led to a gradual normalization of mean arterial pressure and cerebral blood velocity.

Problem: What precautions should be observed when an infant with a chest tube is transported?

The tube can be clamped for a short time while the bottle is elevated and repositioned for transport. During transport the bottles must be kept below the level of the infant's chest unless the tubing is clamped. An alternative is to use a Heimlich valve (Bard Parker) placed in-line, which negates the need for the bottle collection system during transport. The Heimlich flutter valve is connected to the chest tube with the distal end connected to a specimen trap.

SUMMARY

Caring for the infant with respiratory compromise requires the integration of information from multiple sources; clinical assessment of the infant, data from invasive and noninvasive monitors, and interpretation of clinical cues. Understanding the physiological concepts that underlie nursing procedures enables the nurse to provide appropriate, planned, and individualized care to a vulnerable population.

REFERENCES

1. Thiebeault DW: Pulmonary care of infants with endotracheal tubes, *in* Theibeault DW, and Gregory GA, eds., Neonatal Pulmonary Care, Menlo Park, California, 1986, Addison Wesley, p. 388.
2. Kuhns LR, and Poznanski AK: Endotracheal tube position in the infant, Journal of Pediatrics 78, 1971, pp. 991–996.
3. Tordes D, et al.: Endotracheal tube displacement in the newborn infant, Journal of Pediatrics 89(1), 1976, pp. 126–127.
4. Donn SM, and Blane CE: Endotracheal tube movement in the preterm neonate: Oral versus nasal intubation, Annals of Otology, Rhinology and Laryngology 94, 1985, pp. 18–20.
5. Cohen MD: Tubes, wires and the neonate, Clinical Radiology 31, 1980, pp. 249–256.
6. Slovis TL, and Poland RL: Endotracheal tubes in neonates: Sonographic positioning, Radiology 160, 1986, pp. 262–263.
7. Marshall TA, et al.: Physiologic changes associated with endotracheal intubation in premature infants, Critical Care Medicine 12(6), 1984, pp. 501–503.
8. Carrillo PJ: Palatal groove formation and oral endotracheal intubation, American Journal of Diseases of Children 139, 1985, pp. 859–860.
9. Saunders BS, Easa D, and Slaughter RJ: Acquired palatal groove in neonates, Journal of Pediatrics 89(6), 1976, pp. 988–989.
10. Duke PM, et al.: Cleft palate associated with prolonged orotracheal intubation in infancy, Journal of Pediatrics 89(6), 1976, pp. 990–991.
11. Gowdar K, et al.: Nasal deformities in neonates, American Journal of Diseases of Children 134, 1980, pp. 954–957.
12. Pettett G, and Merenstein GB: Nasal erosion with nasotracheal intubation, Journal of Pediatrics 87(1), 1976, p. 149.
13. Jung AL, and Thomas GK: Stricture of the nasal vestibule: A complication of nasotracheal intubation in newborn infants, Journal of Pediatrics 85(3), 1984, pp. 412–414.
14. Boice JB, Krous HF, and Foley JM: Gingival and dental complications of orotracheal intubation, Journal of the American Medical Association 236(8), 1976, pp. 957–958.
15. Moylan FMB, et al.: Defective primary dentition in survivors of neonatal mechanical ventilation, Journal of Pediatrics 96(1), 1980, pp. 106–108.
16. Marshak G, and Grundfast KM: Subglottic stenosis, Pediatric Clinics of North America 28, 1981, pp. 941–948.
17. Strong RM, and Passy V: Complications in neonates, Archives of Otolaryngology 103, 1977, pp. 329–335.
18. Johnson DE, et al.: Management of esophageal and pharyngeal perforation in the newborn infant, Pediatrics 70(4), 1982, pp. 592–595.
19. Clarke TA, et al.: Esophageal perforations in premature infants and comments on the diagnosis, American Journal of Diseases of Children 134, 1980, pp. 367–368.
20. Talbert JL, et al.: Traumatic perforation of the hypopharynx in infants, Journal of Thoracic and Cardiovascular Surgery 74(1), 1977, pp. 152–156.
21. Goodwin SR, Graves SA, and Haberkern CM: Aspiration in intubated premature infants, Pediatrics 75(1), 1985, pp. 85–88.
22. Harris H, Wirtschafter D, and Cassady G: Endotracheal intubation and its relationship to bacterial colonization and systemic infection of newborn infants, Pediatrics 56(6), 1976, pp. 816–823.
23. Grylack LJ, and Anderson KD: Diagnosis and treatment of traumatic granuloma in tracheobronchial tree of newborn with history of chronic intubation, Journal of Pediatric Surgery 19(2), 1984, pp. 200–201.
24. Martin RJ, Fanaroff AA, and Skalina ME: The respiratory distress syndrome and its management, *in* Fanaroff AA, and Martin RJ, eds., Behrman's Neonatal-Perinatal Medicine, St. Louis, 1983, C.V. Mosby, p. 438.
25. Andriani J, and Griggs T: An improved endotracheal tube for pediatric use, Anesthesiology 15, 1954, p. 466.
26. Kubota V, et al.: Tracheo-bronchial angles in infants and children, Anesthesiology 64, 1986, pp. 374–376.
27. Fewell J, Arrington R, and Seibert J: The effect of head position and angle of tracheal bifurcation on bronchus catheterization in the intubated neonate, Pediatrics 64(3), 1979, pp. 192–194.
28. Richards SD: A method for securing pediatric endotracheal tubes, Anesthesia and Analgesia 60(4), 1981, pp. 224–225.
29. Fletcher MA, MacDonald MG, and Avery GB: Atlas of Procedures in Neonatology, Philadelphia, 1983, J.B. Lippincott, pp. 220–223.
30. Heller RM, and Cotton RB: Early experience with illuminated endotracheal tube in premature and term infants, Pediatrics 75(4), 1985, pp. 664–666.
31. Everts E, et al.: Nonradiographic determination of tracheal tube position in children: Initial clinical impressions, Abstracts from the 9th World Congress of Anaesthesiologists, Washington, DC, May 1988.

32. Cassady G: Transcutaneous monitoring in the newborn infant, Journal of Pediatrics 103(6), 1983, pp. 837–848.

33. Rooth G, Huch A, and Huch R: Transcutaneous oxygen monitors are reliable indicators of arterial oxygen tension (if used correctly), Pediatrics 79(2), 1987, pp. 283–286.

34. Peabody JL: Historical perspective of noninvasive monitoring, Journal of Perinatology 7(4), 1987, pp. 306–308.

35. Peabody JL, and Emery JR: Noninvasive monitoring of blood gases in the newborn, Clinics in Perinatology 12(1), 1985, pp. 147–160.

36. Boyle RJ, and Oh W: Erythema following transcutaneous PO_2 monitoring, Pediatrics 65(2), 1980, pp. 333–334.

37. Golden SM: Skin craters—a complication of transcutaneous oxygen monitoring, Pediatrics 67(4), 1981, pp. 514–516.

38. Pierce JR, and Turner BS: Physiologic monitoring, *in* Merenstein GB, and Gardner S, eds., Handbook of Neonatal Intensive Care, St. Louis, 1985, C.V. Mosby, p. 126.

39. Herrell N, et al.: Optimal temperature for the measurement of transcutaneous carbon dioxide tension in the neonate, Journal of Pediatrics 97, 1980, p. 114.

40. Cabal L, et al.: Factors affecting heated transcutaneous PO_2 and unheated transcutaneous PCO_2 in preterm infants, Critical Care Medicine 9, 1981, p. 298.

41. Bucher HU, et al.: Transcutaneous carbon dioxide tension in newborn infants: Reliability and safety of continuous 24 hour measurement at 42° C, Pediatrics 78(4), 1986, pp. 631–635.

42. Brunstler I, Enders A, and Versmold HT: Skin surface PCO_2 monitoring in newborn infants in shock: Effect of hypotension and electrode temperature, Journal of Pediatrics 100(3), 1982, pp. 454–457.

43. Anderson JV: The accuracy of pulse oximetry in neonates: Effects of fetal hemoglobin and bilirubin, Journal of Perinatology 7(4), 1987, pp. 309–319.

44. Fanconi S: Reliability of pulse oximetry in hypoxic infants, Journal of Pediatrics 112(3), 1988, pp. 424–427.

45. Ramanathan R, Durand M, and Larrazabal C: Pulse oximetry in very low birth weight infants with acute and chronic lung disease, Pediatrics 79(4), 1987, pp. 612–617.

46. Jennis MS, and Peabody JL: Pulse oximetry: An alternative method for the assessment of oxygenation in newborn infants, Pediatrics 79(4), 1987, pp. 524–528.

47. Barrington KJ, Finer NN, and Ryan CA: Evaluation of pulse oximetry as a continuous monitoring technique in the neonatal intensive care unit, Critical Care Medicine 16(11), 1988, pp. 1147–1153.

48. Hay WW: Physiology of oxygenation and its relation to pulse oximetry, Journal of Perinatology 7(4), 1987, pp. 309–319.

49. Cunningham MD, Shook LA, and Tomazic T: Clinical experience with pulse oximetry in managing oxygen therapy in neonatal intensive care, Journal of Perinatology 7(4), 1987, pp. 333–335.

50. Emery JR: Skin pigmentation as an influence on the accuracy of pulse oximetry, Journal of Perinatology 7(4), 1987, pp. 329–330.

51. Turner BS: Current concepts in endotracheal suctioning, Journal of the California Perinatology Association 3(1), 1983, p. 104.

52. Cunningham ML, Baun MM, and Nelson RM: Endotracheal suctioning of premature neonates, Journal of the California Perinatal Association 4(1), 1984, p. 49.

53. Raval D, et al.: Changes in transcutaneous PO_2 during tracheobronchial hygiene in neonates, Perinatology-Neonatology, August 1980, p. 41.

54. Cabal LA, et al.: Cardiac rate and rhythm changes during airway suctioning in premature infants with RDS, Journal of the California Perinatal Association 4(1), 1984, pp. 45–48.

55. Brandstater B, and Muallem M: Atelectasis following tracheal suction in infants, Anesthesiology 31(5), 1969, p. 468.

56. Kuzenski BM: Effect of negative pressure on tracheobronchial trauma, Nursing Research 27(4), 1978, pp. 260–263.

57. Storm W: Transient bacteremia following endotracheal suctioning in ventilated newborns, Pediatrics 65(3), 1980, pp. 487–490.

58. Vaughan RS, Menke JA, and Giacoia GP: Pneumothorax: A complication of endotracheal tube suctioning, Journal of Pediatrics 92(4), 1978, pp. 633–634.

59. Rudy EB, et al.: The relationship between endotracheal suctioning and changes in intracranial pressure: A review of the literature, Heart & Lung 15(5), 1986, pp. 488–494.

60. Perlman JM, and Volpe JJ: Suctioning in the preterm infant: Effects on cerebral blood flow velocity, intracranial pressure, and arterial blood pressure, Pediatrics 72(3), 1983, p. 329.

61. Fanconi S, and Duc G: Intratracheal suctioning in sick preterm infants: Prevention of intracranial hypertension and cerebral hypoperfusion by muscle paralysis, Pediatrics 79(4), 1987, pp. 538–543.

62. Anderson KD, and Chandra R: Pneumothorax secondary to perforation of sequential bronchi by suction catheters, Journal of Pediatric Surgery 11(5), 1976, pp. 687–693.

63. Hodge D: Endotracheal suctioning and the infant: A nursing care protocol to decrease complications, Neonatal Network 9(5), 1991, pp. 7–15.

64. Acherman MH: The use of normal saline instillations in artificial airways: Is it useful or necessary? Heart & Lung 14(5), 1985, pp. 505–506.

65. Nugent J, Matthews B, and Goldsmith J: Pulmonary care, *in* Goldsmith J, and Karotkin E, eds., Assisted Ventilation of the Neonate, Philadelphia, 1988, W.B. Saunders, p. 92.

66. Cabal L, et al.: New endotracheal tube adaptor reduces cardiopulmonary effects of suctioning, Critical Care Medicine 7, 1979, p. 352.

67. Zmora E, and Merritt TA: Use of side-hole endotracheal tube adaptor for tracheal aspiration, American Journal of Diseases of Children 134, 1980, p. 250.

68. Ballard JL, Musia MJ, and Myers MG: Hazards of delivery room resuscitation using oral methods of endotracheal suctioning, Pediatric Infectious Disease 5(2), 1986, pp. 198–200.

69. Van Dyke RB, and Spector SA: Transmission of herpes simplex virus type 1 to a newborn infant during endotracheal suctioning for mechanical aspiration, Critical Care Medicine 3(2), 1984, pp. 153–156.

70. Proceedings of the Conference on the Scientific Basis of In-Hospital Respiratory Therapy, Atlanta, Georgia, November 14–16, 1979, American Review of Respiratory Diseases 122, 1980, pp. 1–16.

71. Carlo WA, and Chatburn RL: Neonatal Respiratory Care, Chicago, 1988, Yearbook Medical Publishers, pp. 118–120.

72. Meyers C: Pulmonary physiotherapy, *in* Schreiner R, and Kisling JA, eds., Practical Neonatal Respiratory Care, New York, 1982, Raven Press, p. 384.

73. Nugent J, Hanks H, and Goldsmith J: Pulmonary care, *in* Goldsmith J, and Karotkin A, eds., Assisted Ventilation of the Neonate, Philadelphia, 1988, W.B. Saunders, pp. 97–102.

74. Murphy JF: The ketchup bottle method, New England Journal of Medicine 300(20), 1979, pp. 1155–1157.

75. Etches PC, and Scott B: Chest physiotherapy in the newborn: Effect on secretions removed, Pediatrics 62(5), 1978, pp. 713–715.

76. Finer NN, and Boyd J: Chest physiotherapy in the neonate: A controlled study, Pediatrics 61(2), 1978, pp. 282–285.

77. Fox WW, Schwartz JG, and Shaffer TH: Pulmonary physiotherapy in neonates: Physiologic changes and respiratory management, Journal of Pediatrics 92, 1978, p. 977.

78. Holloway R, et al.: Effect of chest physiotherapy in blood gases of neonates treated by intermittent positive pressure respiration, Thorax 24, 1969, pp. 421–426.

79. Curran CL, and Kachoyeanos MK: The effects on neonates of two methods of chest physical therapy, Maternal Child Nursing 4, 1979, pp. 309–313.

80. Purohit DM, Caldwell C, and Levkoff AH: Multiple rib fractures due to physiotherapy in a neonate with hyaline membrane disease, American Journal of Diseases of Children 129, 1975, p. 1103.

81. Hagedorn MI, Gardner SL, and Abman SH: Respiratory disease, *in* Merenstein GB, and Gardner SL, eds., Handbook of Neonatal Intensive Care, St. Louis, 1985, C.V. Mosby, p. 324.

82. Gregory SEB: Air leak syndromes, Neonatal Network 5(5), April 1987, pp. 40–46.

83. Ryan CA, et al.: Contralateral pneumothoraces in the newborn: Incidence and predisposing factors, Pediatrics 79(3), 1987, pp. 417–421.

84. Hill A, Perlman JM, and Volpe JJ: Relationship of pneumothorax to occurrence of intraventricular hemorrhage in the premature newborn, Pediatrics 69(2), 1982, pp. 144–149.

85. Baton DG, Hellman J, and Nardis EE: Effect of pneumothorax-induced systemic blood pressure alteration on the cerebral circulation in newborn dogs, Pediatrics 74(3), 1984, pp. 350–353.

5 Historical and Present Application of Positive Pressure Ventilation

V. L. Cassani III, RNC, MS, NNP
Captain, Army Nurse Corps
William Beaumont Army Medical Center
El Paso, Texas

As we enter the era of surfactant replacement therapy and use of extracorporeal membrane oxygenation to enhance survival and hopefully decrease morbidity in babies afflicted with respiratory distress syndrome (RDS), it is important to reflect on the progress made in the past quarter century in the application of positive pressure ventilation. As has often been stated, those who are not aware of history are doomed to repeat it. Having a clear grasp of the development of mechanical ventilation in the newborn will foster rational application of the technique by practitioners. Clinicians also need to understand the pioneering changes made in the social milieu by our predecessors that have enabled neonatal intensive care to flourish.

This chapter discusses not only the historical development of newborn mechanical ventilation, but also provides the reader with a clear understanding of some of the underlying physiologic principles of positive pressure ventilation. The effects of applying newly acquired scientific knowledge to the clinical arena are also highlighted.

HISTORICAL PERSPECTIVE

The first recorded report of death secondary to respiratory failure in newborns was during the reign of Emperor of China, H Wang T (2698–2599 BC). There were also incidents mentioned in Eber's Papyrus (1552 BC) as well as in the Bible (II Kings 4; 34–35) of a resuscitation of a newborn.[1–4]

Birth asphyxia and respiratory failure of newborns continued to attract the attention of medical scholars throughout the ages. Hippocrates (400 BC) published the technique of endotracheal intubation, but this technique did not become a standard of care until the mid-twentieth century.[4] Robert Boyle (1670 AD) reported the results of resuscitation of asphyxiated kittens, and Chaussier (1806) described endotracheal intubation of asphyxiated infants.[1,2] In the late 1880s, Alexander Graham Bell designed and built a body-enclosing ventilator for newborn resuscitation; a similar device was described in the *Boston Medical and Surgical Journal* by O. W. Doe in 1889. Respiratory failure of the newborn remained an apparently unsolvable problem until a serendipitous cascade of events was set in motion by several key findings during the 1950s and 1960s. The result was the advent of neonatal intensive care.[5–7]

The opinions or assertions are the private views of the author and are not to be interpreted as reflecting Department of the Army or Department of Defense policies.

The knowledge of physiologic principles necessary to ventilate newborns adequately had developed slowly. La Place first described the phenomenon of surface tension in 1806 in a treatise on the movement of the planets and stars.[5,8] This phenomenon was widely studied by physicists and chemists during the succeeding century, but physiologists did not apply the information until the 1920s.[5] In 1929, Von Neergaard demonstrated the principle of alveolar surface tension at an air-liquid interface. He included this information in his discussion of lung elasticity and mechanics.[9] Twenty-five years later this information was applied by Macklin to infer the presence of surface-active material in alveoli.[10] Subsequent work by basic researchers whose work was supported by the Medical Research Laboratories of the U.S. Army Chemical Center and the British Chemical Defense Experimental Establishment helped unravel the mystery of surfactants.[5]

In 1955, Pattle demonstrated that stable foam (foam unaffected by antifoam treatment) was found in the trachea of rabbits with lung edema. Pattle attributed the stability to an insoluble mucous surface layer that formed the original lining of the alveoli. He further reasoned that if the alveolar surface tension were that of an ordinary liquid, the pressure balance between the capillaries and the alveoli would exert enough pressure to fill the alveoli with capillary transudate. Therefore, the mucous protein layer must mitigate the surface tension.[11]

In 1957, Cook and coworkers demonstrated markedly decreased pulmonary compliance in newborns with respiratory distress, and Clements first described the changing surface tension of lung extracts at varying surface areas. The surface tension decreased as the surface film was compressed, thus confirming Macklin's supposition.[12,13]

Avery and Mead took this elegant observation of Clements and in 1959 applied it to their patients dying of hyaline membrane disease

(HMD).[14] They measured an elevated surface tension in the lung extracts of infants who died of HMD when compared with infants who died from other causes. This suggested to Avery and Mead that HMD resulted not from the presence of hyaline membranes (the supposed etiology) but from a lack of surface-active material and increased surface tension during expiration, which led to atelectasis.

Thus, a morbid condition that had had 13 different labels finally had a proposed etiology—*absence* of surface-active material. These researchers provided the rationale for continuous positive airway pressure (CPAP) in 1959. It remained for several other pieces of the puzzle to come together before this became an accepted form of treatment in the 1970s.

The Wedding of Basic Science and Clinical Practice

These findings of Clements, Avery, Mead, Pattle, and others prompted a renewed focus on RDS research in an attempt to characterize surfactant, determine where it came from, and utilize these findings to improve the outcome of infants suffering from RDS.[5,12] At the International Congress of Pediatrics in 1959, several concerns regarding survival were voiced, including avoiding birth asphyxia and providing adequate metabolic support. Another concept discussed at the congress was important to future development and application of mechanical ventilation: the idea that grunting must come from the glottis. It had previously been assumed that grunting resulted from bronchial or bronchiolar obstruction and that therefore the infant's condition would improve with clearing of the obstruction.[3,6]

Clements, Pattle, Thomas, Klaus, Gluck, Hallman, and others continued basic research to characterize the components of surfactants during the 1960s.[5,15] The different biochemical components of surfactants were slowly elucidated, and, coincidentally, the behavior of surfactants *in vitro* was described.[15,16]

As the story of surfactant composition and behavior was unfolding, the site of surfactant production was being identified. Buckingham and Avery in 1962 noted that the appearance of surfactant coincided with the appearance of lamellar bodies in the Type II alveolar cells.[17] Klaus and coworkers stated that the surface-active lining of the lung develops during the process of lamellar transformation of the mitochondria in the alveolar epithelial cell.[18] When direct and indirect evidence was assembled by these basic researchers, the site of surfactant production and release was clearly identified as Type II alveolar cells.[19–21]

How was all this basic science benefiting infants afflicted with RDS? The properties, components, and time of appearance of surfactants were important to know and understand so that the patients at risk for developing RDS could be identified and a plan for treatment could be developed.

During the 1950s and early 1960s, newborn care was quite different from what it is today. Delivery room care was provided by obstetricians and labor and delivery nurses. Well-baby care was provided by pediatricians, but it was not reimbursed by insurance companies. Intensive care units did not exist, and there was no economic incentive for hospitals to develop neonatal intensive care units because insurers did not provide reimbursement for any newborn care.

Laboratory support was rudimentary. Direct measurement of arterial oxygen tension (PaO_2) via a Clarke electrode was not available.[21,22] Incubators did not have access ports so that a warm environment could be maintained while the infant received care. Blood pressure monitoring was unheard of; total parenteral nutrition did not exist. Drug pharmacokinetics in the newborn was a rudimentary science. As with other things, necessity was the mother of invention.

Gluck and coworkers initiated the first neonatal intensive care unit in 1960.[23]

Stahlman described a neonatal intensive care unit with a blood gas machine containing a Clarke electrode for measuring an infant's PaO_2 directly in the unit.[24] Health care providers successfully passed legislation requiring insurance reimbursement for newborn care.[22] Severinghaus contributed an arterial blood gas machine to measure pH, arterial carbon dioxide tension ($PaCO_2$), and PaO_2 on microsamples of blood.[6,25] Gluck and coworkers evolved a means of predicting RDS with amniocentesis.[23]

A means of obtaining blood samples through umbilical vessel catheterization was described.[26] Incubators with the ability to provide constant thermoneutral environments were added to the armamentarium.[27,28] Direct measurement of blood pressure and heart rate in infants was developed. Thus, the wedding of basic researchers and clinical practitioners resulted in the rapid development of neonatal intensive care. However, there were many lessons to be learned along the way.

The first description of providing patient controlled ventilation to newborns was made by Donald and Lord in 1953.[29] Use of mechanical ventilation was reserved for treating moribund infants with intractable respiratory insufficiency because there was limited success (less than 10 percent lived) and the procedure was technically difficult.[30–34] Stahlman and associates described the use of positive pressure ventilation in treating RDS in 1962.[34]

Despite the renewed interest in applying positive pressure ventilation to treat RDS, the method was adopted slowly because experimental data in animals and adults showed that the increased intra-alveolar pressure obtained was transmitted to the thorax and impeded venous return and cardiac output.[35] It remained for the clinicians to develop and evaluate methods of applying positive pressure ventilation to infants with decreased pulmonary compliance and to apply a scientific, physiologically based solution to the problem.

The Beginnings of Neonatal Ventilatory Support

In 1962, several centers began providing ventilation to newborns with respiratory insufficiency.[22] Success varied, with one center reporting a 60 percent survival rate while others had lower rates.[22,30,36] The variability was understandable, because each unit was adapting adult ventilators and designing their own equipment. In addition, the patients selected for treatment were moribund by the time therapy was started, and the staff providing care was venturing into uncharted waters.[22,25]

Standards of care were developed as the care was being provided. The ability to rapidly evaluate and adjust therapy was lacking because microtechnique measurement of PaO_2, $PaCO_2$, pH, bicarbonate, and base excess did not exist.[22,25] Much remained to be learned.

Reports of these early attempts at ventilation stimulated further debate about the efficacy of this treatment.[35-37] In the milieu of health care in the 1960s, the use of mechanical ventilation was *not* an accepted method of treatment of RDS despite the early success of Donald and Lord and the promising results of Thomas and coworkers.[29,30]

The primary debate centered around the teleologic arguments and inferences made concerning the physiologic effects of mechanical ventilation, which some authors argued contributed to the progressive acidosis of the infants who died.[35,38,39] The basic error in logic was that positive pressure ventilation impeded the cardiac return and output of the patient.[35,36,38,39] The assumption that the lung compliance and resistance of the infant with RDS was the same as adults without interstitial and intra-alveolar pulmonary edema, peribronchiolar and perivascular hemorrhage, or terminal airway and alveolar collapse required many years and meticulous studies to refute.[5,6]

In addition, development of the adjuncts to therapy as well as a physiologically based method of ventilation required accumulation of scientific knowledge acquired from basic and clinical research.[5-7] Not only did this information need to be obtained; it also needed to be shared among clinicians.[5] This was a significant problem, because the condition was still not labeled consistently, thus inhibiting interchange of information among clinicians because literature searches were needed to cross-reference 13 different labels to obtain all current information on the problem.

The Seeds of Future Therapy

Coincident with the initial reports of Smith, Daily, and Papodopulus, the stage was being set to develop the information and support necessary to move forward.[5-7,31] In 1963, Tooley, Clements, Klaus, and colleagues conducted a clinical trial of *surfactant replacement therapy* in Kandang Kerbau Hospital in Singapore. Although the therapy did initially improve the physiologic state of the infants, it did not improve the long-term outcome. The investigators attributed the poor outcome to an inadequate mechanism for delivering the surfactant, lack of adequate monitoring, and inability to measure blood gases and provide thermoneutrality.[6,40] This experiment was an attempt to marry the clinical acumen of Tooley and Klaus with the scientific data that numerous investigators had acquired regarding surface-active materials.

Application of the lessons learned in Singapore led to development of clinical research facilities to rapidly overcome the limitations of the clinicians. The subsequent development of instruments to measure blood gases and blood pressure and regulate temperature resulted in improved outcomes.[5-7] Still, the solution to the problem of providing adequate mechanical ventilation remained elusive.

All mechanical ventilators utilized were either modifications or home-built adaptations of adult ventilators. Treatment included paralyzing the infant and providing nutrition via gastrostomy tube.[30] The development of an infant ventilator awaited the serendipitous alignment of resources and personnel.

In 1968, an anesthesiologist was assigned full-time to the nursery at the University of California, San Francisco (UCSF), but not as an anesthesiologist. George Gregory had no responsibilities other than conducting ventilatory research and providing care to the moribund patients in the nursery. He had developed an interest in RDS as a medical student at UCSF in 1961. As a resident, he had worked extensively with the pediatric staff during the development of intensive care for newborns. Following his fellowship, Gregory was assigned to the intensive care nursery by the Anesthesia Department chairman.[5,6]

Along with Tooley, Phibbs, Kitterman, and members of the nursing staff such as Lilly Yoshida, he labored to develop better methods of care. One of their concerns was to treat RDS with the knowledge developed by Von Neergaard, Macklin, Pattle, Mead, Avery, Clements, and others. From the information that grunting improved the metabolic status of infants with RDS, Gregory and colleagues reasoned that applying continuous positive airway pressure would *improve* their metabolic and ventilatory status by maintaining lung volume and not impairing cardiac output.[25,41]

Previous work had shown that compromised infants were relatively hypovolemic and hypoproteinemic, so the infants at UCSF had these problems corrected by meticulous volume replacement.[6] In addition, Gregory and colleagues had shown that only 20 percent of the airway pressure applied to the infants with RDS was transmitted to intrathoracic structures.[42]

The staff continued to experiment with intermittent positive pressure ventilation, but without consistent success. Ventilating patients with the Bird Mark VIII with a J-circuit or a Bournes LS1000, the group attained a survival rate of only 20 percent. There were several reasons for this poor outcome. At respiratory rates of 20 or less, these ventilators did not provide a con-

tinuous flow of fresh gas to patients or maintain continuous positive pressure. Ventilation at more rapid rates (60/minute or greater) maintained both continuous positive pressure and an almost continuous provision of fresh gas. However, the infants were unable to be weaned from rapid rates without compromise.[6,25]

In 1968, Gregory and colleagues decided to try an alternative therapy—CPAP—for any infant with RDS who was breathing spontaneously. This therapy delivers a continuous flow of fresh, humidified gas with a selected fraction of inspired oxygen (FiO_2) while maintaining a continuous distending pressure on the infants' lungs. Sixteen of the 20 patients treated survived.[31] Their preliminary results were reported at the meeting of the Society for Pediatric Research in 1970, and their final results were reported in 1971. This success was marked, especially considering the 70 percent survival rate of infants weighing less than 1.5 kg. The four infants who died had complications of patent ductus arteriosus (PDA).[6,31] Later progress was the direct result of this change in therapy.

A cadre of nurses with special skills and abilities in the recently developed intensive care nursery provided CPAP and other therapy. These staff nurses, who learned along with the pediatricians, could monitor heart rate and blood pressure, manage thermoregulation, manipulate complex electronic equipment, and safely manage umbilical arterial and venous catheters while anticipating problems and identifying patients developing these problems.

When Gregory reported the preliminary data and mode of therapy at the Society for Pediatric Research in 1970, he piqued the interest of many of his colleagues in the audience. Included in this group were Robert Kirby, an Air Force anesthesiologist, and Robert de Lemos, an Air Force pediatrician.

Kirby and de Lemos applied the information presented by Gregory and his colleagues and by Thomas and coworkers and other researchers to the problem of providing adequate mechanical ventilation.[30] The adaptation of adult mechanical ventilators to the neonatal population had been singularly unsuccessful. Various centers had modified Bennett PR-2, Bird Mark VIII, MA-1, or Bournes LS1000 ventilators. These ventilators did not provide a continual flow of gas during spontaneous breathing but only during mandatory mechanical breaths.

Kirby and de Lemos reasoned that the benefits of Gregory's CPAP system should be incorporated into mechanical ventilation. Kirby designed a pneumatically driven, time-cycled, pressure-limited ventilator that delivered a continual flow of gas, CPAP, and intermittent mandatory ventilation (IMV) to the patient being ventilated.[39] Intermittent mandatory ventilation became a mainstay of neonatal mechanical ventilation in the 1970s and early 1980s.

The treatment of RDS had progressed from attempting to maintain the baby's lung volume by attaching a towel clip around the xiphoid process and suspending it from the incubator roof with a rubberband to applying the knowledge of physiologic principles of surface-active materials by maintaining CPAP.[43] Gregory and his colleagues had brought to fruition the knowledge accumulated by Von Neergaard, Gruanwald, Macklin, Radford, Clements, Avery, Mead, and Tooley. However, the benefits of this new therapy proved to be a double-edged sword. To wield it effectively would require the accumulation of clinical data in controlled trials.

Positive Pressure Ventilation: Improving Outcome Through Technologic Development

For mechanical ventilation of the newborn, 1970 and 1971 were watershed years. Kirby and de Lemos described IMV; Daily, Smith, and coworkers published their series, "Mechanical Ventilation of the Newborn Infant: III, IV, V," in *Anesthesiology*; and Gregory and colleagues reported their data on CPAP.[31–33,39,44–46] Whether the therapy was warranted, however, continued to be a subject of debate. It remained for clinical researchers to develop the principles of mechanical ventilation and its applications.

There were many problems to overcome. The small tidal volumes (V_T) required by infants (25 cc or less) were difficult to regulate accurately in modified adult ventilators designed to deliver greater than 1,000 cc. In addition, there was an effort to mimic the ventilatory pattern of infants with RDS by designing infant ventilators capable of patient-triggered frequencies of 100 breaths per minute (bpm) or more. These capabilities were not possible, given the technical limitations of the equipment. Carbon dioxide retention was markedly increased when ventilator failure resulted in uncoordinated attempts at spontaneous ventilation without machine cycling and no gas flow to the patient.[45]

Gregory and associates' application of CPAP resulted in markedly improved survival, but some infants continued to require ventilatory support with modified adult ventilators.[31–33] Because of their inherent limitations, these ventilators were not always able to correct the abnormalities of atelectasis, reduced functional residual capacity (FRC), ventilation/perfusion ($\dot{V}_A/\dot{Q}_C$) abnormalities, and right-to-left intrapulmonary shunting.

These limitations were overcome when IMV was introduced. Intermittent mandatory ventilation provided a continuous flow of gas in excess of the infant's minute ventilation for spontaneous breathing as well as a means of delivering mandatory breaths by occluding the gas outflow tract, resulting in inflation of the infant's lungs. Thus, there was a means of providing the level of support infants required by varying from totally manual to completely spontaneous breathing. Intermittent mandatory ventilation enabled clinicians to select ventilatory patterns for specific purposes with minimal physiologic consequences such as hypercarbia.[45,46]

Therapy's Transition

As NICUs began to proliferate and mechanical ventilation evolved, a common language for discussing therapy became necessary. Many authors coined new phrases to describe therapy, and confusion started to creep into scientific discussions. A precise language was necessary to ensure accurate exchange of information among clinicians.

There was and continues to be confusion about the differences among controlled and assisted ventilation, intermittent positive pressure ventilation (IPPV), IMV, time-cycled ventilators, positive end-expiratory pressure (PEEP), and CPAP. An understanding of these differences is essential for rational application of therapy.

Intermittent positive pressure ventilation, a therapy developed to treat adults with nearly normal lung parenchyma, provides intermittent gas flow under pressure through the ventilator circuit. Therefore, spontaneous breathing between mechanical breaths results in rebreathing of previously exhaled gases.[45,46]

Controlled ventilation, which allows the clinician to determine the ventilatory pattern, results when the rate of respiration is determined by the rate of the ventilator without patient-initiated breaths. To achieve controlled ventilation, paralytic agents are administered to block voluntary respiratory effort, or deliberate hyperventilation is employed.[46]

Assisted ventilation, which clinicians attempted to utilize without success in the neonatal population, is mechanical ventilation that the patient triggers with each inspiratory attempt, which establishes the ventilator rate and pattern. This technique requires a sophisticated triggering device that detects air flow through the circuit as the patient inspires in order to initiate the mechanical breath.[46] As noted previously, assisted ventilation led to significant morbidity secondary to asynchronous breathing and resultant hypercarbia.[45]

Intermittent mandatory ventilation, the conceptual breakthrough of Kirby and de Lemos, provides a continuous flow of gas through the ventilator circuit even when the ventilator is not delivering a mechanical breath. This is a departure from intermittent positive pressure ventilation, which provides gas flow only during the mechanical breath. Positive pressure breaths are thus delivered on a predetermined schedule while the patient continues to breathe voluntarily and receive fresh, humidified gas at a predetermined airway pressure with a selected FiO_2. This allows the infant to breathe efficiently, independent of the mandatory ventilations, and prevents development of biochemical disruptions such as respiratory acidosis.

Time-cycled ventilators end the inspiratory phase of the mechanical breath after a preset time has passed. This cycling occurs regardless of the volume of gas delivered or pressure buildup within the ventilator circuit.[43]

Pressure-limited ventilators end the inspiratory phase when a preset pressure is reached within the ventilator circuit. The inspiratory phase ends regardless of the volume of gas delivered during the inspiration.[47]

Volume-limited ventilators end the inspiratory phase when a preset volume of gas is delivered. This volume is delivered regardless of the pressure reached within the ventilator circuit.[47] Not all of the volume of gas is delivered to the patient; some is lost in the dead space and compliance of the circuit.

Continuous positive airway pressure (CPAP), also called continuous distending airway pressure, continuous distending pressure, and several other names, maintains lung volume in patients with high alveolar surface tension by applying airway pressure sufficient to overcome the tendency for alveolar closure. There are several methods of providing CPAP, including use of an endotracheal tube, head-enclosing box, face mask, and nasal prongs.

These devices may be attached to a ventilator circuit or anesthesia bag with an underwater pressure relief valve.[47] All ventilation is supplied by the patient's voluntary breaths.

Positive end-expiratory pressure (PEEP), maintains positive airway pressure during expiration and between mandatory breaths of the ventilator. It is not synonymous with CPAP. While employing CPAP, pressure remains constant during the patient's voluntary respirations; PEEP is the residual airway pressure maintained at the end of a positive pressure ventilation.

Peak inspiratory pressure (PIP) is the maximal inspiratory pressure generated with each mechanical breath of the ventilator. Pressure is selected and preset on the ventilator. The mechanical breath will not be delivered at a higher pressure than the preset PIP.[47]

Neonatal IMV ventilators incorporate both time and pressure limits to establish the amount of gas delivered during the inspiratory phase of the mechanical breath. The inspiratory time limits the amount of time the positive pressure breath is delivered. The PIP limits the maximal airway pressure generated during the mechanical breath.

Clearly, neonatal positive pressure ventilation has evolved rapidly during the past 29 years and has become more technically complex. This brief discussion of some of the concepts should serve as a guide for clearer understanding of the principles; it is not intended to supplant the extensive treatises available on design and function of mechanical ventilators.[48]

Readers are encouraged to become familiar with the specific mode of operation of the mechanical ventilators employed in their units. Particular attention should be paid to the safe operation and monitoring of the ventilator used. Clinicians should be acutely aware of the limitations of particular products.

Pulmonary Physiology: A Quick Review

In order to have an understanding of the basic principles of ventilation, it is important to understand some concepts of pulmonary physiology. After the review of physiology, the science and art of marrying physics and physiology will be discussed.

Practitioners are often intimidated by the myriad of terms used in discussing mechanical ventilation and pulmonary physiology: dead space (D), dynamic and static compliance, resistance, FRC, (V_T), ventilation of the alveoli per unit time $(\dot{V}_A)$, perfusion $(\dot{Q})$, elastic recoil, surface tension, mean airway pressure $(\overline{Paw})$, transpulmonary pressure, air trapping, FiO_2, partial pressure of oxygen in alveolar gas (P_AO_2), ventilation-to-perfusion ratio $(\dot{V}_A/\dot{Q}_C)$, arterial blood gases, and many others. These words can blend together to form an incomprehensible foreign language to the novice. It is one of the rites of passage in the NICU to master this new lexicon. To smooth the way, discussion focuses here on the practical aspects of pulmonary physiology as they apply to NICU patients. A word of caution: All concepts interrelate in a *dynamic* system that requires a broad understanding.

Ventilation is the bulk flow of gas per unit time into and out of the alveoli to effect oxygen uptake and carbon dioxide elimination. Most practitioners refer to carbon dioxide elimination as ventilation and reserve the term oxygenation for oxygen uptake. These two concepts are intertwined to the extent that an increase in **alveolar minute ventilation** $(\dot{V}_A)$—that is, the volume of gas moved into the alveoli per unit time—will increase oxygen content and carbon dioxide elimination within certain limits.

Alveolar ventilation is *not* equal to the volume of gas inspired with each breath (the **tidal volume** or V_T) multiplied by the number of breaths per minute (f). It is the V_T minus the **respiratory dead space** (V_D), the volume of the anatomic passages between the external environment and the alveoli, which do not function in gas exchange, times the number of inspirations per minute; that is, [47,48]

$$\dot{V}_A = V_T - V_D \times f$$

FIGURE 1 ▲ Physiologic lung volumes

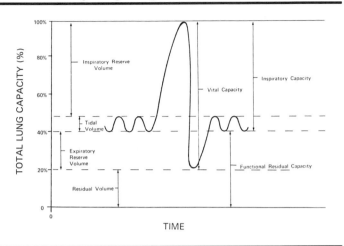

In addition to the volumes defined, another physiologic volume is important to understand: **functional residual capacity (FRC)**. This refers to the point at which the elastic recoil of the lungs and chest wall balance out. It is the lung volume that exists at the end of expiration. This is the volume that allows continual oxygen uptake and carbon dioxide elimination—even when there are no active inspirations. Functional residual capacity is difficult to establish and maintain in patients with RDS because the surface tension in the alveoli of these babies is four times greater than that of normal subjects; therefore atelectasis with resultant hypoxemia and hypercarbia supervenes. Functional residual capacity and other physiologic volumes are illustrated in Figure 1.

Surface tension results from the intermolecular attraction of structures at a surface. When air and liquid interface, as in the alveoli, the intermolecular attraction among liquid molecules exceeds the forces of attraction between air and liquid molecules. These forces work to minimize the area of interface between air and liquid, and this accounts for the lung's retractive forces, which are calculated according to the La Place relationship:

$P = \frac{2\,ST}{r}$. (Pressure [P] is equal to two times the surface tension [ST] divided by the radius [r] of the alveolus.) According to this relationship, the surface tension must increase as the alveolar radius decreases. Lung surfactants act at low lung volume and small alveolar radii to minimize these forces of attraction and stabilize the alveolus before it collapses.[45,47,49]

Minimizing surface tension at the end of expiration helps maintain FRC by preventing atelectasis. Thus, the goal of maintaining oxygenation and ventilation is achieved when atelectasis is prevented and the elastic recoil of the lung is balanced.[46,47,49]

The lung naturally returns to the smallest resting volume because of its property of **elastic recoil** and the surface tension at the air-liquid interface. This tendency of stretched objects to return to their resting state results in a balance of chest wall (both tissue and bony rib cage tissue) and lung elastic recoil that returns the lung to FRC at end expiration in the absence of pathology.[49,50] Figure 2 illustrates this concept.

This ability to distend the chest wall and increase the volume of the thorax depends on

FIGURE 2 ▲ Elastic recoil of the lung and chest wall

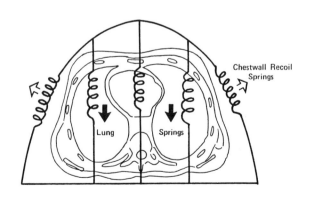

Adapted with permission from: Harris T: Physiologic Principles *in* Goldsmith J, and Karotkin E, eds., Assisted Ventilation of the Neonate, Philadelphia, 1981, W.B. Saunders.

FIGURE 3 ▲ Pressure-volume curves of normal and diseased newborn lungs

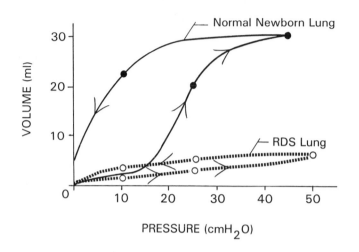

Adapted from: Harris T: Physiologic Principles *in* Goldsmith J, and Karotkin E, eds., Assisted Ventilation of the Neonate, Philadelphia, 1981, W.B. Saunders, Reprinted with permission.

the **compliance** of the system. The relationship of unit change in volume per unit increase in intrathoracic pressure expresses the compliance and thus is a measure of the ability to increase the lung volume with minimal work.

Compliance is expressed both in static and dynamic terms. **Static compliance** is measured by holding volume constant, at different levels, and measuring the pressure within the system needed to maintain the volume. **Dynamic compliance** is measured at the top of inspiration and the bottom of expiration.[50] In the absence of pathology, the compliance of the lung is marked. A change in volume is achieved with a minimum change in pressure. Distensibility is quite apparent, as demonstrated in Figure 3. **Lung compliance** (C_L) is equal to change in volume (ΔV) divided by change in pressure (ΔP):

$$C_L = \frac{\Delta V}{\Delta P}$$

It is important to appreciate this concept of compliance, because patho-physiology of the lung directly affects compliance and thus requires the clinician to adjust the ventilatory therapy employed.

As the lung becomes diseased, compliance decreases markedly, and the pressure required to achieve V_T rises. An example of pathophysiology that changes lung compliance is the RDS compliance curve in Figure 3. This is a snapshot of a dynamic system that is constantly changing. Therefore, the astute clinician will be alert for any improvement or deterioration in lung disease that will dictate a change in compliance and thus an adjustment in ventilation.

Unrecognized changes in lung compliance can drastically alter the FRC of the patient. If compliance improves and the airway pressure remains the same, overdistension of the lung can occur. Conversely, as the disease state worsens and compliance deteriorates, atelectasis occurs if airway pressure remains the same. These concepts are represented in Figure 4.

FIGURE 4 ▲ Compliance curves at various FRCs

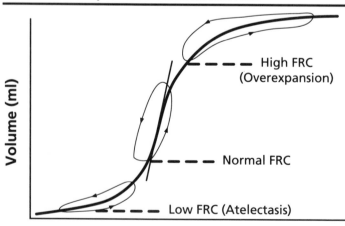

Adapted from: Harris T: Physiologic Principles *in* Goldsmith J, and Karotkin E, eds., Assisted Ventilation of the Neonate, Philadelphia, 1981, W.B. Saunders, Reprinted with permission.

Compliance changes are not restricted to infants with RDS. They occur in all diseases of the newborn lung, including pneumonia, sepsis caused by Group B *ß-hemolytic streptocci*, meconium aspiration syndrome, fluid overload, and PDA.

As the curve in Figure 4 shows, C_L is greatest (the largest change in volume occurs with the least change in pressure) when normal FRC is maintained. This information can be applied clinically by evaluating chest wall excursion, and hence lung expansion, with each ventilator cycle. As C_L improves, chest wall excursion increases. At that point, ventilatory support can be decreased to avoid overdistension and its concomitant deleterious effects, such as decreased cardiac output and surfactant production.[14,50-54]

Reduced cardiac output results from increased intrathoracic pressure causing splinting, which impedes venous return to the right atrium.[52] Surfactant production and release are influenced by the mechanical distension of the lungs, and researchers have inferred that lung overdistension diminishes surfactant production and release.[55]

As lung compliance changes over time, so does resistance. **Resistance** results from friction, such as the viscous resistance of the lungs, as well as resistance to the gas flow in airways and the ventilator circuit.[47,56,57] Airway resistance is directly proportional to the length of the tube through which the gas is flowing and inversely proportional to the fourth power of the radius of the tube, if the flow is laminar. If the flow is turbulent, resistance increases by the gas flow rate's square. In addition, resistance depends primarily upon the cross-sectional area of the smallest diameter tube in the system.[47,57] Therefore, as the radius decreases and tube length increases, the pressure required to drive the gas may rise by a factor of 16 just to overcome the resistance of the system and move gas through it.

The anatomical structures and ventilatory appliances that increase resistance include nasal passages, glottis, trachea, bronchi, and endotracheal tube. Application of CPAP has been reported to both increase and decrease airway resistance.[42,58] Some data indicate that system resistance is increased by endotracheal tubes, but increasing FRC decreases resistance.[58]

As can readily be appreciated, resistance depends on a number of interrelated and dynamic variables, including airway diameter, endotracheal tube diameter, and gas flow rates. Clinicians must be alert to changes in resistance that result from secretion accumulation in the airway, which can increase the work of breathing.

Resistance and compliance interrelate to determine the **time constant** of the lung: a measure of how quickly pressure generated in the proximal airway results in a 63 percent pressure change in the alveoli. The time constant is a calculated value obtained by multiplying resistance by compliance. It is expressed symbolically as:

$$Time\ constant\ (seconds) = $$
$$Resistance\ (cm\ H_2O/liter/second) \times$$
$$Compliance\ (liters/cm\ H_2O)$$

It is important to appreciate that as either the resistance or compliance changes, the time constant changes as well. Thus, an increase in resistance results in a prolonged time constant and a need to adjust ventilation therapy.[50,51]

Perfusion ($\dot{Q}$) is the flow per unit time of blood through the lung. This is usually expressed as liters per minute.

The ventilation-to-perfusion ratio ($\dot{V}_A/\dot{Q}_C$) expresses the relationship between the alveolar ventilation and the blood flow to the lung's capillaries. If the alveolus is ventilated but not perfused, then the ratio will be different, and PaO_2 will be diminished. Conversely, if the alveolus is not ventilated but is perfused, an intrapulmonary right-to-left shunt will supervene.

Matching of ventilation and perfusion at the alveolar level is the goal of ventilation therapy. Through meticulous adjustment of ther-

FIGURE 5 ▲ The Final Common Pathway of Both Hypoventilation and Hypoperfusion

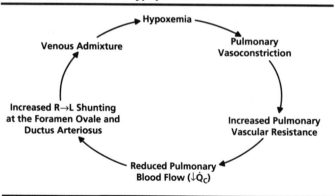

apy, the consequences of atelectasis and right-to-left shunting may be avoided, and FiO_2, which affects PaO_2, can be diminished while PaO_2 is maintained.[49,50]

Numerous pathophysiologic mechanisms affect both $\dot{V}_A$ or $\dot{Q}_C$. However, these conditions all display a final common pathway in their effects on either $\dot{V}_A$ and $\dot{Q}_C$. Pathophysiologic states that decrease $\dot{V}_A$ include: hypoventilation; apnea; lung restriction from (1) extrinsic factors such as mass effects or (2) intrinsic factors due to space-occupying changes/lesions within the lung; atelectasis or lung volume reduction; airway obstruction due to aspiration, infection, or bronchospasm; and gas trapping and alveolar overdistension. Mechanisms that impact on $\dot{Q}_C$ include: pulmonary hypoperfusion; pulmonary hyperperfusion due to left-to-right shunting; and venous admixture or right-to-left shunting from (1) intrapulmonary shunting in which ventilation to a segment of lung is zero but perfusion persists or (2) extrapulmonary or intracardiac shunting (shunting at the atrial or ductal level).[50]

Hypoventilation may result from extreme prematurity, abnormalities of the muscles of respiration (including phrenic nerve palsy, spinal cord injury, myasthenia gravis, and Werding-Hoffman syndrome), drug intoxication, birth asphyxia, and tetanus neonatorum. Apnea can be caused by seizures, Ondine's

curse, hypoxic-ischemic encephalopathy, intracranial hemorrhage, sepsis, or apnea of prematurity.

Extrinsic lung restriction results from congenital diaphragmatic hernia, tumor, chylothorax, and pneumothorax. Intrinsic lung restriction may be caused by congenital malformations such as lobar emphysema, cystic adenomatoid malformation, and lymphangiectasis and by pulmonary interstitial emphysema (PIE), bronchopulmonary dysplasia (BPD), pulmonary edema, pulmonary hemorrhage, and Wilson-Mikity syndrome.

Airway obstruction may be due to laryngomalacia, choanal atresia, Pierre-Robin syndrome, macroglossia, micrognathia, nasopharyngeal tumor, subglottic stenosis, aspiration pneumonia, or malpositioned endotracheal tube.[50] All these conditions result in decreased $\dot{V}_A$ that may result in decreased PaO_2 and increased $PaCO_2$ if they are not recognized and appropriate intervention initiated.

Pulmonary hypoperfusion supervenes when persistent pulmonary hypertension of the newborn (PPHN) results from increased pulmonary vascular resistance secondary to hypoxemia and acidosis.[50,59] Patent ductus arteriosus and ventricular septal defect are two causes of pulmonary hyperperfusion that can lead to pulmonary edema, resulting in hypoxemia and increased pulmonary vascular resistance, which eventually leads to pulmonary hypoperfusion. Venous admixture also results in hypoxemia and acidosis, which increases pulmonary vascular resistance (PVR).

No matter what the pathophysiology causing the alteration in ventilation or perfusion, the ultimate result is the same vicious cycle. This final common pathway is seen in Figure 5. The infant is at risk for slipping into this final common pathway if the prodromal signs of decreased alveolar ventilation or decreased perfusion, such as increased $PaCO_2$, decreased pH, decreased PaO_2, ductal shunt, hypotension, hyperinflation, decreased C_L, or decreased cardiac output, are not recognized. Clinicians direct their intervention at improving alveolar ventilation ($\dot{V}_A$) and perfusion ($\dot{Q}_C$) to maintain $PaCO_2$, PaO_2, and pH within normal limits, thus minimizing capillary fluid leaks. Preventing capillary fluid leaks helps improve lung compliance and reduce the infant's ventilatory requirements.

When compliance changes, the transpulmonary pressure necessary to increase lung volume also changes. **Transpulmonary pressure** is the difference in pressure between the alveolus and the intrapleural space. When compliance decreases, the transpulmonary pressure necessary to increase lung volume must increase. In other words, the pressure gradient generated across the lung must increase to compensate for the lung's stiffness. However, as intra-alveolar pressure is increased with CPAP, the lung may become overdistended, and air trapping may occur.[49,50]

Air trapping, which can cause significant rises in $PaCO_2$, results from alveolar overdistension and can lead to proximal airway collapse prior to complete emptying of the V_T. Because the V_T is not completely exhaled, the carbon dioxide released in the alveolus is not exhausted but instead remains available for reuptake into the capillary blood flowing by the alveolus. The judicious use of CPAP and mechanical ventilation can improve physiologic aberrations; inappropriate use results in further complications.

The patient's clinical status is improved by establishing and maintaining FRC by adjusting the CPAP or IMV parameters to titrate the **mean airway pressure** ($\overline{Paw}$) within the ventilator circuit. All the components of ventilation already discussed—V_T, frequency (f), gas flow, PIP, PEEP, inspiratory time (I_T)—inter-relate to determine $\overline{Paw}$. As with any

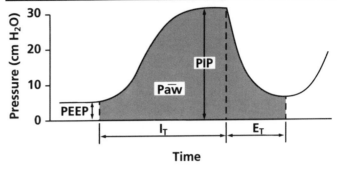

FIGURE 6 ▲ The positive pressure ventilator cycle

PIP—Peak Inspiratory Pressure
PEEP—Positive End-Expiratory Pressure
I_T—Inspiratory Time
E_T—Expiratory Time
$\overline{Paw}$—Mean Airway Pressure (the total area under curve—shaded)

Adapted from: Coulter D: Neonatal Transport Manual, 1981, University of Utah; Cassani III VL: Neonatal Transport Manual, 1985, Washoe Medical Center. Reprinted with permission.

dynamic fluid system, an adjustment in one parameter influences the others. Mean airway pressure is the algebraic sum of the PIP, PEEP, I_T, flow rate of the gas through the ventilator circuit, and rate of mechanical ventilation (f). It is the average pressure transmitted to the airways over a series of ventilator cycles. Mean airway pressure is the area under the pressure-time curve of the ventilator cycle, as illustrated in Figure 6 and expressed algebraically as:

$$\overline{Paw} = \frac{(f)\ (I_T)\ (PIP) + [60 - (f)\ (I_T)]\ (PEEP)}{60}$$

As any clinician in neonatal intensive care can tell you, there are numerous ways of altering the components of $\overline{Paw}$. If the rate of mechanical ventilation is held constant, $\overline{Paw}$ may be increased by increasing inspiratory flow rate, PIP, and PEEP or reversing the inspiratory-to-expiratory (I:E) ratio.[60] This is a powerful tool for managing patients with RDS.

MEAN AIRWAY PRESSURE: WHERE THE MONEY IS

Mean airway pressure has a pivotal role in maintaining FRC and $\dot{V}_A$ during mechanical ventilation. Clinical researchers have evaluated the effects of altering breaths per minute,

FIGURE 7 ▲ Ventilator changes that increase mean airway pressure

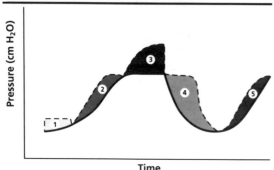

1. Positive end-expiratory pressure higher
2. Inspiratory flow rate increased
3. Peak inspiratory pressure higher
4. Inspiratory time longer
5. Increased ventilator rate

Adapted from: Coulter D: Neonatal Transport Manual, 1981, University of Utah; Cassani V: Neonatal Transport Manual, 1985, Washoe Medical Center. Reprinted with permission.

PIP, PEEP, and pressure waveform on oxygenation of infants with RDS.[60,61–69] Reynolds and coworkers, as well as Smith and colleagues, have shown that increasing bpm and PIP within certain limits improves oxygenation.[60–65] Changes in inspiratory flow rate, and hence the pressure waveform of the ventilator, also alter oxygenation.[63] Fox and associates demonstrated that increasing PEEP improved oxygenation of infants with RDS.[66] Reversing the inspiration-to-expiration ratio (I:E) has also improved oxygen content in some patients.[61,62,68]

When evaluated on an individual basis, these data would appear to conflict. However, the underlying principle that weaves through all of these studies is that altering P̄aw changes oxygenation and ventilation in newborns with RDS. Each of the parameters evaluated by these researchers—PIP, PEEP, I:E ratio, f, and gas flow—directly affects P̄aw. In the dynamic system of an infant with RDS and a continuous flow ventilator, changes in any one of these components may result in a significant change in P̄aw.

Boros and coworkers, in an elegantly designed study, independently varied I:E ratio, PEEP, and inspiratory flow rate during IMV.[67] Oxygenation improved with severe RDS as P̄aw increased when any of the three variables were manipulated. These investigators argued that P̄aw has a central role in maintaining FRC and that manipulation of the ventilator variable is only important because of its direct effect on P̄aw.

Diagramatically, this concept is simple. As shown in Figure 7, changes in (1) inspiratory flow rate, (2) PIP, (3) I:E ratio, (4) ventilator rate, and (5) PEEP change the shape of the pressure waveform. However, the P̄aw, which is the area under the curve of the pressure waveform, may be the *same* when one of these parameters is decreased while another is increased.

Before this underlying principle was recognized, great debates raged among clinicians about what parameters were important to manipulate when providing IMV and weaning the infant from mechanical ventilation. Clinicians at one center would advocate rapid rate ventilation with low PIPs; those at another would employ lower ventilatory frequencies with higher PIPs. As the understanding of the physics and physiology became clearer, it was apparent that both methods of ventilation were successful because they both maintained FRC by increasing P̄aw to the point necessary to overcome the resistive forces of the atelectatic lung.

These are not the only manipulations that can affect P̄aw. Changing the diameter of the endotracheal tube or ventilator circuit tubing will also change P̄aw.[70] This is a fluidic system that changes from moment to moment. As the infant's lung disease lessens, compliance improves, the time constant of the lung lengthens, and the upstroke of the inspiratory cycle will rise rapidly. The PIP will be reached more rapidly, and the ventilator will deliver more V_T with each breath.[70,71] This is synonymous with a change to a more "square wave" ventilatory pattern, and it results in increased minute ventilation.[56,70] Thus, an increase in P̄aw will occur as compliance improves.

This may be beneficial, up to a point. Mirro

TABLE 1 ▲ Criteria for Initiating Mechanical Ventilation

1. Respiratory acidosis with pH of <7.25
2. Severe hypoxemia (PaO$_2$ <50 mmHg) despite FiO$_2$ greater than 0.8
3. Apnea complicating the clinical course of respiratory distress syndrome

and associates have recently demonstrated that increased P$\bar{a}$w in normal lungs decreases cardiac output (CO) in a linear relationship, whereas increased P$\bar{a}$w in diseased lungs reduces heart, kidney, and intestinal blood flow despite arterial blood pressure remaining the same.[72] Thus, application of mechanical ventilation requires continual adjustments in therapy.

Patient Application: More Art Than Science

As mentioned previously, Gregory and coworkers rekindled interest in applying positive pressure in treating RDS.[31] Daily and associates and Smith and coworkers demonstrated that mechanical ventilation, judiciously applied, improved the outcome of infants with RDS.[32,33,44,64,65] After these findings were published, there was an avalanche of articles and books on the subject.[39,46,60,72,73] The discussions ranged from proper techniques for modifying adult ventilators for neonatal application to the introduction of IMV.[33,39,45,52,64,65,74]

As sophistication in applying mechanical ventilation developed, three basic mechanical ventilator variants evolved: (1) negative pressure ventilators, derivatives of the "iron lung" utilized for poliomyelitis victims; (2) positive pressure volume-cycled ventilators; and (3) positive pressure ventilators that are pressure limited and time-cycled.[24,75,76] A detailed review of ventilator design, controls, and fact sheets is available in the literature.[46-48]

Inherent limitations in both the negative pressure and volume-cycled ventilators have resulted in their limited use.[46] Since the mid 1970s, the neonatal ventilators produced for use in the United States have been pressure limited and time cycled. Therefore, this discussion focuses on application of pressure-limited, time-cycled ventilators for treatment of neonatal respiratory failure.

Mechanical ventilation is employed to accomplish effective gas exchange.[48,77] Yet the optimal application of mechanical ventilation remains a controversial topic 35 years after Donald and Lord first described the technique in newborns.[29] One problem is that clinicians have become victims of their own initial success.

When first introduced, mechanical ventilators were employed for treating infants weighing more than 1,500 gm. As clinicians became more adept, survivors weighing less than 1,000 gm became the rule rather than the exception.[71,77] Therefore, the patient population receiving mechanical ventilation became larger and more diverse physiologically. Organized, blinded, randomized, controlled studies of mechanical ventilation in newborns have been difficult to establish because of this diversity as well as the ethical dilemma of utilizing control groups. Reports of initial successes led to widespread use of mechanical ventilation, and the crush of events has pushed the application of technology forward. Scientific inquiries have, unfortunately, not been performed to evaluate all the arguments of some very expert clinicians.

After Gregory's evaluation of CPAP, Reynold's studies seemed to indicate that prolonged inspiratory time and lower PIP would improve oxygenation and decrease the likelihood of sequelae.[31,60-62] Mannino and collaborators demonstrated improved survival with fewer sequelae through early mechanical ventilation, without prior application of CPAP, when compared to infants receiving conventional management of RDS.[74] The criteria for initiating mechanical ventilation changed. Use of CPAP as an initial treatment of RDS and meconium aspiration syndrome gave way to use of IMV for initial therapy.[48,78] Coincidentally, students of mechanical ventilation appreciated the need for tailoring therapy to treat either an atelectatic or obstructive disease process.[48,78,79]

Because these are the two primary problems faced in the NICU, the remainder of this discussion focuses on managing atelectatic and obstructive airway problems in neonates with respiratory failure. Respiratory failure, as defined here, is limited to impaired pulmonary gas exchange. Physiologic alterations in gas exchange from primary lung disease result in hypercarbia and acidosis. Patients require mechanical ventilation to correct these problems and prevent further compromise. Table 1 delineates commonly accepted criteria for initiating mechanical ventilation in these patients.

Atelectatic processes requiring IMV include RDS and sepsis caused by Group B *ß-hemolytic streptococci*. These problems result in decreased FRC and diminished gas exchange.[48,78,80]

Currently there are two basic approaches to managing respiratory failure caused by atelectasis in neonates. Both manipulate $\overline{Paw}$ to achieve adequate gas exchange and minimize hypoxemia and acidosis. Adherents of slow rate IMV recommend that I_T be 1 second or longer and that PIP be as high as 35 cm H_2O in infants weighing more than 1,500 gm.[48,78-80] Positive end-expiratory pressure is applied to assist with "recruitment" of atelectatic alveoli; FiO_2 is adjusted to maintain a PaO_2 of 50–70 mmHg. Intermittent mandatory ventilation is 20–30 bpm, and flow through the ventilator circuit is 8–12 liters per minute.

As hypoxemia and acidosis are corrected, the infant is weaned from ventilation until the FiO_2 is less than 0.6. At that point, I_T is lengthened while IMV and PIP are decreased as tolerated to maintain PaO_2 at 50–70 mmHg.[48,78,81]

These manipulations result in a decrease in $\overline{Paw}$ as the lung disease improves. Thus, hyperinflation and increased dead space are avoided as FRC is maintained. This ensures adequate gas exchange and avoids right-to-left intrapulmonary shunts and impaired CO.[48,78,81] This mode of therapy is not, however, without sequelae. Protein leaks in perialveolar epithelium have been demonstrated following use of high PIPs.[82]

Pulmonary interstitial emphysema, pneumothorax, and BPD have been reported in up to 35 percent of patients receiving this form of IMV.[83-87] Based on these observations, as well as the findings of Stewart and associates that increases in PEEP more consistently increase PaO_2 and $\overline{Paw}$, Bland and Sedin as well as others have become proponents of rapid rate, low inflation pressure ventilation.[88,89]

Advocates of high-frequency IMV utilize ventilatory rates of 60–120 bpm, PIPs of less than 35 cm H_2O, PEEPs of 4–9 cm H_2O, and inspiratory times of 0.15–0.25 seconds. Following stabilization of gas exchange and improvement of lung disease, the infant is weaned from FiO_2, PIP, and PEEP as tolerated.[89] Rate is kept constant. This method of ventilation is based on the assumption that the results of previous work by Reynolds, which showed improved gas exchange through prolonging inspiratory time, would not hold true if PEEP had been employed.[60-62] In addition, Heicher and coworkers demonstrated a decreased incidence of pulmonary air leaks when rapid rate, low PIP, and low V_T ventilation was employed to treat RDS.[90] Drummond and associates have shown this to be effective therapy for PPHN.[91]

Bland and Sedin have reported excellent respiratory gas exchange utilizing low peak inflation pressure with rapid ventilation rates.[89] However, this method of ventilation makes the patient particularly susceptible to progressive air trapping, which can lead to increases in respiratory dead space and resultant hypercarbia.[92] As the air trapping increases FRC, thoracic hyperinflation may lead to pneumothorax or thoracic splinting and decreased cardiac output. It is therefore important to wean PIP and PEEP when compliance improves in order to avoid air trapping.[92]

Both methods of ventilation—slow rate and high-frequency IMV—have their risks and benefits. It is important to remember that both manipulate $\overline{Paw}$ to maintain adequate gas exchange during respiratory failure secondary to atelectasis. Positive end-expiratory pressure is employed for alveolar "recruitment" and stabilization to maintain FRC. Minute ventilation is maintained through the use of PIP, I_T, and f. The minute ventilation is similar in both methods; they are just achieved in a different manner by varying PIP, I_T, and f.

Obstructive airway problems are encountered in retained fetal lung fluid, meconium aspiration syndrome, and PIE. They are characterized by severe $\dot{V}_A/\dot{Q}_C$ mismatch from uneven distribution of alveolar ventilation. Alveolar ventilation is disrupted by space occupying lesions or particulate matter in the terminal bronchioles adjacent to the alveolar structure in the form of meconium plugs, amniotic fluid, or distended air dissections in the peribronchiolar parenchyma. Although alveolar inflation usually occurs with each ventilator cycle, complete deflation to FRC does not.

Expiration is impeded by the lesions, and air trapping results in alveolar overdistension and increased FRC. The air trapping is caused by the partial airway obstruction, airway collapse when closing volume is reached before FRC, or an exhalation time that is insufficient to allow complete emptying of the alveoli.[50] The risk of alveolar rupture and pneumothorax as well as reduced CO increases with air trapping. Therefore, ventilator therapy is designed to achieve adequate gas exchange while minimizing air trapping.[47,48,50,78]

Because, overall, the time constant of the lung is prolonged during obstructive airway disease, despite normal compliance, clinicians advocate using a prolonged I_T of 0.4–1 second and an f of 30–60 bpm. This relatively slow f will allow for maximal exhalation of gas from

TABLE 2 ▲ Maneuvers To Improve Oxygenation and Ventilation

To Improve Oxygenation (PaO_2)		
Maneuver	Effect	Risk
1. ↑ FiO2	↑ PaO_2	?BPD with prolonged exposure
2. ↑ PEEP or ↑ CPAP	Recruitment of atelectatic areas— ↓ intrapulmonary shunt	Air leaks
	↑ FRC	↑ CO_2 retention with hyperinflation
	↑ $P\overline{aw}$	↓ Venous return and cardiac output
3. ↑ PIP	↑ FRC	Air leaks
	↑ $P\overline{aw}$	?BPD
4. ↑ I_T	↑ $P\overline{aw}$	Air leaks
		↓ Venous return and cardiac output
		↑ CO_2 retention 2° to ↓ expiratory time
		?BPD
To Improve Ventilation ($PaCO_2$)		
Maneuver	Effect	Risk
1. ↑ PIP	↑ FRC	Air leaks
	↑ $P\overline{aw}$	?BPD
2. ↑ PEEP or ↑ CPAP	↑ FRC	↓ V_T → ↓ minute ventilation
	↑ $P\overline{aw}$	↓ Venous return and cardiac output
		Air leaks
3. ↑ PEEP or ↑ CPAP	↑ V_T	↓ PaO_2
4. ↓ I_T	↑ E_T	↓ PaO_2
5. ↑ Rate (f)	↑ Minute ventilation	↓ PaO_2

the alveolus before the next positive pressure breath, minimizing air trapping.[79]

In patients with obstructive airway disease, there are some lung units that are not obstructed and have normal resistance and time constants. The alveolar pressures of these areas will eqilibrate with the $P\overline{aw}$ more rapidly and be preferentially ventilated with each positive pressure breath. Therefore, V_T and minute ventilation within these lung units will increase and help maintain gas exchange while minimizing air trapping.[48,78,79] In order to minimize overdistension and pneumothorax in these lung units, PIP should be increased only to the point of achieving chest excursion.

Some clinicians advocate minimal or no

TABLE 3 ▲ Side Effects of Tolazoline Infusion

Hypotension
Hypertension
Edema
Oliguria
Hematuria
Gastrointestinal bleeding
Pulmonary hemorrhage
Seizures

application of PEEP in order to prevent alveolar overdistension and rupture; others have employed PEEP without a significant increase in air leaks.[93] In all likelihood, application of PEEP maintains the patency of the obstructed airways and facilitates emptying of the alveoli.[59,94]

Unfortunately, a significant number of infants with obstructive airway problems develop a superimposed problem of persistent pulmonary hypertension of the newborn (PPHN). This problem appears to respond to very aggressive ventilator therapy, including hyperventilation to correct the hypoxemia and acidosis.[59,93] Some centers have reported successful outcomes for these infants without utilizing hyperventilation.[94] However, all have utilized some form of vasoactive therapy to achieve adequate pulmonary and systemic perfusion.[59,91,93–97]

Hyperventilation is employed to maintain the pH above 7.5 and the $PaCO_2$ below 25 mmHg.[59,91] This therapy is associated with a decrease in pulmonary artery pressure and right-to-left shunt through the PDA.[59,93]

Table 2 summarizes the current information regarding manipulation of mechanical ventilation to improve oxygenation and ventilation.

ADJUNCTS TO
MECHANICAL VENTILATION

Cardiotonic therapy is utilized to decrease PVR and/or maintain mean arterial blood pressure. Vasodilators used to decrease pulmonary vascular resistance include tolazoline, nitroprusside, and prostaglandins. Each has been shown to be beneficial in *some* patients.[59,91,95–100]

However, clinical response is quite variable and requires close, careful observation and preparation prior to and during therapy.

Tolazoline hydrochloride (Priscoline), an alpha-adrenergic blocking agent, has been employed as an adjunctive therapy in infants with PPHN to achieve pulmonary vasodilation and decrease pulmonary vascular resistance. Data from two reports published in the 1950s and 1960s seemed to demonstrate improvement in oxygenation of neonates with PPHN. However, reevaluation of these data does not support the commonly held belief that tolazoline is a pulmonary vessel vasodilator.[98]

Both Drummond and associates and Stevenson and coworkers have described the pharmacologic effects of tolazoline in the neonatal population with PPHN.[91,101] Their data indicated that administration of 1–2 mg/kg of tolazoline hydrochloride over ten minutes and an infusion of 1–2 mg/kg/hour resulted in an increase in PaO_2 of more than 20 mmHg on the first arterial blood gas in 10 of 15 infants with RDS, 13 of 15 infants with meconium aspiration syndrome, and 4 of 9 infants with other pulmonary diseases. The tolazoline decreased pulmonary artery pressure below systemic arterial pressure in 2 of 5 patients.[91,101] Apgar scores, diagnosis, or pretolazoline arterial blood gas values did not predict response to tolazoline.[101]

The overall survival of these infants did not correlate with response to tolazoline infusion, although survivors did have a greater increase in PaO_2 when compared with nonsurvivors. This effect may be achieved at the expense of having the patient display the side effects listed in Table 3.

Because tolazoline is excreted unchanged in the urine, its half-life depends on urinary output and varies from 3.3 to 33 hours.[102] The wise clinician will avoid starting an infusion on an oliguric patient. In order to temporize the side effects of hypotension and decreased cardiac output, a cardiotonic infusion and colloid volume support may be necessary.

Sodium nitroprusside, a direct acting vasodilator, achieves its effect through action on vascular smooth muscle. Reduction of preload and afterload contributes to improvement of cardiac output, left ventricular function, tissue perfusion, and urinary output. These effects are achieved after blood volume expansion and initiation of a cardiotonic drip to ameliorate systemic hypotension.

Benitz and associates report a therapeutic effect of sodium nitroprusside in infants with RDS and a survival rate in infants with PPHN similar to that reported by Drummond for tolazoline infusion.[91,97] These investigators recommend starting the infusion at 0.25 μg/kg/minute and advancing the rate to a maximum of 6 μg/kg/minute until a therapeutic effect is achieved.[97] Adverse effects are listed in Table 4.

The half-life of nitroprusside is considerably shorter than that of tolazoline. Thus, it is recommended as the first-line choice when treating PPHN because the drug will clear from the patient's system within minutes.[97]

Prostaglandins, metabolites of arachidonic acid, decrease pulmonary artery pressure and increase pulmonary blood flow in experimental animals. PGI_2 is a nonspecific vasodilator; PGD_2 acts specifically on pulmonary smooth muscle in fetal and newborn animals. However, this specificity was not replicated in human neonates who received infusions of 0.1–10 μg/kg/minute. In these human studies, a nonspecific vasodilation occurred.[99]

The deleterious effects of hypotension are ameliorated by providing cardiotonic pressure support and colloid volume expansion. When infusing PGI_2, PGD_2, or PGE_2, infants should be observed for pyrexia, apnea, and diarrhea as well as hypotension. All prostaglandins are rapidly metabolized, and their effects clear minutes after discontinuing the drug infusion.[100]

Shock and myocardial dysfunction result in decreased cardiac output and all its coincident

TABLE 4 ▲ Adverse Effects of Nitroprusside Infusion

Hypotension
Tachycardia
Cyanide poisoning (theoretical)
Abolition of intrapulmonary autoregulation
Metabolic acidosis
Tachyphylaxis
Thyroid suppression

problems such as acidosis, hypoxemia, hypoglycemia, hypocalcemia, and hypovolemia. Sympathomimetic amines are employed to improve cardiac output. Included in this armamentarium are dopamine, dobutamine, and isoproterenol.

Dopamine, an intermediate metabolic precursor of norepinephrine and epinephrine, has a dose-dependent effect on heart rate and contractility. This is achieved through $alpha_1$, $beta_1$, and $beta_2$ stimulation to achieve dopaminergic effects at doses ranging from 2 to 20 μg/kg/minute. Lower doses result in increased renal blood flow and decreased peripheral vascular resistance. Doses of 5–10 μg/kg/minute provide a positive inotropic effect, increase contractility, and stimulate β_1 receptors. Increasing the dosage above 10 μg/kg/minute results in dose-related rises in systemic vascular resistance through α_1 stimulus.

Side effects include tachycardia, arrhythmia, hypertension, and gangrenous skin sloughs from IV infiltration. The half-life of dopamine is two minutes, so these side effects may quickly be corrected by discontinuing the infusion.[96,97,102] Sloughs may be prevented with instillation of phentolamine at the site of infiltration.

Some clinicians mistakenly believe that dopamine achieves its effect by increasing peripheral and central vasoconstriction. Data available from animal and human studies indicate that dopamine has an inotropic effect and causes *central vasodilation* at doses less than 4 μg/kg/minute.[103] This is why it is essential to ensure adequate intravascular volume prior to initiating therapy.

Dobutamine, a synthetic β_1 selective agonist, increases myocardial contractility and heart rate. It has no effect on renal blood flow and increases peripheral vascular resistance only minimally. It is administered as a continuous infusion at rates of 0.5–10 µg/kg/minute and has a half-life similar to dopamine. Side effects include arrhythmias and intrapulmonary shunting. There are reports that combining dopamine and dobutamine maintains CO and systemic arterial pressure with a minimal increase in peripheral vascular resistance.[96,102–104]

Isoproterenol, a synthetic catecholamine, stimulates both beta$_1$ and beta$_2$ receptors to increase myocardial activity while decreasing peripheral vascular resistance through vasodilation. Thus, left ventricular afterload reduction may be achieved while heart rate and cardiac output increase and renal blood flow remains unchanged or decreases. Isoproterenol's use is limited by its marked chronotropic effect with the accompanying increase in myocardial oxygen consumption. In addition, the vasodilation may result in decreased central venous pressure and hypotension.

The patient on isoproterenol must be closely monitored for tachycardia and hypotension, the two most common side effects. Atrial and ventricular arrhythmias have also been noted with its use. All these effects are more marked with this drug than with dobutamine or dopamine.

Isoproterenol is administered intravenously at a dosage varying between 0.05 and 0.5 µg/kg/minute. It clears rapidly after discontinuation of the drip and has a half-life similar to the other catecholamines reviewed.[96,102–104]

Vasodilators and cardiotonic agents are usually employed in the management of critically ill infants with multiple system disease. These infants are able to maintain physiologic function only within a narrow window of opportunity. Developmentally, the cardiovascular system of these patients is structurally and functionally different from those of adults and older children. The myocardium is less organized and unable to demonstrate the classic Frank-Starling response to a volume load.[96] Hence, they maintain CO through alterations in heart rate. Sympathetic innervation is incomplete, and target organs have an increased sensitivity to catecholamines. Because resting cardiac output is maximal cardiac output and endogenous stores of catecholamines are developmentally subnormal, the infant may very rapidly display signs of cardiac failure.[103]

It is incumbent upon all who provide care to these infants to carefully and meticulously monitor heart rate, systemic blood pressure, urinary output, oxygen content, and $PaCO_2$, as well as monitoring crystalloid and colloid fluid loads. Vasodilators and cardiotonic drugs alter preload, afterload, the size of the vascular space, renal blood flow, and peripheral vascular resistance in a milieu that is less than optimal. Meticulous care is necessary to recognize and prevent complications of these drugs before the patient slips into the spiral of cardiac failure, hypoxemia, and acidosis. Which cardiotonic agent to use is a question that cannot be clearly answered with the data currently available. Clinical experience with these drugs and careful review of the available literature are indicated before undertaking such therapy.

Sedation and/or muscle relaxation through neuromuscular blockade remains a controversial topic in neonatal intensive care.[102,105,106] Proponents argue that sedation with morphine has a minimal cardiovascular effect, prompt onset of action, a duration of action of four to six hours, and minimal side effects while achieving the goal of eliminating the infant's "fighting the ventilator." They argue that this results in an improved V_A/Q_C ratio while avoiding the risks associated with pancuronium. Morphine administration results in histamine release and may cause hypotension and circulatory depression in the newborn.[109]

Fentanyl, a synthetic narcotic, is 50–100 times more potent than morphine. It has a rapid onset and brief duration of action when administered in doses of 1–2 µg/kg and produces both analgesia and respiratory depression with minimal cardiovascular effects. Its half-life is 3.6 hours.[110] Certain centers are administering this drug as an infusion to labile infants with PPHN at 0.5–2 µg/kg/hour, titrated to desired effect. Respiratory muscle paralysis, muscle rigidity, and apnea may result from too rapid administration of fentanyl infusion.[111] Prolonged use causes tolerance which requires periodic increases in dosage. Infants treated with fentanyl can demonstrate physical dependency and a dose reduction regime may be required.[112]

Proponents of neuromuscular blockade with pancuronium argue that its use plays a role in improving oxygenation while reducing barotrauma and intracranial hemorrhage.[102,106] Runkle and Bancalari have demonstrated improved oxygenation for infants with meconium aspiration syndrome and PPHN but not for infants with RDS who received this therapy.[105] Reduction of barotrauma and air leak has been reported.[107] However, Pollitzer and coworkers, in a randomized controlled trial, demonstrated no difference in the incidence of air leaks between the paralyzed and control groups.[108]

Similarly, there have been reports advocating use of pancuronium to reduce the incidence of intracranial hemorrhage as well as reports indicating an increased risk of intracranial hemorrhage with pancuronium use.[102] Currently, no objective data reliably predict which, if any, infants benefit from pancuronium administration. This therapy has traditionally been administered as a therapeutic trial to severely hypoxemic infants and continued if PaO$_2$ improves.

Pancuronium bromide, a long-acting, competitive neuromuscular blocking agent, blocks transmission by competition with acetylcholine at the neuromuscular junction. It has a rapid onset of 2–4 minutes and a prolonged half-life of 60–90 minutes, which is increased in infants

with acidosis, hypokalemia, or decreased renal function and those receiving aminoglycosides. Dosage varies from 0.06 to 0.09 mg/kg administered as an IV push.[102,106]

Side effects include tachycardia, hypotension following vascular pooling, soft tissue edema from capillary leaks, contractures, and pressure sores.[106] The most potentially catastrophic hazard is covert extubation. Therefore, careful observation and monitoring of oxygenation and changes in heart rate and a meticulous general physical exam are warranted. Because paralysis obscures the clinical signs of seizures, some centers advocate loading these infants with phenobarbital and maintaining therapeutic levels of this drug until the infant is weaned from the paralytic agent.

Newer nondepolarizing neuromuscular blockers with minimal cardiovascular effects are now available. These neuromuscular blockers include atracurium, alcuronium, and vecuronium. They are available to be used as continuous infusions and have a half-life of 20–64 minutes. Dosage, for continuous infusion, varies from 1–2 µg/kg/minute for vecuronium to 6–8 µg/kg/minute for atracurium.[110]

Use of vasodilators, cardiotonic agents, and paralytic agents is not restricted to infants with PPHN. Application of any of these modalities in ventilated newborns must be weighed against the risks inherent in the therapy. Careful review of the data available on these agents should guide clinicians in their application of the planned intervention. Arguments for employing any of these therapies have not always been supported by clinical data.[96,97,105] Benitz and associates demonstrated a beneficial effect when nitroprusside was utilized in low-birthweight infants with RDS rather than in infants with PPHN.[97] Paralysis of infants with RDS results in acute cardiopulmonary effects and a variable response in oxygenation.

SUMMARY

Mechanical ventilation of newborns is a

recently developed technique for treating respiratory failure. It requires meticulous application of basic physiologic principles and careful titration of therapy to maintain adequate gas exchange. Early reports of success have resulted in widespread use of the technique without blinded, controlled trials to demonstrate efficacy of a particular technique. Clinicians have applied the technique to treat atelectatic and obstructive diseases of the newborn respiratory system. Various adjuncts to therapy include vasodilators, cardiotonic agents, and paralytic agents. Sequelae include pulmonary interstitial emphysema, air leaks, and bronchopulmonary dysplasia.

DEDICATION

This chapter is dedicated to Jennifer Marie Day and all the other babies who proved the efficacy of IMV.

REFERENCES

1. Strang LB, ed.: Neonatal Respiration: Physiology and Clinical Studies, Philadelphia, 1977, J. B. Lippincott.
2. Milner AD, and Martin RJ, eds.: Neonatal and Pediatric Respiratory Medicine, Philadelphia, 1985, J. B. Lippincott.
3. Stern L, ed.: Hyaline Membrane Disease, Pathogenesis and Pathophysiology, New York, 1984, Grune and Stratton.
4. Kirby RR, and Greybar GB, eds; Intermittent mandatory ventilation, International Anesthesiology Clinics 18(2), 1980, whole issue.
5. Comroe JH: Retrospectroscope: Insights into Medical Discovery, Menlo Park, California, 1977, Von Gehr.
6. Gregory GA: Personal communication, October 7, 1987.
7. Sunshine P: Personal communication, October 7, 1987.
8. La Place PS: Traite'de Me'canique Ce'leste, 5 vols, Paris, 1798–1827, Crapelet, Courcier.
9. von Nerrgaard K: Neve auffassungen uber einen grundbegriff der atemmechanik. Die retraktionskraft der lunge, abhangig von der oberflachenspunnung in den alveoleh, English translation *in* Comroe JH, Jr, ed., Pulmonary and Respiratory Physiology: Benchmark Papers in Human Physiology, Part I, Stroudsberg, Pennsylvania, 1976, Dowden, Hutchinson and Ross, pp. 214–234.
10. Macklin CC: The pulmonary alveolar mucoid film and the pneumocytes, Lancet 1, 1954, pp. 1099–1104.
11. Pattle RE: A test of silicone anti-foam treatment of lung oedema in rabbits, Journal of Pathology Bacteriology 72, 1956, p. 203.
12. Cook C, Sutherland J, and Segal S: Studies of respiratory physiology in the newborn infant, III: Measurements of mechanics of respiration, Journal of Clinical Investigation 36, 1957, p. 440.
13. Clements JA: Surface tension of lung extracts, Proceedings of the Society of Experimental Biology and Medicine 95, 1957, p. 170.
14. Avery ME, and Mead J: Surface properties in relation to atelectasis and hyaline membrane disease, American Journal of Diseases of Children 17, 1959, p. 517.
15. Klaus MH, Clements JA, and Havel RJ: Composition of surface-active material isolated from beef lung, Proceedings of the National Academy of Science 47, 1961, p. 1858.
16. Thannhauser SJ, Benotti J, and Boncoddo NF: Isolation and properties of hydrolecithin (dipalmityl lecithin) from lungs, its occurrence in the sphingomyelin fraction of animal tissues, Journal of Biological Chemistry 166, 1946, p. 669.
17. Buckingham S, and Avery ME: Time of appearance of lung surfactant in the foetal mouse, Nature 193, 1962, p. 688.
18. Klaus M, et al.: Alveolar epithelial cell mitochondria as a source of the surface-active lung lining, Science 137, 1962, p. 750.
19. Gil J, and Reiss OK: Isolation and characterization of lamellar bodies and tubular myelin from rat lung homogenates, Journal of Cellular Biology 58, 1973, p. 152.
20. Williams MC, and Mason RJ: Development of the type II cell in the fetal rat lung, American Review of Respiratory Diseases 115 (supplement), 1977, p. 37.
21. Campiche MA, et al.: An electron microscope study of the fetal development of human lung, Pediatrics 32, 1963, p. 976.
22. Sunshine P: Personal communication, October 10, 1987.
23. Gluck L: Personal communication, February 22, 1988.
24. Stahlman M: Treatment of cardiovascular disorders of the newborn, Pediatric Clinics of North America 11(2), 1964, p. 363.
25. Gregory GA: Personal communication, October 10, 1987.
26. Kitterman JA, Phibbs RH, and Tooley WH: Catheterization of umbilical vessels in newborn infants, Pediatric Clinics of North America 17, 1970, p. 895.
27. Hey E, and Mount L: Temperature control in incubators, Lancet 2, 1966, p. 202.
28. Hey E, and O'Connell B: Oxygen consumption and heat-balance in the cot-nursed baby, Archives of Disease in Childhood 45, 1970, p. 335.
29. Donald I, and Lord J: Augmented respiration studies in atelectasis neonatorum, Lancet 1, 1953, p. 9.
30. Thomas DV, et al.: Prolonged respirator use in pulmonary insufficiency of newborn, Journal of the American Medical Association 193(3), 1965, p. 183.
31. Gregory GA, et al.: Treatment of the idiopathic respiratory distress syndrome with continuous positive airway pressure, New England Journal of Medicine 284(24), 1971, p. 1333.
32. Daily WJR, et al.: Mechanical ventilation of newborn infants: III, Historical comments and development of a scoring system for selection of infants, Anesthesiology 34(2), 1971, p. 119.
33. Smith PC, and Daily WJR: Mechanical ventilation of newborn infants: IV, Technique of controlled inter-

mittent positive-pressure ventilation, Anesthesiology 34(2), 1971, p. 127.

34. Stahlman MT, Young WC, and Payne G: Studies of ventilatory aids in hyaline membrane disease, American Journal of Diseases of Children 104, 1962, p. 526.

35. Cournand A, et al.: Physiological studies of the effects of intermittent positive pressure breathing on cardiac output in man, American Journal of Physiology 152, 1948, p. 162.

36. Swyer PR: An assessment of artificial respiration in the newborn, *in* Problems of Neonatal Intensive Care Units, Report of the Fifty-ninth Ross Conference on Pediatric Research, Columbus, Ohio, 1965, Ross Laboratories.

37. Harrison VC, Hesse H deV, and Klein M: The significance of grunting in hyaline membrane disease, Pediatrics 41, 1968, p. 549.

38. Kirby RR: Mechanical ventilation of the newborn: Pitfalls and practice, Perinatology-Neonatology, July-August 1981, p. 47.

39. de Lemos RA, and Kirby RR: Early development: Intermittent mandatory ventilation in neonatal respiratory support, International Anesthesiology Clinics 18(2), 1980, p. 39.

40. Tooley WH: Hyaline membrane disease: Telling it like it was, American Review of Respiratory Disease 115(6), 1977, p. 19.

41. Heese H deV, Harrison VC, and Klein M: Intermittent positive pressure ventilation in hyaline membrane disease, Journal of Pediatrics 76, 1970, p. 183.

42. Gregory GA, et al.: The time course changes in lung function after a change in CPAP, Clinical Research 25 (abstract), 1977, p. 193.

43. Love J, and Tillery N: New treatment for atelectasis of the newborn, American Journal of Diseases of Children 86, 1953, p. 423.

44. Daily WJR, Sunshine P, and Smith PC: Mechanical ventilation of newborn infants: V, Five years' experience, Anesthesiology 34(2), 1971, p. 132.

45. Kirby RR, et al.: Continuous-flow ventilation as an alternative to assisted ventilation in infants, Anesthesia and Analgesia 51(6), 1971, p. 871.

46. Kirby RR: Design of mechanical ventilators, *in* Thibeault DW, and Gregory GA, eds., Neonatal Pulmonary Care, Menlo Park, California 1979, Addison-Wesley.

47. Kirby RR, Smith RA, and Desautels DA, eds.: Mechanical Ventilation, New York, 1985, Churchill-Livingstone.

48. Carlo WA, and Martin RJ: Principles of neonatal assisted ventilation, Pediatric Clinics of North America 33, 1986, p. 221.

49. Mines AH: Respiratory Physiology, New York, 1981, Raven Press.

50. Harris TR: Physiological principles, *in* Goldsmith JP, and Karotkin EH, eds.: Assisted Ventilation of the Neonate, Philadelphia, 1981, W. B. Saunders.

51. Suter PM, Fairley HB, and Isenberg MD: Optimum end-expiratory airway pressure in patients with acute pulmonary failure, New England Journal of Medicine 292(6), 1975, p. 284.

52. Kumar A, et al.: Continuous positive pressure ventilation in acute respiratory failure, New England Journal of Medicine 283(26), 1970, p. 1430.

53. Richards CC, and Backman L: Lung and chest wall compliance of apneic paralyzed infants, Journal of Clinical Investigation 40(1), 1961, p. 73.

54. Polgar G: Opposing forces to breathing in newborn infants, Biology of the Newborn 11, 1967, p. 1.

55. Truog WE: Surface active material: Influence of lung distension and mechanical ventilation on secretion, Seminars in Perinatology 8(4), 1984, p. 51.

56. Polgar G, and String ST: The viscous resistance of the lung tissues in newborn infants, Journal of Pediatrics 69, 1966, p. 787.

57. Briscal WA, and Dubois AB: The relationship between airway resistance, airway conductance and lung volume in subjects of different age and body size, Journal of Clinical Investigation 37, 1958, p. 1279.

58. Saunders RA, Milner AD, and Hopkins IE: The effects of continuous positive airway pressure on lung mechanics and lung volume in the neonate, Biology of the Neonate 29, 1976, p. 178.

59. Fox WW, and Duara S: Persistent pulmonary hypertension in the neonate: Diagnosis and management, Journal of Pediatrics 103(4), 1983, p. 505.

60. Reynolds EOR: Pressure waveform and ventilator setting for mechanical ventilation in severe hyaline membrane disease, International Anesthesiology Clinics 12(4), Winter 1974, pp. 259–280.

61. Reynolds EOR: Effects of alterations in mechanical ventilator settings on pulmonary gas exchange in hyaline membrane disease, Archives of Disease in Childhood 46, 1971, p. 152.

62. Herman S, and Reynolds EOR: Methods for improving oxygenation in infants mechanically ventilated for severe hyaline membrane disease, Archives of Disease in Childhood 48, 1973, p. 612.

63. Owen-Thomas JB, Ulan OA, and Swyer PR: The effect of varying inspiratory gas flow rate on arterial oxygenation during IPPV in the respiratory distress syndrome, British Journal of Anesthesiology 40, 1968, p. 493.

64. Smith PC, Schaeh E, and Daily WJR: Mechanical ventilation of newborn infants: II, Effects of independent variation of rate and pressure on arterial oxygenation, Anesthesiology 37(5), 1972, p. 498.

65. Smith PC, Daily WJR, and Fletcher G: Mechanical ventilation of the newborn infant: I, The effect of rate and pressure on arterial oxygenation of infants with respiratory distress syndrome, Pediatric Research 3, 1969, p. 244.

66. Fox WW, et al.: The PaO_2 response to changes in PEEP in RDS, Critical Care Medicine 5, 1977, p. 226.

67. Boros SJ, et al.: The significance of mean airway pressure, Journal of Pediatrics 91, 1977, p. 794.

68. Spahr A, et al.: Hyaline membrane disease, American Journal of Diseases in Children 134, 1980, p. 373.

69. Erickson J, et al.: The influence of ventilatory pattern on ventilation, circulation and oxygen transport, Acta Anaesthesiologica Scandinavica 64, 1977, p. 149.

70. LeSouef PN, England SJ, and Gryan AC: Total resistance of the respiratory system in preterm infants with and without an endotracheal tube, Journal of Pediatrics 104(1), 1984, p. 108.

71. Cunningham MD: Methods of monitoring pulmonary function, Clinics in Perinatology 13(2), 1986, p. 299.

72. Mirro R, et al.: Relationship between mean airway pressure, cardiac output, and organ blood flow with normal and decreased respiratory compliance, Journal of Pediatrics 111, 1987, p. 101.

73. Meyer HBP, et al.: Ventilatory support of the newborn infant with respiratory distress syndrome and respiratory failure, International Anesthesiology Clinics 12(4), Winter 1974, pp. 81–110.

74. Mannino F, et al.: Early mechanical ventilation in RDS, Pediatric Research 10(1), 1976, p. 464.

75. Hakanson DO: Volume ventilators, *in* Goldsmith JP, and Karotkin EH, eds, Assisted Ventilation of the Neonate, 2nd ed., Philadelphia, 1988, W.B. Saunders, pp. 171–189.

76. Fox WW, Shutack JG, and Spitzer AR: Positive pressure ventilation: Pressure and time-cycled ventilators, *in* Goldsmith JP, and Karotkin EH, eds, Assisted Ventilation of the Neonate, 2nd ed., Philadelphia, 1988, W.B. Saunders, pp. 146–170.

77. Bhat R, and Zikos-Labropoulou E: Resuscitation and management of infants weighing less than 1000 grams, Clinics in Perinatology 13(2), June 1986, p. 285.

78. Krauss AN: Assisted ventilation: A critical review, Clinics in Perinatology 7(1), 1980, p. 61.

79. Reynolds EOR: Treatment of respiratory failure, *in* Thibeault DW, and Gregory GA, eds., Neonatal Pulmonary Care, Menlo Park, California 1979, Addison-Wesley.

80. Stark AR, and Frantz ID: Respiratory distress syndrome, Pediatric Clinics of North America 33(3), 1986, p. 533.

81. Mannino F, and Gluck L: Treatment of RDS, *in* Thibeault DW, and Gregory GA, eds., Neonatal Pulmonary Care, Menlo Park, California 1979, Addison-Wesley.

82. Egan EA, Olver RR, and Strong LB: Changes in non-electrolyte permeability of alveoli and absorption of lung liquid at the start of breathing in the lamb, Journal of Physiology (London) 244, 1975, p. 161.

83. Northway WH, Rosan RC, and Porter DY: Pulmonary disease following respiratory therapy of hyaline membrane disease, bronchopulmonary dysplasia, New England Journal of Medicine 276, 1967, p. 357.

84. Rhodes PG, et al.: Minimizing pneumothorax and bronchopulmonary dysplasia in ventilated infants with hyaline membrane disease, Journal of Pediatrics 103(4), 1983, p. 634.

85. Thibeault DW, et al.: Pulmonary interstitial emphysema, pneumomediastinum, and pneumothorax occurrence in the newborn infant, American Journal of Diseases of Children 126, 1973, p. 611.

86. Watts JL, Ariagno RL, and Brady JP: Chronic pulmonary disease in neonates after artificial ventilation: Distribution of ventilation and pulmonary interstitial emphysema, Pediatrics 60(3), 1977, p. 273.

87. Ackerman MB, et al.: Pulmonary interstitial emphysema in the premature baboon with hyaline membrane disease, Critical Care Medicine 12(6), 1984, p. 512.

88. Stewart AR, Finer NN, and Peters KL: Effects of alterations of inspiratory and expiratory pressures and inspiratory/expiratory ratios on mean airway pressure, blood gases, and intracranial pressure, Pediatrics 98, 1981, p. 957.

89. Bland R, and Sedin E: High frequency mechanical ventilation in the treatment of neonatal respiratory distress, International Anesthesiology Clinics 21(3), 1983, p. 125.

90. Heicher DA, Kasting DS, and Harrod JR: Prospective clinical comparison of two methods for mechanical ventilation of neonates: Rapid rate and short inspiratory time versus slow rate and long inspiratory time, Journal of Pediatrics 98, 1981, p. 957.

91. Drummond WH, et al.: The independent effects of hyperventilation, tolazoline, and dopamine on infants with persistent pulmonary hypertension, Journal of Pediatrics 98, 1981, p. 603.

92. Perez-Fontan JJ, et al.: Dynamics of expiration and gas trapping in rabbits during mechanical ventilation at rapid rates, Critical Care Medicine 14(1), 1986, p. 39.

93. Fox WW, Berman LS, and Downes JJ: The therapeutic application of end-expiratory pressure in meconium aspiration syndrome, Pediatrics 56, 1975, p. 214.

94. Wong JT, et al.: Management of infants with severe respiratory failure and persistence of the fetal circulation, without hyperventilation, Pediatrics 76(4), 1985, p. 488.

95. Bacsik RD: Meconium aspiration syndrome, Pediatric Clinics of North America 24(3), 1977, p. 463.

96. Drummond WH: Use of cardiotonic therapy in the management of infants with PPHN, Clinics in Perinatology 11(3), 1984, p. 715.

97. Benitz WE, et al.: Use of sodium nitroprusside in neonates: Efficacy and safety, Journal of Pediatrics 106(1), 1985, p. 102.

98. Ward RM: Pharmacology of tolazoline, Clinics in Perinatology 11(3), 1984, p. 703.

99. Soifer SJ, and Heymann MA: Future research directions in persistent pulmonary hypertension of the newborn, Clinics in Perinatology 11(3), 1984, p. 745.

100. Turner GR, and Levin DL: Prostaglandin synthesis inhibition in persistent pulmonary hypertension of the newborn, Clinics in Perinatology 11(3), 1984, p. 581.

101. Stevenson DK, et al.: Refractory hypoxemia associated with neonatal pulmonary disease: The use and limitations of tolazoline, Journal of Pediatrics 95(4), pp. 595–599.

102. Goetzman BW, and Milstein JM: Pharmacologic adjuncts, *in* Goldsmith JP, and Karotkin EH, eds, Assisted Ventilation of the Neonate, 2nd ed., Philadelphia, 1988, W.B. Saunders, pp. 272–283.

103. Driscoll DJ: Use of inotropic and chronotropic agents in neonates, Clinics in Perinatology 14(4), 1987, p. 931.

104. Yeh TF: Drug Therapy in the Neonate and Small Infant, Chicago 1985, Year Book Medical Publishers.

105. Runkle B, and Bancalari E: Acute cardiopulmonary effects of pancuronium bromide in mechanically ventilated newborn infants, Journal of Pediatrics 104, 1984, p. 614.

106. Costarino AT, and Polin RA: Neuromuscular relaxants in the neonate, Clinics in Perinatology 14(4), 1987, p. 965.

107. Greenough A, et al.: Pancuronium prevents pneumothoraces in ventilated premature babies who actively expire against positive pressure inflation, Lancet 1(1), 1984, p. 1.

108. Pollitzer MJ, et al.: Pancuronium during mechanical ventilation speeds recovery of lungs of infants with hyaline membrane disease, Lancet 1, 1984, p. 346.

109. Roscow C, et al.: Hemodynamics and histamine release during induction with sufentanil or fentanyl, Anesthesiology 60(5), 1984, pp. 489–491.

110. Wood M, and Wood AJJ: Drugs and Anesthesia, Pharmacology for Anesthesiologists, Baltimore, 1990, Williams and Wilkins.

111. Billmire D, et al.: Use of IV fentanyl in the outpatient treatment of pediatric facial trauma, Journal of Trauma 25, 1985, pp. 1079–1080.

112. Bell SG, et al.: Use of fentanyl for sedation of mechanically ventilated neonates, Neonatal Network 6(2), 1987, pp. 27–31.

6 Complications of Assisted Ventilation in the Neonate

Anne McCormick, RN, MS
Perinatal Nursing Consultant
Lincolnwood, Illinois

Karen Braune, RNC, MSN
University of Alabama at Birmingham
Birmingham, Alabama

The number of neonates surviving respiratory distress in the neonatal period has increased significantly because of advancements in mechanical ventilation. Technological developments, along with expert medical, nursing, and respiratory therapy care, have decreased the mortality statistics of the past. Unfortunately, serious acute and chronic complications accompany this mode of therapy, and nurses must be aware of these concerns in order to provide comprehensive care.

Complications of assisted ventilation include infection, pulmonary air leaks, tracheobronchial injury, intracranial hemorrhage, bronchopulmonary dysplasia, and retinopathy of prematurity. This chapter discusses pulmonary air leaks, bronchopulmonary dysplasia (BPD), and retinopathy of prematurity (ROP), formerly referred to as retrolental fibroplasia (RLF). These three entities have particular implications for nursing care. In reviewing these general complications, it is important to remember that infection remains one of the leading causes of mortality and morbidity in infants receiving mechanical ventilation.[1]

PULMONARY AIR LEAKS

Pulmonary air leaks, or extra-alveolar or extraneous air syndromes, are the most common serious complication of assisted ventilation in the neonate.[1,2] The incidence of pulmonary air leaks in ventilated infants varies from unit to unit, ranging anywhere from 16 to 48 percent.[3,4] The overall incidence of pulmonary air leaks has been found to be higher in extremely low-birthweight infants.[5] The common occurrence of these disorders among infants makes it imperative that nurses be able to identify, assess, and intervene appropriately. In order to correctly identify the occurrence of these entities, then provide early intervention, it is paramount that all nurses working in neonatal units have a thorough understanding of relevant anatomy (Figure 1) and physiology. The cone shaped newborn thorax consists of much cartilage, resulting in it being more flexible than an adult

FIGURE 1 ▲ Relationship of vital structures within the neonatal chest

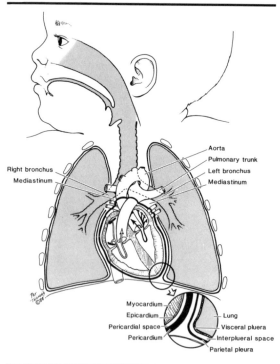

The area between these two pleurae, the interpleural space, provides a lubricated surface for the lung to inflate and deflate. The pulmonary interstitium, the connective tissue that surrounds the alveoli and capillary vessels, forms perivascular sheaths that are connected to mediastinal connective tissue, continuous with the pericardial and retroperitoneal connective tissue.

Pulmonary air leaks occur when the alveoli are overdistended during ventilation, which results in alveolar rupture with gas escaping into normally nonventilated tissues. Depending upon which tissues are affected, one of the following disorders will result: pulmonary interstitial emphysema (PIE), pneumomediastinum, pneumothorax, pneumopericardium, and pneumoperitoneum. Of these, PIE, pneumomediastinum, and pneumothorax are the most common forms.[2]

Intra-alveolar pressure is high during positive pressure ventilation. The connective tissue sheaths surrounding the pulmonary blood vessels attempt to expand with the alveoli while the vessels remain the same size. This results in unbalanced forces developing across the base of the alveolus proximal to the pulmonary capillary bed. Alveoli then rupture.

After rupture occurs, the air moves from the alveolus into loose connective tissue sheaths surrounding the arterioles, traveling along these sheaths to the hilum of the lung. The interstitial air can dissect through connective tissue around blood vessels or along the lymphatics, resulting in pulmonary interstitial emphysema. From the hilum, the escaped air can move into the mediastinum (pneumomediastinum) or the thoracic cavity, rupturing through the visceral pleura (pneumothorax). If the air moves along the great vessels to the pericardial sac, a pneumopericardium is formed. When the air dissects down from the mediastinum through the sheaths of the aorta and vena cava into the peritoneal cavity, pneumoperitoneum occurs.

Lung distention is proportional to pressure and to the length of time that pressure is exert-

thorax. The posterior portion consists of 12 thoracic vertebrae and the ribs; the anterior position consists of the sternum and costal cartilage. The 11 separations between the ribs are called intercostal spaces.

The mediastinum is located within the thoracic cage behind the sternum and between the pleural spaces. Here, vital structures are gathered in rather close proximity, so pathologic changes in one structure are likely to affect the others. The heart lies in the anterior mediastinum. Its surface is covered by a tissue layer referred to as the epicardium, which in turn is covered by the pericardium. The space between these two layers is called the pericardial sac. Connective tissue sheaths suspend the heart.

The trachea lies midline in the neck. Any shifts of viscera within the thorax may displace both the larynx and the trachea.

The visceral pleura covers the surface of the lung; the parietal pleura covers the thoracic cage, diaphragm, and lateral wall of the mediastinum.

FIGURE 2 ▲ Pulmonary interstitial emphysema and pneumoperitoneum. This film demonstrates bilateral PIE with the characteristic cyst "bubbles" resulting in a spongelike appearance. Common branching is also present. The free air in the right abdominal area clearly indicates a pneumoperitoneum.

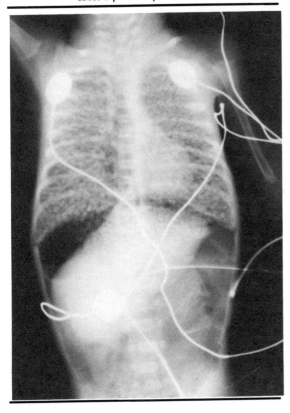

ed. Overdistention of alveoli can occur after the application of high pressure for short periods of time or low pressures for long periods of time.[6]

Pulmonary Interstitial Emphysema

As gas is trapped in the interstitium or lymphatics of the lung, pulmonary interstitial emphysema (PIE), results. This free interstitial air decreases lung compliance, tidal volume, and alveolar ventilation. The decrease in ventilation results in a significant drop in oxygen pressure and retention of carbon dioxide. The interstitial air can also impair cardiac output and increase pulmonary vascular resistance. Two forms of air collection can occur: (1) intra-

pulmonary pneumatosis, in which air is trapped in the interlobular septa, and (2) intrapleural pneumatosis, in which subpleural blebs occur.

Pulmonary interstitial emphysema is generally related to the use of high peak ventilatory pressures. Preterm and very low-birthweight infants are at an increased risk for developing PIE because they have more extensive connective tissue in their immature lungs, which is more likely to trap the ruptured air.[7] In this population, PIE is associated with mortality and serious morbidity.[8] An infant who has developed PIE generally undergoes a marked deterioration and requires increased oxygen and ventilatory adjustments. Diagnosis is by radiologic examination: The film is characterized by coarse reticular patterns of both linear and cystlike translucencies extending out from the hilum. Part or all of the lung may be affected. Figure 2 demonstrates a classic chest radiograph of PIE.

Various interventions have been proposed, from conservative treatment to surgical removal of the affected lobe(s). Increased oxygen, often to 100 percent, is required. Reducing the peak inspiratory and positive end-expiratory pressures may be helpful.[8]

Unilateral PIE results in overdistention of the affected lung, mediastinal displacement, compression atelectasis of the contralateral lung, and ventilation/perfusion inequalities. Intermittent mandatory ventilation with an extremely short inspiratory time (0.10–0.15 seconds) has been found to be effective.[9] Selective intubation of the unaffected bronchus has also been proposed.[10,11] This procedure results in an occlusion of the affected lobe or lung, allowing resorption of interstitial air and effective ventilation of the uninvolved lung. The procedure is difficult, however, and includes the risks of severe acidosis, bradycardia, and infection of the involved lung.[11] High-frequency oscillatory and jet ventilation (see Chapters 7 and 8) have been used successfully for PIE.

Interstitial emphysema commonly can progress to pneumothorax; approximately 50

FIGURE 3 ▲ Pneumomediastinum. In an anterior-posterior view such as this, pneumomediastinum is characterized by free air around the heart. The wide lateral areas of free air with a distinct border represent the "spinnaker sail sign."

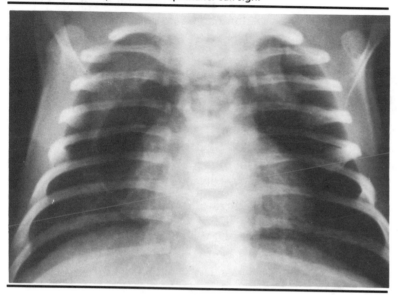

Figure 3 demonstrates a pneumomediastinum.

Usually a pneumomediastinum will resolve spontaneously. If the gas moves to the area above the hemidiaphragm, a lung can become compressed and displaced. In these cases, the gas is aspirated.

Pneumothorax

Pneumothorax is a very common occurrence during assisted ventilation. Incidence is reported as high as 35 percent among ventilated infants.[12] It results when air from the ruptured alveoli enters the pleural cavity from the mediastinum or from the rupture of subpleural blebs. Nurses should be aware that infants with respiratory distress syndrome commonly develop a pneumothorax just when the severity of their disease is decreasing and lung compliance is increasing.[13]

A spontaneous pneumothorax is a leak into the intrapleural space between the lung and chest wall. It is usually not serious, and infants are frequently asymptomatic.[1] A tension pneumothorax, on the other hand, involves an interpleural collection of air above atmospheric pressure, which collapses the affected side of the lung, shifting the mediastinum to the opposite side and causing the heart vessels to compress. Risk factors for developing a tension pneumothorax include early gestational age, respiratory distress syndrome (RDS), mechanical ventilation with high pressures, and the previous occurrence of PIE and/or pneumomediastinum.

Tension pneumothorax produces abrupt signs and symptoms. As the lung collapses, hypoxia and hypercapnia occur; circulatory collapse can result as mediastinal structures are compressed and venous return impeded. Nurses

percent of pneumothoraces are associated with it.[1] The formation of a pneumothorax can, however, result in a decompression of the PIE, improving patient outcome. Unfortunately, the incidence of chronic lung disease among survivors remains high.

Pneumomediastinum

Pneumomediastinum is generally not a significant problem because the air present in the mediastinum usually does not have enough tension to cause any circulatory distress. If the tension does increase drastically, it can dissect into the neck, producing subcutaneous emphysema, or rupture into the thoracic cavity to produce a pneumothorax.

The most common signs of a pneumomediastinum are tachypnea, muffled heart sounds, and cyanosis. Diagnosis is by x-ray examination, which shows a halo around the heart. Air collections are usually central and can elevate and surround the thymus and great vessels. Air present below the thymus, for example, lifts the thymus from the heart and produces the characteristic "windblown spinnaker sail sign."

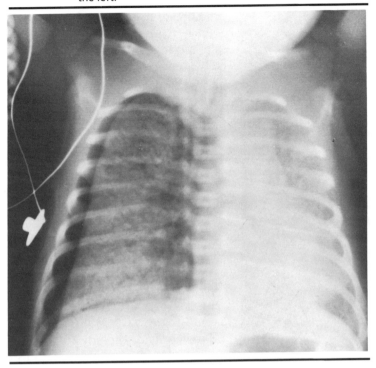

FIGURE 4 ▲ Pneumothorax. In this unilateral pneumothorax, the right lung is underexpanded, and there is a mediastinal shift to the left.

should be alert for sudden cyanosis with decreased blood pressure, heart rate, and pulse pressure. Diminished breath sounds, bulging of the affected side, and a shift of heart sounds are common. The abdomen becomes tense and distended. In severe cases, the liver is easily palpable and the spleen depressed by the diaphragm.

Transillumination of the neonatal chest provides a rapid preliminary diagnosis in critical situations when immediate intervention is necessary. A normal lung and pleura absorb light; a pneumothorax produces illumination. Confirmation by x-ray examination should be obtained as soon as possible. The collapsed lung is easily identifiable, as is the mediastinal shift. Figure 4 shows the x-ray film of an infant with a pneumothorax.

Rapid intervention is possible by needle aspiration. One or more chest tubes are placed, if necessary, for aspiration of reaccumulating air, and are connected to continuous suction. The suction is maintained until bubbling and air fluctuation in the tube have ceased.

Continued ventilatory management usually consists of reducing ventilator pressures and volume while increasing oxygen concentration. Because it has been found to decrease the rate of air leakage through the pneumothorax, high-frequency ventilation has been proposed as an alternative to conventional ventilation for these infants.[14] The short inspiratory times utilized in this method result in ventilation of areas with the lowest resistance, avoiding ruptured areas producing the leak; a shorter duration of pressure is applied to the ruptured area, reducing peak pressure and barotrauma. In addition, the reduced mean airway pressure and possible decreased mean alveolar pressure that result from high-frequency ventilation reduce the pressure driving the gas through the pneumothorax.

A good percentage of infants with PIE and a single pneumothorax will develop a contralateral pneumothorax; infants who do not exhibit PIE on chest x-ray film at the time of the first pneumothorax will usually not experience a second one.[15] Intraventricular hemorrhage has also been associated with pneumothorax. The pathogenic mechanism involved is an abrupt increase in cerebral blood flow at the time of pneumothorax.[16]

Pneumopericardium

When the interstitial air moves along the great vessels and ruptures into the pericardial sac, a pneumopericardium is produced. The degree of severity can vary from asymptomatic to cardiac collapse from cardiac tamponade resulting from gas tension. Pneumopericardi-

FIGURE 5 ▲ Pneumopericardium. The heart is entirely circled by a halo of free air.

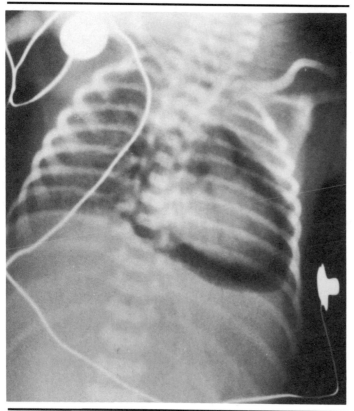

um is not common and seldom occurs spontaneously, usually accompanying other forms of air leaks.[12] The majority of cases occurs during the first days of therapy.[17]

Bradycardia, cyanosis, and muffled or absent heart sounds are common signs. Decreased stroke volume produces hypotension; metabolic acidosis occurs as a result of diminished tissue perfusion. Decreased arterial and pulse pressures also occur.

Diagnosis is confirmed by anterior and lateral chest films. Large air volumes are usually seen surrounding the heart, producing a halo appearance. The appearance of gas under the inferior surface of the heart is the diagnostic radiographic sign (Figure 5).[17] When pneumomediastinum is also present, a pericardial line is produced by the pericardium, outlined by air on either side.[12]

Infants without cardiac tamponade require close observation for deterioration of their condition. Increased oxygen concentrations and reduced mean alveolar pressure may be required. Infants with cardiac tamponade must undergo immediate pericardial taps to remove the accumulated air. If air reaccumulates, a pericardial catheter is inserted; care is similar to that for chest tubes used for a pneumothorax. The catheter is usually removed within 72 hours to prevent pericarditis.

Pneumoperitoneum

A pneumoperitoneum can be related to either pulmonary or bowel disease. When it originates from the thorax, it is directly related to ventilator therapy and is associated with pneumomediastinum and pneumothorax.[2]

Figure 2 demonstrates the radiological film; air, appearing as a dark cloud, is present in the peritoneum. Vision of the bowel is often occluded.

It is necessary to determine whether the cause of a pneumoperitoneum is respiratory or gastrointestinal, because the latter cause would require surgical intervention. Gastrointestinal perforation is generally indicated by delayed gastric emptying, bloody stools, sepsis, vomiting, and absence of respiratory disease. In contrast, diagnosis of pneumoperitoneum due to an air leak is based on extraneous air in the peritoneum and usually in the chest, absence of peritoneal fluid in the peritoneum, and normal bowel wall thickness. Paracentesis with lavage or an upper GI series may be helpful in the differentiation. If the aspirated gas shows a high oxygen pressure, a pulmonary origin is indicated.

Intervention may not be necessary unless respiratory status is seriously compromised or

TABLE 1 ▲ Assisted Ventilation: Causes of Overdistention

High peak inspiratory pressures (>25 cm H_2O)
High PEEP (>5 cm H_2O)
High CPAP (>8 cm H_2O)
Prolonged inspiratory time (>0.3 seconds)
Short expiratory time (<0.3 seconds)
Reverse inspiratory:expiratory (I:E) ratios
Inadvertent positive expiratory pressure

Adapted from: Thibeault DW: Pulmonary barotrauma: Interstitial emphysema, pneumomediastinum, and pneumothorax *in* Thibeault DW, and Gregory G, eds., Neonatal Pulmonary Care, Newark, New Jersey, 1987, Appleton-Century-Crofts, chapter 20.

venous return to the heart impeded. In these cases, a soft drainage catheter connected to low suction can be utilized.

Prevention

Because pulmonary air leaks are caused by alveolar rupture created by overdistention, minimizing the causes of overdistention should reduce the incidence of pulmonary air leaks. These causes are listed in Table 1.

During ventilation, the degree of alveolar distention is directly related to the peak inflation pressure, the inspiratory time, and the end-expiratory pressure. Prolongation of the inspiratory time causes more overdistention than does increased peak pressure. If the I:E ratio exceeds 1:2, gas trapping can occur, causing further distention.[18]

Preventive care, then, consists of keeping the inspiratory time as low as possible and ventilating infants with a fast rate and low tidal volume. An understanding of neonatal pulmonary mechanics is essential in providing appropriate therapy for infants requiring mechanical ventilation. Care in determining parameters must be meticulous. This can be difficult, however, because of the nature of the underlying illness and the individuality of infant response.

Nursing Implications

The nursing role in caring for infants with pulmonary air leaks involves awareness of potential development, prompt identification, early intervention, astute management, and parental support. Because of the critical nature of these disorders, it is imperative that nurses caring for these infants be well qualified, experienced, and thoroughly understand the relevant anatomy and physiology. Orientation programs, including a comprehensive review of the principles involved, must be followed by ongoing staff development programs. Primary care providers, whether physicians or nurse practitioners, should routinely share the findings of their diagnostic workups with the nursing staff.

Infants at risk for developing pulmonary air leaks include those who have been resuscitated or have aspirated meconium, preterm infants with RDS, and especially those on mechanical ventilation. Fifty percent of ventilated infants with pulmonary hypertension experience pulmonary air leaks.[19]

Prompt intervention is based on immediate identification of signs and symptoms. Although in many cases they may be nonspecific, the cardinal signs (Table 2) should alert the nurse to the probable development of an air leak.

A complete respiratory assessment (see Chapters 3 and 4) with evaluation of all equipment is fundamental following the development of any

TABLE 2 ▲ Clinical Signs of Pulmonary Air Leaks

Interstitial Emphysema	Deterioration of patient's status Increased oxygen requirements, cyanosis
Pneumomediastinum	Tachypnea, occasionally cyanosis Muffled heart sounds
Pneumothorax	Cyanosis, grunting, flaring, abdominal distension Diminished breath sounds on affected side Mediastinal shift Decreased BP, HR, RR Decreased pulse pressure or EKG amplitude
Pneumopericardium	Abrupt cyanosis, pallor Severely muffled or inaudible heart sounds Decreased BP, decreased pulse pressure

TABLE 3 ▲ Proposed Stages of Bronchopulmonary Dysplasia

Stage I	2–3 days	Acute respiratory disease
Stage II	4–10 days	Regeneration • regeneration and proliferation • ulceration and membrane formation in bronchioles
Stage III	10–20 days	Development of chronic lung disease • extensive repair with phagocytosis • alveolar collapse • bronchiolar metaplasia • interstitial fibrosis
Stage IV	More than 1 month	Chronic disease • obliterative bronchiolitis with interstitial fibrosis • peribronchiolar fibrosis • epithelial proliferation, bronchiolar metaplasia

Adapted from: Korones SB: Complications, *in* Goldsmith JP, and Karotkin A, eds., Assisted Ventilation of the Neonate, Philadelphia, 1987, W.B. Saunders, Chapter 13; and Northway WH, Rosan RC, and Porter DT: Pulmonary disease following respiratory therapy for hyaline membrane disease, New England Journal of Medicine 27, 1967, pp. 357–368.

signs and symptoms. The primary care provider should be immediately notified to ensure prompt diagnosis and management. The head of the infant's bed can be elevated 30–40° to localize the air in the upper chest and keep the abdominal organs away from the diaphragm.[3]

Equipment for transillumination, needle aspiration, and chest tube placement should be readily available for all infants at risk for pulmonary air leaks. The care of infants requiring these modes of intervention is described in detail in the literature.[3,20,21]

The sudden deterioration of an infant is quite upsetting to parents, especially if they are present when the air leak occurs. An experienced, supportive staff member should remain with them when they are asked to leave the unit while emergency procedures are performed. Explanations should be complete, yet simple. Parental contact with the infant should resume at the earliest time, with the primary nurse explaining equipment and procedures. Chest tubes and drainage apparatus can be particularly frightening to parents. Questions regarding any pain the infant may be experiencing need to be handled delicately yet honestly.

BRONCHOPULMONARY DYSPLASIA

The major chronic complication associated with mechanical ventilation in the neonate is bronchopulmonary dysplasia (BPD), a chronic lung disease occurring primarily in preterm infants who have experienced respiratory disease. Most cases of BPD are preceded by respiratory distress syndrome (RDS), but it has been known to occur in association with other disorders.

Bronchopulmonary dysplasia is related to increased mortality and morbidity among patients in neonatal units today. Long-term hospitalizations, the difficulties involved in transfers and discharges, and the emotional consequences to staff and families take their toll in severe financial and social problems for families and others caring for these patients.

Bronchopulmonary dysplasia was first described in 1967 by Northway and colleagues, who reported a series of lung changes in preterm infants with RDS who had experienced mechanical ventilation with high concentrations of oxygen.[1,22] Four stages based on roentgenographic changes were identified (Table 3).

Since this initial description, the diagnosis of BPD is not based solely on roentgenographic changes, but relates to a chronic pulmonary disease process following respiratory failure. Not all infants exhibit the four stages described by Northway; therefore, hyperinflation is usually the predominant x-ray finding. Reported incidence can vary due to differences in patient populations, management techniques, length of therapy, and terminology. Hence, there is often significant disparity in reported incidence. During the 1970s the estimated incidence was 30–40 percent of infants on mechanical ventilation; it is now 10–20 percent of those who receive ventilation and survive.[1,23]

When BPD was initially described, high oxygen concentration was considered the main cause of the pulmonary lesion. It is now known

FIGURE 6 ▲ Advanced stage of bronchopulmonary dysplasia. The lungs are hyperflated; strands, streaks, and patches are seen throughout. Cardiomegaly is present.

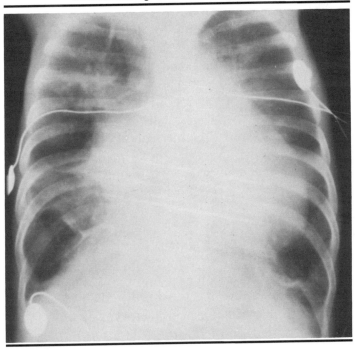

to be caused by numerous factors, each affecting patients individually. Common risk factors include an immature lung, lung injury, oxygen toxicity, mechanical ventilation with high pressures, and a long course of respiratory therapy. Other contributing factors include genetic predisposition, pulmonary air leaks, pulmonary edema, patent ductus arteriosus (PDA), and small-airway reactivity. Of all these factors, an immature lung is considered the most important predisposing factor in the development of chronic lung disease.[24,25]

Clinical Presentation

The diagnosis of BPD is based upon clinical and radiographic characteristics. Most of those who develop BPD are preterm infants with RDS requiring mechanical ventilation during the first few days of life.

Instead of showing an improvement in respiratory status, the infant developing BPD requires high oxygen and pressure parameters. Chest films change from the typical RDS appearance to show coarse, granular infiltrates dense enough to obscure cardiac borders—giving a "white out" appearance. A PDA can commonly occur during this acute period, as can PIE or pneumothorax. These complications may prolong the need for respiratory assistance with the use of high oxygen concentrations and pressures that can cause further lung tissue damage.

Although the infant's condition may seem to improve, it is not possible to wean him from oxygen or the ventilator. Carbon dioxide retention increases, with wheezing and cyanosis common. The chest film generally has a bubbly appearance as cyst formation begins as well as hyperinflation.

By one month of age, infants with BPD are clearly identified: They always require supplemental oxygen and often mechanical ventilation. Increased oxygen and ventilator requirements, cardiomegaly, bacterial and viral infections, and poor growth characterize this chronic period. Infants may die from respiratory failure or other complications.

Because not all infants with BPD exhibit the stages of radiographic changes described in Table 3, diagnosis depends on the changes seen in the advanced stage.[23] Typical characteristics include large, irregular cysts alternating with strands of radiodensity due to atelectasis, fibrosis, and hyperinflation. Figure 6 demonstrates a chest film showing this stage.

Infants with BPD are in respiratory failure with some degree of hypoxia and hypercapnea. The hypercapnea is related to the alveolar hypoventilation. The decrease in pulmonary function is related to airway obstruction, fibrosis, atelectasis, and emphysema present in this disease.[23] These infants usually have an increase in airway resistance, which causes a decrease in compliance; both result in increased work of breathing.[23,26,27] In severe cases, the functional residual capacity is increased. A grossly abnormal ventilation-to-perfusion ratio exists. The severity of the pulmonary disease will determine oxygen requirements.

Pathology

The clinical presentation of BPD reflects significant disruption of the integrity of the respiratory epithelium, local inflammatory reaction, exudation of fluids and proteins, opportunistic infection, and healing accompanied by disordered growth and scarring.[28] Every tissue of the lung is affected by BPD. The early stages consist of cellular necrosis, edema, and inflammation. Pulmonary dysfunction and fibrosis result. Accumulated interstitial fluid promotes fibroblast growth. The endothelial and epithelial damage can interfere with normal development as smooth muscle hyperplasia develops around the pulmonary vessels. Later, as bronchiolitis occurs, the bronchi and bronchioles become scarred. The airways become obstructed or obliterated.

Over an extended period, the lung responds to this necrotizing process with regenerative efforts. New alveoli lining cells grow, accompanied by a fibroproliferative response. The entire process continues with necrosis, fibrosis, and new growth in an edematous environment.[29]

Management

Management of infants with BPD focuses on providing sufficient ventilation to maintain adequate blood gases while preventing progression of the existing pulmonary damage. Infants with BPD always require oxygen beyond one month of age and often mechanical ventilation. Oxygen is the most essential medication for this infant.[30]

Oxygen therapy. Oxygen must be administered in a well-controlled manner to maintain arterial gases within the desired range. The oxygen concentration is based upon arterial blood measurements, which can become difficult to obtain in patients in the later stages of BPD. Because transcutaneous monitoring may not be useful in older (>1 month) infants with severe BPD, pulse oximetry monitoring is recommended. It is essential to check oxygenation during feedings and other care provisions when hypoxia can occur. Attempts to wean the infant too soon can result in poor growth and pulmonary hypertension.[31]

Ventilation. Mechanical ventilation is individually patterned for the needs of each infant. The main strategy is to improve ventilation of poorly perfused tissues without distending the fairly normal ones. Weaning is difficult and requires gradual adjustments. When the infant can maintain adequate arterial oxygen and carbon dioxide pressures (PaO_2 and $PaCO_2$) with peak pressures less than 25 and a fraction of inspired oxygen (FiO_2) lower than 0.5, the rate can be lowered to allow the infant to do more breathing on his own.[23] Oxygen concentrations may have to be increased; a mild hypercapnea is permissible. Infants with BPD exhibit diminished CO_2 responsiveness and inefficient respiratory drive. Using normal PCO_2 values as criteria for ventilator weaning will prolong the weaning process and promote chronic lung injury. It is recommended that the $PaCO_2$ be allowed to rise moderately as long as oxygenation is adequate and pH is ≥7.25. This increases respiratory drive and provides an opportunity for reducing ventilatory support.[28]

Extubation is attempted when blood gases are adequate for 24 hours with continuous positive airway pressures (CPAP) of 2–4 cm of H_2O pressure and/or intermittent mandatory ventilation is ≤10 breaths per minute.[28]. Extubation may be complicated by inspiratory stridor due to tracheal scarring. Tracheal stenosis may occur after extubation as collagen in the scar tissue contracts. When the respiratory status worsens for no readily apparent reason, airway lesions of the trachea and bronchial tree should be suspected. Bronchoscopy can be helpful in diagnosing airway abnormalities responsible for unclear radiographic and clinical findings.[32]

Nutrition. Appropriate nutrition is essential for the infant with BPD because the lung tissue is healing and developing. Nutritional management is complex, however, because of low birthweight, feeding intolerance, and potential fluid overload. These infants tolerate fluid increases poorly and tend to accumulate interstitial fluid in the lungs. Fluid restriction is absolutely warranted in very low-birthweight infants because peribronchial edema can be a factor in airway damage.[22] Fluid intake is limited to the minimal amount necessary for metabolic requirements. Upon admission, 60–100 ml/kg/day is usually administered. As the infant grows, this may be increased to 140 ml/kg/day, depending upon the infant's condition.[26] Signs of fluid overload must be watched for carefully.

Feeding difficulties are quite common in these infants. Tube feedings are frequently necessary to prevent aspiration from bulbar dysfunction. Baseline caloric requirements, which average 50–70 calories/kg/day, are increased in these infants because of their higher metabolic rates.[27] Increased activity levels, increased work of breathing, and tissue repair needs may result in requirements of 120–150 calories/kg/day.[26,27,31] Because fluids must be restricted, caloric density can be achieved through the addition of medium-chain triglycerides and glucose polymers. The risks involved in this form of supplementation include (1) increased oxygen consumption associated with increased energy intake and resulting in hypoxia and (2) increased carbon dioxide production from glucose metabolism.[26] Malnutrition and failure to thrive are common developments of the disease. Osteopenia, another complication, can occur because of low calcium and vitamin D intake.[31]

Medications. Continued research on pharmacological intervention is necessary, but the role of medications is already known to be crucial to outcome. After BPD has developed, diuretics are used to treat pulmonary edema, decreased lung compliance, and increased airway resistance. Furosemide is generally the drug of choice, 1–3 mg/kg is given IV, IM or orally and repeated every 6–7 hours as needed.[28] Furosemide promotes diuresis with clearance of interstitial pulmonary water improving airway resistance, conductance, and compliance.[33] Prolonged use causes depletion of chloride, potassium, and sodium resulting in metabolic alkalosis, blunted CO_2 responsiveness, and growth failure. It is recommended to give the infant periodic respites from furosemide and correct electrolyte conditions—especially chloride—with potassium chloride, sodium chloride, and ammonium chloride. Other significant complications of chronic diuretic therapy are nephrolithias, bone demineralization, and metabolic acidosis. Spironolactone, a thiazide diuretic, can be given when the patient is refractory to furosemide in doses of 0.8–1.6 mg/kg PO every 12 hours.[28]

Infants with BPD have indications of hyperactive airway disease, and bronchodilators have sometimes been found to have a beneficial effect. The clinical effects are measured by a drop in oxygen requirements and a reduction in ventilator support.[34]

Of the available bronchodilators, methylxanthines have been found beneficial, because they decrease pulmonary resistance and increase compliance, especially when combined with diuretics.[35] Methylxanthines prevent dyspneic attacks, which can occur during physiotherapy.[27] Improved ventilatory effects include increasing minute ventilation, increased diaphragmatic contractibility, and bronchodilatation. Administration of theophylline may also increase respiratory drive which is one indication for administering these agents prior to extubation.

Theophylline dosage must be carefully calculated because infants with BPD have a prolonged theophylline half-life, and monitoring of serum levels is essential during administration. The therapeutic level for caffeine is 10–20 mg/liter; for theophylline, it is 10–12 mg/liter the first week of life and 15–20 mg/liter thereafter.[33] Side effects include vomiting, irritability, diarrhea, tachycardia, and seizures. Caffeine shows fewer side effects and is generally better tolerated than theophylline.

Bronchodilators in aerosol form decrease airway resistance and increase conductance, resulting in a reversal of the acute bronchospasm seen in BPD. They can be administered via the ventilator for intubated infants. Isoproterenol and albuterol (Ventolin) have been used frequently. Because airway obstruction is at least partly reversible with bronchodilators, they provide an opportunity for early intervention to reduce the progression of the disease.[23]

The administration of steroids has been attempted in ventilator-dependent infants to facilitate weaning from the respirator and to reduce the length of ventilation therapy. The beneficial effects of steroids include enhancing surfactant synthesis, reducing inflammation in injured airways, reducing bronchospasm, stabilizing membranes, and reducing pulmonary edema.[22]

Criteria which have been used to identify infants who could benefit from steroid therapy are: postnatal age 2–6 weeks, no progress on the ventilator for 5 days, absence of complications (sepsis, PDA, pneumothorax), and x-ray evidence of early BPD. These infants receive dexamethasone 0.25 mg/kg every 12 hours for 3 days. If the infant responds (weans from the ventilator or has substantial decrease in ventilator parameters) dexamethasone is tapered over approximately a month. A suggested regime is 0.5 mg/kg/day for 3 days; 0.3 mg/kg/day for 3 days; then reduction every 3 days by 10 percent until the dose is 0.1 mg/kg/day; then 0.1 mg/kg/day every other day for 1 week, then discontinue the drug. If the infant does not respond, the drug can be discontinued after the third day without adrenal suppression.[28,36]

Potential complications of steroid therapy include sepsis, glucose intolerance, hypertension, and adrenal suppression. Further research is needed to define precise indications and complications of this therapy.[28]

Oxidant damage to tissue can result either from the direct administration of oxygen or from the release of free oxygen radicals. Exposure of the lung to oxygen produces endothelial and alveolar Type I cell damage; the resultant edema and loss of integrity of the alveolar capillary barrier interferes with pulmonary mechanics and inactivates surfactants.[29] To prevent such damage from oxygen therapy, the administration of antioxidant agents has been proposed.

Vitamin E, the major lipid antioxidant, protects cell membranes. Deficiencies can lead to enhancement of susceptibility to oxygen injury; supplementation reverses or prevents deficiencies. Administration of vitamin E in pharmacologic doses has not been helpful in preventing BPD, but deficiencies should be prevented because they may contribute to the disease's progression.

Vitamin A is necessary for epithelial cell integrity and differentiation. Severe deficiencies result in respiratory tract changes, including basal cell proliferation and necrosis of the epithelial lining resulting in squamous metaplasia. Infants with BPD have been observed to have low levels of vitamin A, so it has been advocated as a treatment. Clinical trials of vitamin A administered to low-birthweight infants resulted in decreased morbidity, reduced incidence of BPD, and a progressive decrease in ventilatory parameters.[37] It appears that vitamin A promotes regenerative healing from lung injury. To prevent depletion of vitamin A, blood levels should be monitored to ensure that a deficiency does not exist.[34]

There have not been many reports on the use of antihypertensive agents in patients with BPD. When indicated, hydralazine is the drug of choice because it is associated with improvement in pulmonary hypertension.[33]

Prevention

The most effective means of preventing BPD

would be to eradicate RDS or at least reduce its severity. More research is clearly indicated in this problem area. Currently available preventive measures include administering tocolytic agents for preterm labor and enhancing surfactant synthesis *in utero*. Administration of surfactant after birth may reduce the incidence of BPD. Preliminary studies indicate that surfactant can significantly improve survival in infants with RDS, without the occurrence of BPD (Chapter 9).[38] Because BPD develops early in life, other nursery preventive measures should be instituted shortly after birth. These include attention to fluid management and respiratory support.

Fluid intake must be carefully monitored and restricted, especially if a patent ductus arteriosus (PDA) exists. Very low-birthweight infants who are at risk for BPD have a high incidence of PDA. The left to right shunt secondary to the PDA increases pulmonary circulation, which reduces compliance and delays weaning from the ventilator. Aggressive treatment of the PDA with indomethacin (0.2 mg/kg every 8 hours for 3 doses) or surgical ligation is recommended to prevent prolonged ventilator dependency.[28] Early administration of diuretics has been attempted to prevent progression of BPD, but induced diuresis has not been found to be effective.[33]

Before the BPD diagnosis, efforts must be directed toward minimizing the oxygen concentration and decreasing the pressures and length of mechanical ventilation while maintaining an adequate PaO_2.[26] The goal is to achieve adequate ventilation with the lowest possible peak pressure and mean airway pressure. An inspiratory time of 0.3–0.5 seconds is usually adequate, with flow rates between 5 and10 liters/minute.[23] To avoid peak pressures over 30 cm H_2O, oxygen pressure can often be tolerated in the lower range of normal—as long as the pH is greater than 7.25 and perfusion is good.[28,34] Ventilator adjustments must be made meticulously to prevent overdistention. Whenever positive end-expiratory pressure (PEEP) is decreased, peak pressure also should be decreased to maintain a constant tidal volume. Weaning the infant off the ventilator as soon as possible is a major priority.

Discharge and Outcome

Approximately 25–35 percent of infants with severe BPD die. However with the mortality rate of BPD decreasing, preparing for care at home becomes a priority.[28] If infants can be given the required supplemental oxygen at home, the duration of hospitalization can be significantly reduced. Before discharge, careful assessment of parental adjustment and abilities along with resources available to the family should be carried out. The infant should be assessed for feeding abilities, medications required, respiratory status, amount of oxygen, and method of oxygen delivery.[39]

After discharge home, major improvements are often seen, including weight gain and better developmental skills.[27,31] Significant risks are present after discharge, and death may occur from sudden infant death syndrome or respiratory infections.[23,31] There are few long-term studies on survivors. Respiratory infections with wheezing are quite common, and there is a high incidence of ear infections.[31] Abnormal pulmonary function is experienced for the first year of life and in some cases through the preschool years.[23]

Nursing Implications

Care of infants with BPD in its earlier stages is similar to that of infants with RDS. It is essential that nurses providing this care have an astute awareness of the risk factors involved in the development of BPD, preventive measures, and signs and symptoms of the disease.

Once BPD has been diagnosed, care is supportive. These infants' numerous problems necessitate that the care provider be extremely patient and sensitive to each infant's particular needs. Consistency in providers is critical in identifying and implementing the individual infant's requirements for care. Because these infants require such long hospitalization, family support and discharge planning are high priorities in the nursing care plan.

Respiratory care. Oxygen concentrations and ventilator settings must be carefully maintained. Blood gases are monitored as necessary. Pulse oximetry has been found to be more helpful than transcutaneous monitoring for these patients.[40] Weaning is gradual; the alert nurse is able to detect subtle responses to changes in therapy as they occur. The infant must be closely observed for episodes of bronchospasm and any occurrence documented thoroughly and reported. Chest physiotherapy is provided as required for secretions.

Nutritional support. Preventing fluid overload is a major priority from the beginning. Once feedings have started, they are increased slowly as the infant tolerates them. Preventing aspiration is also a major goal; if regurgitation is severe, gastrostomy feedings may be required. Accurate daily assessments of weight, calories, intake, output, specific gravity, and urine and stool reducing substance results are important in evaluating growth. Metabolic demands can be minimized by organizing care to allow for rest periods free from interruption.

Infection control. Infants with BPD are very susceptible to infection. Their increased susceptibility is secondary to prematurity, poor nutritional status, and prolonged need for intubation. Aseptic technique must be assured at all times. Any equipment that comes in contact with the infant must be properly cleaned.

Developmental intervention. Modifying the infant's environment to remove or reduce noxious stimuli is essential for optimal growth and development. Noises, bright lights, and other negative influences should be reduced. Procedures should be performed as efficiently as possible; infants should be allowed recovery time following each of them. Sleep/wake cycles must be identified and care organized

according to the individual infant's schedule. If an infant must be disturbed, a gentle waking period is recommended to reduce negative stimuli.

Tactile, kinesthetic, vestibular, and auditory forms of stimulation appropriate for the infant's gestational age should be provided. Rooting and sucking reflexes can be encouraged by gentle stroking of the lips with finger and nipple. Encouraging the infant to suck on a nipple during gavage feedings is now a standard procedure. Positioning the infant is critical to decrease flattening of the head and promote normal rotation of the extremities.

Parental education and support. Care of the families of infants with BPD is one of the most challenging and difficult aspects of neonatal nursing. Consistent care providers are essential in helping the family adapt to the long-term hospitalization and the various therapies the infant will undergo. Regularly scheduled conferences are good for presenting the infant's current status to the family, and helping them express their concerns, fears, and feelings. Resource team members such as social workers and chaplains are very useful for providing support.

Discharge planning. With improving survival rates, more infants are being discharged home. The primary nurse's role is critical in assuring a safe and smooth transition for the family. The home environment, available resources, abilities of each family member, and their readiness to assume care for the infant all need to be assessed thoroughly. Necessary skills need to be taught well before discharge to enable the responsible parties to feel confident in performing them. Allowing the family to provide care for extended periods before discharge alleviates anxiety about taking the infant home. If home nursing services are to be utilized, group conferences with the nurse(s) involved will provide continuity in care.

Following discharge, continued consultation with staff members should be readily available in addition to support given at follow-up appointments.

RETINOPATHY OF PREMATURITY

Retinopathy of prematurity (ROP) is a disease of the retinal vasculature which consists of abnormal proliferation of small retinal vessels. Over time, ROP can regress or progress to severe proliferation and retinal detachment.[41] As with many complications of prematurity, ROP continues to puzzle all who care for tiny infants. More than 40 years have passed since the initial reports of retrolental fibroplasia, and still the exact cause or causes of this tragic problem are unknown.

Contrary to earlier thinking, ROP is no longer considered to be solely related to hyperoxia. The sickest and smallest premature infants in intensive care units now appear to be at great risk for this destructive eye disorder—regardless of how carefully oxygen utilization is monitored.

Once referred to as retrolental fibroplasia (RLF), ROP was first described in 1942 by Terry, who reported finding fibrous tissue behind the lens in the eyes of premature infants.[42] Several factors were implicated. Genetics, premature closure of the ductus arteriosus and foramen ovale, hyperoxia or hypoxia, relative hypothermia, or defective endocrine factors were all thought to be possible causes of ROP.

Retinopathy of prematurity reached epidemic proportions by 1953, and many studies implicated excessive use of oxygen. As a result, the standard practice in neonatal units was to avoid exceeding a 40 percent oxygen concentration.[43] It was also recommended that oxygen administration be limited to times of clinical need and given only for as brief a period as possible.[44] Thus, testing hypotheses that would require oxygen therapy varying from the current standard became ethically difficult, if not impossible. As a result, a real tragedy began to unfold. Many babies died due to a lack of sufficient oxygen. The previously declining mortality rate began to rise, and the incidence of cerebral palsy increased.[45,46] The incidence of ROP did decline, but it never completely vanished.

By the mid-1960s, neonatal care units once again incorporated the use of appropriate oxygen, along with other advances in care, to increase survival rates. Every attempt was made to monitor the state of oxygenation of these infants. The risk of ROP was thought to be minimized with the careful monitoring of PaO_2 levels.

Incidence and Etiology

The incidence of ROP is again rising despite (or perhaps because of) advances in neonatal medicine during the last decade, including more sophisticated oxygen monitoring capabilities. The number of infants blinded each year is now estimated to be comparable to that reported from 1943–1953.[47] However, the babies affected now are much smaller than those affected in the earlier years.

Because of this rise, the simple theory that uncontrolled use of oxygen causes ROP is now disputed. The increased incidence of ROP might be attributed to the increasing survival rate of the very low-birthweight infant, improved awareness of the disease and the diagnosis, or advanced methods of prolonged ventilatory support. These factors, as well as many other problems that plague the premature infant, have led most to consider that oxygen therapy is no longer the sole etiology. In fact, oxygen therapy is not a factor at all in some infants who develop ROP.

Along with hyperoxia and prematurity, other causes for ROP have been investigated. Hypoxia, in particular, has been implicated. Both animal and clinical studies have shown ischemia to be an important factor.[48,49] Other high-risk factors suggested include blood transfusions, exchange transfusions, hypercarbia, hypocarbia, apnea requiring bag and mask ventilation, sepsis, intraventricular hemorrhage, and exposure to bright light.[49-51] Many other possible causes have been reported, but as yet, none has proven to have a direct relationship with ROP.

FIGURE 7 ▲ Zones and clock hours of ROP. Three zones define location of retinal involvement; extent of disease is shown as hours of the clock: **Zone I:** Extends from the disc to twice the distance from the disc to the center of the macula (an arc of 60°). **Zone II:** Extends from the edge of Zone I to the nasal ora serrata (at 3 o'clock in the left eye), and to an area near the temporal anatomic equator. **Zone III:** Is the residual crescent of retina anterior to Zone II. This is the zone last vascularized in the eye of a premature infant and is most frequently involved with retinopathy of prematurity (ROP).

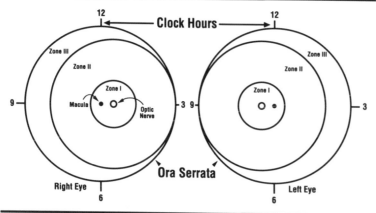

From: Archives of Opthalmology 102, August 1984, pp. 1130–1134; Retinopathy of Prematurity, An International Classification, Ross Laboratories, Columbus, Ohio. Reprinted with permission.

The most common association is serious neonatal illness which compromises the fragile embryonic process of retinal development.[51]

Reported incidence of the disease varies. Although differences in predisposing factors play the greatest role in this variance, the explanation for the remarkably divergent frequencies of ROP among institutions is uncertain.

Prematurity is the single greatest risk factor for ROP. There is an inverse relationship between birthweight/gestational age and the incidence of ROP. In infants who weigh less than 1,000 gm at birth, there is a reported incidence of 38–54 percent compared to 5–15 percent among babies weighing 1,000–1,500 gm at birth. Cicatricial disease (the severe form of ROP) develops in about 22–42 percent of the smaller babies and less than 3 percent of the larger babies.[52] Cicatricial disease is rare in babies with birthweights of more than 1,500 gm.

The magnitude of the damage resulting from ROP is more apparent when looking at the actual number of very low-birthweight infants affected. Based on calculations by Dale Phelps, MD, the projected incidence of ROP in the late 1980s would be about 30 percent.[47] Using the U.S. Health projected birth rate (27,000 infants) of infants who weigh less than 1,500 gm at birth and survival rates as Phelps indicated, the number of infants affected with ROP is about 8,000 for the late 1980s. As many as 2,600 of these babies will have some degree of permanent eye damage, and 650 are anticipated to be legally blind each year.

Pathophysiology and Classification

Vascularization of the retina begins in the fourth month of fetal development and is not completed until the ninth month of gestation or shortly after birth. Once it is complete, oxy-

TABLE 4 ▲ Stages of ROP

Stage	Description
1	Demarcation line: formation of a flat line within the plane of the retina from abnormal branching of vessels; separates posterior vascularized retina from anterior avascularized retina
2	Ridge: demarcation line has progressed in height and width (above the plane of the retina); no vessel growth in the ridge; retinal surface remains intact
3	Ridge with extra retinal fibrovascular proliferation: vessels entering the ridge are dilated and engorged, sometimes with hemorrhage on or adjacent to the ridge, sometimes with retinal buckling; may be mild, moderate, or severe
4	Subtotal retinal detachment: A. macula remains attached B. macula detached
5	Complete retinal detachment

Adapted from: The Committee for Classification of Retinopathy of Prematurity: An international classification of retinopathy of prematurity, Pediatrics 74, 1984, pp. 127–133; and McPherson A, Hittner H, and Kretzer F: Retinopathy of Prematurity: Current Concepts and Controversies, Toronto, 1986, B.C. Decker, p. 18.

gen has no toxic effects on the retinal vessels. If hyperoxygenation (PaO_2 exceeding 100 torr) occurs prior to complete vascularization, retinal vessels may constrict. If this constriction is severe enough, complete occlusion may occur and the vascular growth from the occlusion to the periphery will proceed abnormally. Most retinal changes the ophthalmologists see resolve spontaneously and cause little or no visual impairment. However, some infants do develop cicatricial disease and may later develop glaucoma and micro-ophthalmia.[53]

In 1984, the International Classification of Retinopathy of Prematurity was developed; it clarifies the location, extent, and severity of the disease.[54] "Zones" are used to designate the location of pathology and/or the progression of the vascular growth (Figure 7). Retinal vascular growth normally begins at the optic disc and progresses outward to the anterior edge of the retina (ora serrata). There are three zones; the outer zone (zone 3) is the last area of vascularization in the infant's eye.

The extent of ROP is illustrated with the use of "clock hours" or sectors (Figure 7). This provides a more explicit description of disease location in each eye by showing the number of sectors in which normal or abnormal vasculature is seen.

Previously, four stages specified the advancement of the abnormal vascular response.[54] But to be more explicit, the international classification has expanded its system to elaborate what previously was stage 4 (retinal detachment). ROP ranges from minimal vascular changes with a demarcation line (stage 1) to total retinal detachment (stage 5) (Table 4). The most severe stage present in any sector of either eye is the designated stage for that eye.

Another term, "Plus" disease, is used with stages 2 or 3 to denote increased dilation and tortuosity of the vessels. The iris vessels are engorged, pupillary rigidity is present, and the vitreous has a hazy appearance. "Plus" disease is an ominous sign of progressive vascular incompetence. Retinal detachment may be forthcoming (50 percent of "Plus" disease resolves).

Treatment and Prevention

Most cases of ROP resolve spontaneously and fortunately require no intervention. An indirect ophthalmoscopic exam with scleral depression is necessary to identify ROP. According to the AAP/ACOG Guidelines for Perinatal Care and the CRYO-ROP Cooperative Group, the exam should be performed six to eight weeks after birth for any infant of less than 1,300 gm birthweight or for any infant of less than 1,800 gm birthweight who has oxygen therapy.[55,56]

If ROP is severe and progresses to stage 3 "Plus" disease, the Cooperative Group suggests cryotherapy as the treatment of choice.[56] Cryotherapy is a technique performed by an ophthalmologist in which the avascular area of the retina (from the ridge to the anterior edge of the retina) is frozen. This prevents the abnormal vasoproliferation from proceeding.

Cryotherapy was controversial until recently, but it has shown enough promise to be investigated. The multicenter trial by the CRYO-ROP Cooperative Group showed an approximate 50 percent reduction in severe vision loss in infants on whom cryotherapy was performed.[56] Long-term outcome of infants treated with cryotherapy is yet unknown, but for the short term, it has proven to be effective and should now be used for those infants in need of treatment.

The use of vitamin E to prevent ROP remains very controversial. Many studies have been done on its use, some documenting its effectiveness, others its ineffectiveness. There is now evidence that the routine use of vitamin E is associated with significant risks, including sepsis, necrotizing enterocolitis, and death from toxicity.[57] So until the risk-benefit ratio is clearly defined, prophylactic use of vitamin E is not a desirable treatment. In fact, the Committee on Fetus and Newborn of the American Academy of Pediatrics recommended in 1985 that vitamin E not be used prophylactically in infants weighing less than 1,500 gm.[58]

There is conflicting evidence implicating light exposure as a definitive cause of ROP. Glass and associates demonstrated a reduction in the incidence of ROP in preterm infants who were exposed to reduced light levels.[59] Ackerman and coworkers, in an attempt to replicate Glass' study, demonstrated no difference in the incidence in severity of ROP between a historic control group of premature infants and a group of prematures who were shielded from standard nursery lighting.[60] It is prudent to avoid direct bright light exposure in all infants; however, there is no strong evidence which would support patching the eyes of premature infants or justify significant reduction of light in the NICU. Further research on the timing of light reduction, i.e. immediately after birth, may demonstrate a consequential reduction in ROP.[60]

At this time, ROP is not preventable. Certainly, all health care providers should be particularly alert to any indications of hyperoxygenation. There is a report of a decreased incidence of ROP with use of continuous transcutaneous oxygen monitoring, but only in infants weighing more than 1,000 gm.[61] The amount of oxygen required for survival without neurologic sequelae may not always be low enough to avoid problems with the immature peripheral retina.

Nursing Implications

The nurse is responsible for the routine assessment of the infant and the continual management of the oxygen delivery system. Changes in oxygen administration should be made cautiously. Intermittent arterial blood gases and continuous transcutaneous oxygen monitoring ($TcPO_2$) or oxygen saturation monitoring should be used to determine trends in PaO_2. Noninvasive methods are useful if good tissue perfusion is present and equipment is calibrated, maintained, and used properly. Probe placement for the $TcPO_2$ or oxygen saturation monitor should not be on a bony prominence

or a poorly perfused site. Remember that an airtight seal on a $TcPO_2$ probe is necessary to prevent falsely high readings.[62,63]

Special attention should be given to oxygenation during routine care and other nursing procedures. Use of a $TcPO_2$ or oxygen saturation monitor will reduce the risks and shorten the duration of hypoxia and hyperoxia while procedures are performed. Procedures that result in hypoxia or hyperoxia should be limited whenever possible. When a procedure such as intubation or suctioning is necessary, attempting to compensate for physiologic response in oxygenation may be helpful.

In preparation for an eye exam, the ophthalmologist should order some type of mydriatic drops for the purpose of dilating the infant's pupils. The CRYO-ROP Cooperative Group recommends the use of cyclomydril ophthalmic solution (cyclopentolate hydrochloride 1 percent and phenylephrine 2.5 percent) because it reportedly produces fewer systemic effects (hypertension or hypotension) in the newborn, although problems with GI function in the newborn have been reported from the use of cyclopentolate hydrochloride (0.5 percent) solution.[58,59]

To instill these drops, wash your hands, and check each eye for irritation or drainage that may indicate an infection. If the eyes are clear, instill the drops 30–60 minutes before the exam. Instill one drop in each eye, being careful not to touch the dropper to the eye or any surface; repeat in 5–15 minutes. A maximum of three drops may be placed in each eye if the pupils are not dilated. Gently blot excess solution from the eyelid with a tissue.

During the eye exam, carefully monitor the infant's vital signs. The ophthalmologist who is visualizing the eye will be unable to monitor for any ill effects of the exam. Bradycardia is occasionally seen from a vagal response during scleral depression. If this occurs, temporarily stop the exam. Once the heart rate has returned to normal, the exam may continue.

Providing parents with pertinent and accurate information about any retinal changes found on the eye exam is an essential part of good nursing care. Parents should be particularly reassured that mild ROP usually regresses with little or no visual impairment. Should an infant be transferred or discharged prior to having an ophthalmic exam (six to eight weeks postnatal age), parents should be advised of the importance of follow-up. If an infant's eye exam reveals an immature retina or any ROP changes, a follow-up exam is necessary in two to four weeks, depending on the severity of the ROP. Each ophthalmologist's recommendations may vary slightly, but follow-up is essential to verify that the ROP regresses and the retina matures normally.

Parent teaching about this devastating disease should begin early in the infant's hospitalization. Parents should be educated as to the possible serious problems that sometimes develop in these sickest premature infants. Once ROP has developed, it is important to provide the parents with emotional support and continue to give them information about follow-up care. The ophthalmologist should speak with parents to provide additional support and to inform them of expected developments. Early intervention and referral to appropriate programs will improve the quality of life for these infants.

SUMMARY

Past research has yielded much useful information regarding the prevention of lung and eye injury, but obviously more research is indicated in these areas. Multicenter studies have identified beneficial modes of therapy and principles of management, and further research of this type could prove helpful.

Until low birthweight incidence decreases and improved technological advances are utilized uniformly throughout the country, the problems of mechanical ventilation will unfortunately continue. Each infant must receive scrupulous, consistent care to reduce the hazards associated with this therapy.

REFERENCES

1. Korones SB: Complications, *in* Goldsmith JP, and Karotkin A, eds., Assisted Ventilation of the Neonate, Philadelphia, 1987, W.B. Saunders, chap. 13.

2. Thibeault DW: Pulmonary barotrauma: Interstitial emphysema, pneumomediastinum, and pneumothorax, *in* Thibeault DW, and Gregory G, eds., Neonatal Pulmonary Care, Newark, New Jersey, 1987, Appleton-Century-Crofts, chap. 21.

3. Merenstein G, and Gardner SL: Handbook of Neonatal Intensive Care, St. Louis, 1986, C.V. Mosby.

4. Primhak RA: Factors associated with pulmonary air leak in premature infants receiving mechanical ventilation, Journal of Pediatrics 102(5), 1983, pp. 764–768.

5. Wong PY, Bajuk B, and Szymonowicz W: Pulmonary air leak in extremely low birth weight infants, Archives of Diseases in Childhood 61, 1986, pp. 239–241.

6. Kotas RV: The physiologic correlates between lung surface tension forces, lung unit interdependence, and lung liquid balance, *in* Thibeault DW, and Gregory G, eds., Neonatal Pulmonary Care, Newark, New Jersey, 1986, Appleton-Century-Crofts, chap. 5.

7. Reid L, and Rubino L: The connective tissue septa in the fetal human lung, Thorax 14(2), 1959, pp. 138–145.

8. Yu YH, et al.: Pulmonary interstitial emphysema in infants less than 1000 grams at birth, Journal of Pediatrics 22, 1985, pp. 914–917.

9. Meadow WL, and Chermomcha D: Successful therapy of unilateral pulmonary emphysema: Mechanical ventilation with extremely short inspiratory time, American Journal of Perinatology 2(3), 1985, pp. 914–917.

10. Placzek MM, and Young LW: Unilateral pulmonary interstitial emphysema and selective bronchial intubation, American Journal of Diseases in Children 140, 1986, pp. 161–162.

11. Glenski JA, et al.: Selective bronchial intubation in infants with lobar emphysema, American Journal of Perinatology 3(3), 1986, pp. 199–204.

12. Felman H: Complications of air leak, *in* Radiology of the Pediatric Chest, New York, 1987, McGraw-Hill, chap. 6.

13. Martin RJ, et al.: Respiratory problems, *in* Klaus M, and Fanaroff A, eds., Care of the High Risk Neonate, Philadelphia, 1986, W.B. Saunders, chap. 8.

14. Gonzalez F, et al.: Decreased gas flow through pneumothoraces in neonates receiving high-frequency jet versus convention ventilation, Journal of Pediatrics, 1987, pp. 464–466.

15. Ryan CA, et al.: Contralateral pneumothoraces in the newborn: Incidence and predisposing factors, Pediatrics 79(3), 1987, pp. 417–421.

16. Hill A, Perlman JM, and Volpe JJ: Relationship of pneumothorax to occurrence of intraventricular hemorrhage in the premature newborn, Pediatrics 69(2), 1982, pp. 144–149.

17. Lawson EE, et al.: Neonatal pneumothorax: Current management, Journal of Pediatric Surgery 15(2), 1980, pp. 181–185.

18. Hansen RN, and Gest AL: Oxygen toxicity and ventilatory complications of treatment of infants with persistent pulmonary hypertension, Clinics in Perinatology 11(3), 1984, pp. 653–672.

19. Gregory SC: Air leak syndromes, Neonatal Network, April 1987, pp. 40–46.

20. Oellrich R: Pneumothorax, chest tubes, and the neonate, Maternal Child Nursing 10, 1985, pp. 29–35.

21. Streeter NS: High Risk Neonatal Care, Rockville, Maryland, 1986, Aspen, pp.107–162.

22. Northway WH, Rosan RC, and Porter DT: Pulmonary disease following respiratory therapy for hyaline membrane disease, New England Journal of Medicine 27, 1967, pp. 357–368.

23. Bancalari E, and Gerhardt T: Bronchopulmonary dysplasia, Pediatric Clinics of North America 33(1), 1986, pp. 1–23.

24. Truog WE, et al.: Bronchopulmonary dysplasia and pulmonary insufficiency of prematurity, American Journal of Diseases of Children 139, 1985, pp. 351–354.

25. Goetzman BW: Understanding bronchopulmonary dysplasia, American Journal of Diseases in Children 140, 1986, pp. 332–340.

26. Shannan DC, and Epstein M: Bronchopulmonary dysplasia, in Thibeault DW, and Gregory G, eds., Neonatal Pulmonary Care, Newark, New Jersey, 1987, Appleton-Century-Crofts, chap. 28.

27. Monin P, and Vert P: The management of bronchopulmonary dysplasia, Clinics in Perinatology 14(3), 1987, pp. 531–549.

28. Avery G: Bronchopulmonary dysplasia, in Nelson N, ed., Current Therapy in Neonatal and Perinatal Medicine—2, B.C. Decker, Philadelphia, 1990, pp. 188–192.

29. Sinkin RA, and Phelps DL: New strategies for the prevention of bronchopulmonary dysplasia, Clinics in Perinatology 14(3), 1987, pp. 599–620.

30. O'Brodovich HM, and Mellins RB: Bronchopulmonary dysplasia—Unresolved neonatal acute lung injury, American Review of Respiratory Disease 132, 1985, pp. 694–709.

31. Dickerson BG: Bronchopulmonary dysplasia—Chronic pulmonary disease following neonatal respiratory failure, Chest 87(4), 1987, pp. 528–535.

32. Miller RW, et al.: Tracheobronchial abnormalities in infants with bronchopulmonary dysplasia, Journal of Pediatrics 111(5), 1987, pp. 779–782.

33. Blanchard PW, et al.: Pharmacology in bronchopulmonary dysplasia, Clinics in Perinatology 14(4), 1987, pp. 881–910.

34. Escobedo MB, and Gonzales A: Bronchopulmonary dysplasia in the tiny infant, Clinics in Perinatology 13(2), 1986, pp. 315–326.

35. Kao LC, et al.: Oral theophylline and diuretics improve pulmonary mechanics in infants with bronchopulmonary dysplasia, Journal of Pediatrics 111(3), 1987, pp. 439–444.

36. Avery G, et al.: Controlled trial of dexamethasone in respirator-dependent infants with bronchopulmonary dysplasia, Pediatrics 75, 1985, pp. 106–111.

37. Shenai P, et al.: Clinical trials of vitamin A supplementation in infants susceptible to bronchopulmonary dysplasia, Journal of Pediatrics, 1987, pp. 269–277.

38. Bose C, et al.: Improved outcome at 28 days of age for very low birth weight infants treated with a single dose of a synthetic surfactant, Journal of Pediatrics 177, 1990, pp. 947–953.

39. Koops BL, et al.: Outpatient management and follow-up of bronchopulmonary dysplasia, Clinics in Perinatology 11(1), 1985, pp. 101–122.

40. Riedel K: Pulse oximetry: A new technology to assess patient oxygen needs in the neonatal intensive care unit, Journal of Perinatal and Neonatal Nursing 1(1), 1987, pp. 49–57.

41. Phelps D: Retinopathy of prematurity, in Nelson N, ed., Current Therapy in Neonatal-Perinatal Medicine—2, B.C. Decker, Philidelphia, 1990, pp. 350–353.

42. Terry TL: Extreme prematurity and fibroplastic overgrowth of persistent vascular sheath behind each crystalline lens I: Preliminary report, American Journal of Ophthalmology 25, 1942, p. 203.

43. Lanman JT: The control of oxygen therapy for premature infants, Health News 32, 1955, p. 1446.

44. Guy LP, Lanman JT, and Dancis J: The possibility of total elimination of retrolental fibroplasia by oxygen restriction, Pediatrics, 1956, pp. 247–249.

45. Avery ME, and Oppenheimer EH: Recent increase in mortality from hyaline membrane disease, Journal of Pediatrics 57, 1960, p. 553.

46. McDonald AD: Cerebral palsy in children of very low birth weight, Archives of Disease in Childhood, 1963, p. 579.

47. Phelps DL: Retinopathy of prematurity: An estimate of vision loss in the United States—1979, Pediatrics 67, 1981, pp. 924–925.

48. Katzman G, et al.: Comparative analysis of lower and higher stage retrolental fibroplasia abstracted, Pediatric Research 16, 1984, p. 294.

49. Shohat M, et al.: Retinopathy of prematurity: Incidence and risk factors, Pediatrics 72, 1983, pp. 159–163.

50. Lucy J, and Dangman B: A reexamination of the role of oxygen in retrolental fibroplasia, Pediatrics 73(47), 1984, pp. 82–96.

51. Avery G, and Glass P: Retinopathy of prematurity: What causes it? Clinics in Perinatology 15(4), 1985, pp. 917–928.

52. Porat R: Care of the infant with retinopathy of prematurity, Clinics in Perinatology 11, 1984, pp. 123–151.

53. Korones SB, Complications, in Goldsmith J, and Karotkin E, eds., Assisted Ventilation of the Neonate, Philadelphia, 1988, WB Saunders, pp. 245–271.

54. The Committee for Classification of Retinopathy of Prematurity: An international classification of retinopathy of prematurity, Pediatrics 74, 1984, pp. 127–133.

55. American Academy of Pediatrics/American College of Obstetrics and Gynecology: Guidelines for Perinatal Care, 1988, AAP/ACOG, pp. 244–248.

56. The CRYO-ROP Cooperative Group: Multicenter trial of cryotherapy for retinopathy of prematurity, Archives of Ophthalmology 106(1), 1988, pp. 471–479.

57. Johnson L: Relationship of prolonged pharmacologic serum levels of vitamin E to incidence of sepsis, necrotizing enterocolitis in infants with birth weight of 1500 grams or less, Pediatrics 75, April 1985, pp. 619–638.

58. Committee on Fetus and Newborn: Vitamin E and the prevention of retinopathy of prematurity, Pediatrics 76, 1985, pp. 315–316.

59. Glass, et al.: Effects of bright light in the hospital nursery on the incidence of retinopathy of prematurity, New England Journal of Medicine 313( ), 1985, pp. 401–404.

60. Ackerman B, et al.: Reduced incidental light exposure: Effect on the development of retinopathy of prematurity in low birth weight infants, Pediatrics 83, 1989, pp. 958–962.

61. Bancalari E, et al.: Influence of transcutaneous oxygen monitoring on the incidence of retinopathy of prematurity, Pediatrics 79, 1987, pp. 663–669.

62. Aloan CA: Respiratory Care of the Newborn: A Clinical Manual, Philadelphia, 1987, J.B. Lippincott.

63. Cassady G: Transcutaneous monitoring in the newborn infant, Journal of Pediatrics 103, 1983, pp. 837–848.

64. Isenberg S, et al.: Cardiovascular effects of mydriatics in LBW infants, Journal of Pediatrics 105, 1984, p. 111.

65. Isenberg S, et al.: Effects of cyclopentolate eyedrops on gastric secretory function in preterm infants, Ophthalmology 92, 1985, pp. 698–700.

7 High-Frequency Jet Ventilation: Impact on Neonatal Nursing

Tracy B. Karp, RNC, MS, NNP
Primary Children's Medical Center
Salt Lake City, Utah

High-frequency jet ventilation (HFJV) is a new method of providing respiratory support to infants with severe lung failure.[1–3] During the past 20 years, conventional mechanical ventilators used to treat infants suffering from a variety of cardiorespiratory diseases have resulted in an ever-increasing survival rate.[1] Although death occurs in few patients, complications such as bronchopulmonary dysplasia (BPD) and pulmonary air leak syndrome (see Chapter 6) occur in many of the survivors.[4–6] Bronchopulmonary dysplasia has recently been shown to occur in 6–30 percent of infants weighing less than 1,500 gm at birth and at even higher rates in infants weighing less than 1,000 gm at birth.[4] It has been suggested that these complications may be secondary to barotrauma from high levels of positive pressure ventilation and inspired oxygen.[1,7] A more effective ventilation method using less pressure to sustain infants might decrease the mortality from respiratory failure as well as the incidence and severity of complications. High-frequency jet ventilation may be such a method.

HFJV operates at at least four times the normal neonatal respiratory rate and delivers a tidal volume close to or less than anatomical dead space.[1,8,9] The respiratory gas flow is provided by either a jet impulse or a flow interruption system.[10]

All new care methods influence and impact nursing care. This chapter presents the nursing management of infants receiving HFJV. This care is based upon traditional neonatal intensive care concepts, theory related to high-frequency jet ventilation, and our experience with more than 130 neonatal patients at Primary Children's Medical Center during the last eight years.

HISTORICAL PERSPECTIVE

Though HFJV is a recent technique in treating infants and adults with respiratory failure, the idea is not new. In 1915, Henderson and associates reported that panting dogs maintained adequate gas exchange with tidal volumes less than anatomical dead space.[11] Brisco and associates observed in 1954 that alveolar ventilation could be maintained with small tidal volumes.[12]

During the 1970s, HFJV was used successfully to support adults during bronchoscopic or airway surgery and in 1981 to improve survival in adults for whom conventional ventilation was failing because of large pulmonary air leaks.[13–15]

During the early 1980s, HFJV began to be used with infants. The first successful short-term treatment of respiratory distress syndrome (RDS) with high-frequency ventilation using an oscillatory system was reported in 1981.[16] Two years later, other investigators described the successful short-term treatment of intractable respiratory failure and progressive pulmonary air leaks with HFJV.[17] In 1984, Harris and Christensen treated 22 infants with pulmonary interstitial emphysema (PIE) unresponsive to conventional therapy. Sixteen of these infants showed a favorable response to HFJV; 11 survived.[18] Other research demonstrated the ability of both high-frequency oscillation and HFJV to ventilate infants with RDS using less airway pressure than that used in conventional mechanical ventilation (CMV).[19,20]

Thus, by the mid-1980s, there was preliminary evidence showing that HFJV was a technique potentially effective in improving the survival of infants with severe RDS, pulmonary air leak, or intractable respiratory failure.

During the mid- to late 1980s, work continued to validate the efficacy of HFJV as a rescue method. In 1985, the use of an experimental high-frequency jet respirator (Sechrist 900, Sechrist Industries, Inc., Anaheim, California) for respiratory rescue was reported. Three out of 11 infants survived.[21] In 1987, Mammel and colleagues reported their seven-year experience performing HFJV rescue on 70 infants (there were no controls). More than 75 percent had intractable pulmonary air leaks and very severe respiratory failure. Most infants were treated with the Bunnell Life Pulse Ventilator (Bunnell, Inc., Salt Lake City, Utah). A total of 37 percent survived.[22,23]

In another noncontrolled rescue study reported in 1989, 176 infants, most with severe RDS and air leaks in whom conventional ventilation was failing were treated with the Bunnell HFJV. Fifty-four percent of the infants survived, and ventilation and oxygenation were improved with HFJV usage.[24]

Pauly and associates used the Bunnell HFJV to treat nine infants with persistent pulmonary hypertension in whom CMV was failing. Four infants responded. From their limited experi-

ence, these investigators noted that if no improvement occurred within three hours, further improvement was unlikely.[25] Gonzalez and colleagues found less gas flow though pneumothoraces in neonates receiving HFJV (Bunnell) than in those on CMV. They found that gas flow rates out of the chest tubes decreased from 227 ± 96 ml/minute during CMV to 104 ± 59 ml/minute on HFJV.[26]

Because it appeared that HFJV had a role in rescue ventilation, a collaborative controlled study of the treatment of PIE with HFJV was organized in 1987. Keszler and associates reported the preliminary results at the seventh annual conference on high-frequency ventilation of infants in 1990.[27] The purpose of the study was to determine whether HFJV was more effective than CMV in resolving PIE. Sixteen hospitals participated using a randomized protocol with samples stratified according to weight and severity of disease. One hundred and forty-four (144) infants were enrolled with 75 being treated with HFJV and 69, CMV. In general, there was improved success using HFJV in treating PIE across all weight groups with severe disease (61 percent versus 32 percent). Overall survival for both methods was 67 percent, with HFJV having the greatest impact in the 1,000–1,500 gram birthweight group (86 percent versus 58 percent). There was no difference in incidence of grade 3-4 intraventricular hemorrhage between groups.[27]

Another type of high-frequency jet respirator, the Volumetric Diffusive Respirator (VDR-1, Percussionaire Corp., Sands Point, Indiana), has been used to treat neonates. Bodenstein and colleagues treated 79 infants using a rescue protocol; 60 percent survived.[28] In another uncontrolled study, Pfenninger and Gerber treated 8 infants with hyaline membrane disease using the VDR-1. All survived, but there were many equipment problems.[29]

Gaylord and associates performed a rescue study using the VDR-1 with matched historical controls. The study infants and controls were identified by the "Z" scoring system as having a very high mortality risk: Five of the nine infants survived.[30,31] High-frequency jet ventilation has also been used during the surgical resection of congenital tracheal stenosis.[32]

There has been only one reported controlled randomized trial comparing HFJV with conventional ventilation in infants with RDS. Carlo and associates, in 1990, reported a study where they randomly assigned 42 infants with hyaline membrane disease to either HFJV or CMV within 24 hours of life. All were initially placed on CMV. A proximal HFJV was used at a rate of 250 breaths per minute (bpm) with 20 percent less peak inspiratory pressure (PIP) and mean airway pressure (MAP) than CMV. Positive end-expiratory pressure (PEEP) was unchanged. High-frequency jet ventilation was able to provide gas exchange comparable to CMV at less MAP. There was no difference in the incidence of survival, air leak, or BPD.[19,33]

The efficacy of HFJV for the treatment of meconium aspiration syndrome has been studied. Mammel and associates first reported in 1983 a comparison of high-frequency jet ventilation and conventional mechanical ventilation in adult cats given 25 percent meconium instillation. A VS 600 ventilator (Instrument Development Corp., Pittsburgh, Pennsylvania) was used in a crossover design study. They found—at comparable MAP—higher pulmonary vascular resistance, pulmonary artery pressure, and alveolar-arterial oxygen difference in the animals on HFJV compared to those on CMV.[34]

In 1985, Trindale and colleagues compared HFJV (Bunnell) to CMV in piglets given a 20 percent meconium aspiration. They found that HFJV required only 50 percent of the PIP required by CMV to keep the carbon dioxide pressure equal. Neither hemodynamic nor lung mechanical parameters was different.[35] Keszler and associates studied combined jet ventilation in meconium aspirated puppies. They randomly assigned 28 puppies to CMV, HFJV alone (IDS Co.), or

HFJV with background CMV sighs. In their study, HFJV combined with CMV provided the best oxygenation and ventilation at the least MAP and PIP. Standard HFJV was next best, followed by CMV.[36]

By 1991 there was a large body of information supporting the use of HFJV as a rescue tool. Keszler and associates, through the PIE collaborative study, demonstrated that HFJV is a safe, reliable, and effective means of treating PIE when compared to CMV, especially in the 1,000–1,500 gram birthweight group.[27]

The use of HFJV as the method of choice for uncomplicated HMD remains to be proven and may become a moot point with the widespread use of surfactant replacement therapy. There is evidence that HFJV might be beneficial in infants with meconium aspiration syndrome, but unfortunately the work was done using three different machines and three different animal species.[34-36]

PHYSIOLOGY OF HIGH-FREQUENCY JET VENTILATION

HFJV is still being described and explained. Our knowledge of its hows and whys is far from complete. The experimental information now available, however, allows the formulation of a working theoretical framework to guide practice. The purpose of external support of respiration is to enhance oxygen delivery and carbon dioxide removal.

Conventional Versus High-Frequency Jet Ventilation

Conventional mechanical ventilation mimics many normal physiologic processes. Fresh gas is delivered to the lungs as bulk flow in tidal volumes much greater than anatomical dead space. During inspiration, positive pressure is used to force bulk gas flow through the larger airways. Gas moves through the smaller airways and to the alveolar region mostly by passive diffusion.[1]

FIGURE 1 ▲ CO₂ elimination in high-frequency jet ventilation. Relationship between V_T and CO_2 elimination when PEEP was not controlled. Each frequency has significant ($p < 0.01$ to 0.001, ANOVA) V_T effect on CO_2 elimination; at higher V_T levels, CO_2 elimination is decreased (SD not shown). Symbols represent frequencies (bpm) used.

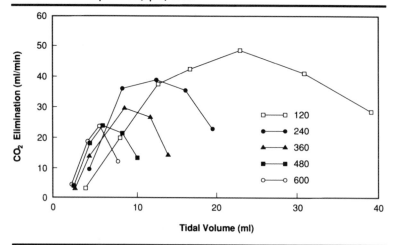

From: Korvenranta H, et al.: Carbon dioxide elimination during high frequency jet ventilation, Journal of Pediatrics 111(1), 1987, p. 109. Reprinted with permission.

Oxygenation during CMV is mostly dependent upon the amount of ambient oxygen (FiO_2) and the MAP used to deliver the gas.[23,37] Many factors affect the MAP, as indicated by the following formula:[38]

$$MAP = \frac{(f)\,(I_T)\,(PIP) + [60 - (f)\,(I_T)]\,(PEEP)}{60}$$

The effect of MAP on oxygenation may be related to enhanced alveolar recruitment and stabilization.[37] However, if effective pulmonary blood flow or perfusion is reduced, the same level of MAP may be detrimental to oxygenation.

Carbon dioxide elimination depends on alveolar ventilation. This can be expressed in the following formula:[37]

$$alveolar\ ventilation = (tidal\ volume - dead\ space) \times frequency$$

Ventilation can be enhanced by increasing either tidal volume or frequency. However, ventilation can be hampered by excessive tidal volume that leads to alveolar distention. High respiratory rates that do not allow sufficient

exhalation time will impair carbon dioxide excretion.[39,40]

Exhalation is a passive event occurring by the natural recoil of the chest. The time necessary to deflate (or inflate) the lung is known as the "time constant." It takes three to five time constants for the lung to empty to functional residual capacity. The time constant is the product of the airway resistance and lung compliance.[37]

*Time constant =
resistance × compliance*

If the time allowed for exhalation is shorter than the time constant, gas trapping will occur.[1] This will lead to alveolar distention and impaired carbon dioxide elimination.[40]

High-frequency jet ventilation can support oxygenation and ventilation.[1,41] Although HFJV and CMV differ in gas flow, tidal volume, and frequency, HFJV may be described using many of the same underlying physiologic principles.

Small volumes of gas under positive pressure are injected by HFJV at rates usually between 250 and 700 bpm. The tidal volumes are usually smaller than or slightly larger than anatomical dead space.[8,42] Inhalation is active, and exhalation is passive.[43]

Oxygenation by HFJV appears to depend on MAP and ambient FiO_2, as with CMV. Often, however, less MAP is required to support the patient.[19,24,33]

High-frequency jet ventilation can effectively eliminate carbon dioxide.[43-45] Tidal volume size and respiratory frequency are two main variables that influence the rate of elimination. Smith and colleagues studied the influence of HFJV rate and tidal volume on carbon dioxide elimination in surfactant-depleted cats using the Bunnell Life Pulse Ventilator. In this study, the highest carbon dioxide elimination occurred at a frequency of 500 bpm when the Delta P (PIP − PEEP) was 15. Carbon dioxide elimination did not improve at 600 bpm.[44]

Korvenranta and colleagues also studied carbon dioxide elimination during HFJV. They utilized an experimental prototype ventilator in a normal lung rabbit model. They found that increasing the tidal volume led to increased carbon dioxide elimination at all frequencies (Figure 1). However, when tidal volume was increased to the point of causing inadvertent PEEP, carbon dioxide elimination decreased despite an increased minute ventilation. If the PEEP was controlled, tidal volume explained 67–95 percent of the variance in carbon dioxide elimination.[45]

Another important factor affecting carbon dioxide elimination is gas trapping in the lung. As in CMV, exhalation is passive and is a function of the time constant of the respiratory system—including the endotracheal tube and the ventilator system.[46] The ability of the gas to leave the lung is, in part, dependent upon sufficient time for exhalation. Weisberger and associates studied the effect of varying inspiratory and expiratory times during HFJV in a surfactant-depleted rabbit model. An experimental HFJV was used with rates of 120, 240, and 480 bpm. As inspiratory time was shortened, increased Delta P was required to keep tidal volume constant. As expiratory time was shortened, air trapping occurred. These investigators concluded that when too short an expiratory time is used in relationship to the expiratory time constant, marked air trapping can occur. They also noted a positive relationship between the compliance of the respiratory system and the degree of air trapping. As compliance was less or worsened, the expiratory time required to avoid air trapping was less. However, they were unable to determine whether absolute expiratory time or the inspiratory-to-expiratory (I:E) ratio was more important in causation of air trapping.[47]

Frantz and Close found elevated lung volumes and alveolar pressure during experimental jet ventilation of rabbits. They discovered that insufficient exhalation time increased lung volumes. The degree of elevation depended on tidal volume and the relationship of actual expiratory time and expiratory time constant.[40]

Johnston and colleagues studied the effect of exhalation time on blood gases during HFJV. The Bunnell Life Pulse was employed at 600 bpm in surfactant-depleted cats. They found that functional residual capacity increased whenever expiratory time was shorter than expiratory time constants. Improved ventilation occurred when sufficient exhalation time was allowed.[43]

Ventilation and oxygenation during HFJV are complex phenomena. There is increasing evidence that tidal volume may be the major determinant of ventilation. Frequency is important, but an optimal range dependent upon disease state probably exists. Adequate exhalation time must be provided to prevent gas trapping.[46] An understanding of the various components of pulmonary mechanics and function, such as time constants, compliance, and resistance, is important for better prediction of response to various HFJV strategies. There is more evidence to indicate that too much of a good thing—in terms of tidal volume and frequency—may result in air trapping that increases the risk of barotrauma, air leak, and poor gas exchange.

Gas Exchange Mechanisms

We know that gas exchange can occur during high-frequency ventilation, even when tidal volume approaches or is less than anatomical dead space.[48–50] Numerous physiologic mechanisms are responsible. Two major mechanisms—convection and diffusion—explain this gas exchange.

Convection. Various types of convective gas movements can occur in both the airways and the terminal respiratory units during HFV. Although the individual volumes of each breath may be less than the anatomical dead space, gas

FIGURE 2 ▲ Pendeluft. Representation of inter-regional gas mixing caused by different time constants in two lung units. The fast (1) time constant unit can be seen to be filling at end expiration. The slow (2) time constant unit fills at the end of inspiration. Tracheal flow is zero at this time, and this effect thus augments alveolar tidal volume.

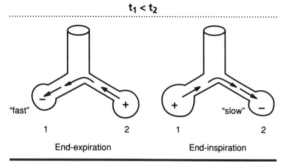

$t_1 < t_2$

From: Wetzel RC, and Gioia FR: High frequency ventilation, Pediatric Clinics of North America 34(1), 1987, p. 20. Reprinted with permission.

FIGURE 4 ▲ Asymmetric velocity profiles

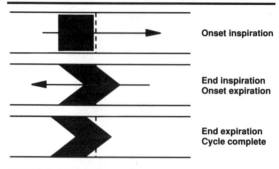

Onset inspiration

End inspiration
Onset expiration

End expiration
Cycle complete

From: Wetzel RC, and Gioia FR: High frequency ventilation, Pediatric Clinics of North America 34(1), 1987, p. 22. Reprinted with permission.

movement can still occur in a bulk fashion. Direct aeration of proximal airways and alveolar units can occur because of short transit times from the main airways.[1] These units may provide a significant portion of the total gas exchange because of local hyperventilation.[49]

Convective mixing and recirculation of gas can occur between neighboring respiratory units during the whole respiratory cycle.[51] This inter-regional mixing or "pendeluft" is due to the different time constants of the respiratory units.

This results in out-of-phase gas movements and facilitates convective exchange (Figure 2).

Convective flow streaming is another means of gas transport. Henderson and colleagues showed that the more energy or speed generating a puff of smoke, the greater the forward movement of the center of the puff (Figure 3).[11] A parabolic-shaped puff or breath is formed from the development of asymmetric velocity profiles. During exhalation, there are blunt flow profiles in the opposite direction, but the elongated center portion does not return to the starting point. At the end of a breath, there is a small net forward movement (Figure 4). After several cycles of HFJV, gas tends to flow down the center or inner core of

FIGURE 3 ▲ The quicker the puff, the sharper the spike. Forward movement of gas in the center and backward movement of gas at the walls.

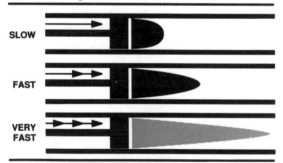

SLOW

FAST

VERY FAST

Adapted by: Harris TR, from Henderson Y, Chillingworth FP, and Whitney JL: Journal of Physiology 38(1), 1915. Reprinted with permission.

FIGURE 5 ▲ Helical pattern of convective streaming during HFJV

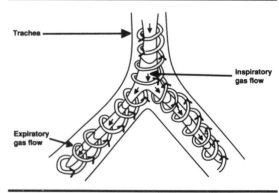

Trachea

Inspiratory gas flow

Expiratory gas flow

Adapted by Solon JF, from: Rausch K via Ellis R, unpublished data, Milpitas, California. Reprinted with permission.

FIGURE 6 ▲ Taylor dispersion. The inspiratory gas front is parabolic, and this provides a greatly increased area over which radial molecular diffusion can occur, as represented by the arrows.

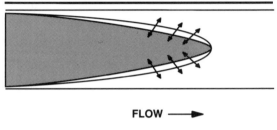

FLOW ⟶

From: Wetzel RC, and Gioia FR: High frequency ventilation, Pediatric Clinics of North America 34(1), 1987, p. 21. Reprinted with permission.

the tube (or airway) and out along the outer walls (Figure 5).[52,53]

Diffusion. Diffusion describes gas exchange by random (Brownian) movement wherever a concentration gradient occurs. This exchange occurs in any part of the lung where there is a gradient—not just in the terminal respiratory units.

Taylor dispersion. In 1954, Taylor described the augmented movement of gas and radial diffusion in situations of parabolic gas flow (such as the high-energy jet spike, Figure 6).[54] This augmented diffusion can occur wherever gas meets, such as in the coaxial flow in the

FIGURE 7 ▲ A representation of which mechanisms of gas transport predominate in given lung regions

1 Convection
2 Taylor Type
3 Velocity Profiles
4 Interregional (Pendeluft)
5 Molecular Diffusion

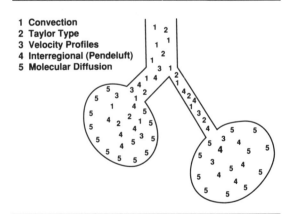

From: Wetzel RC, and Gioia FR: High frequency ventilation, Pediatric Clinics of North America 34(1), 1987, p. 23. Reprinted with permission.

larger airways and convective streaming farther out in the lung. This diffusion process is facilitated by the increased surface area between two gases during high-frequency ventilation (HFV) due to increased viscous drag.[55] Actual gas exchange may be hampered by Taylor dispersion because of the diffusion of carbon dioxide from the expiring gas into the fresh gas. The high-energy jet spikes probably result in the delivery of more total fresh gas to the respiratory units before significant contamination of the inflow gas can occur. This preserves the diffusion gradient needed to move carbon dioxide out of the blood.[56]

Various aspects of convective and diffusive mechanisms of gas transport are probably responsible for the majority of gas exchange during HFV. These mechanisms are not restricted to any one anatomical area. Convective forces are probably more dominant in areas where bulk flow occurs and diffusion in areas where it stops. There must also be areas of overlap and simultaneous operation (Figure 7). Traditional concepts such as bulk flow need to be modified in the context of high-frequency ventilation, but they still have validity in many situations. Tidal volumes greater than anatomical dead space have been measured during HFJV, but these include entrained gases without increased pressure.[46] Bulk flow may also occur as a result of an accumulation of breaths, rather than as an isolated event during a single breath.

Much more research will be necessary before this phenomena is fully described and understood. In order to have generalizable results, investigators must attempt to standardize the process and procedure. Unfortunately, this is unlikely given the current trends in HFV research.

COMPLICATIONS

Although HFJV appears to be efficacious in treating severe pulmonary air leak and respiratory failure, several serious complications have been reported. Some are similar to those seen with conventional ventilation (air leak, BPD, and intracranial hemorrhage). Others, most notably airway damage, may occur with CMV but may be worse with HFJV.[57] Various complications have been attributed to certain machines and ventilation strategies, but few causal relationships have been identified, and generalizations are limited. The same ventilator used with different clinical strategies can produce different degrees of injury.[28,30,58] Airway damage can occur in any infant treated with mechanical ventilation.[57–62] Airway damage spans a wide spectrum.

Air leaks. Air leaks, including pneumothorax, pneumopericardium, pneumoperitoneum, pneumomediastinum, and pulmonary interstitial emphysema, have occurred in infants being treated with HFJV.[56] Pneumopericardium was reported in 13 percent of infants treated with HFJV in a study done in 1987.[22] This compares to a reported incidence of less than 2 percent in infants with RDS.[63] The etiology of air leaks is multifactorial. One factor that may be of greater importance with HFJV than CMV is gas trapping, which may be due to insufficient expiratory time or inadvertent PEEP.[46,64]

Necrotizing tracheobronchitis (NTB). This is a condition of acute inflammation, extensive hemorrhage, tissue necrosis, and erosion of tracheal epithelium with increased thick secretions and mucus plugging.[58,60,63,65] Necrotic debris can slough off the trachea and, together with the thick secretions, lead to total airway obstruction.[62,65,66]

The cause of necrotizing tracheobronchitis is most likely multifactorial.[57] Lack of proper humidification of respiratory gases is considered an important etiologic factor.[60,61] Early models of HFJV systems provided humidification by a variety of methods, both singly and in combination. Humidity was provided to the entrainment gas by traditional cascade systems supplemented by the infusion of varying amounts of normal saline or one-half normal saline directly into the jet stream.[34,62] The Bunnell system humidifies the jet pulses with a built-in heated liquid system that supplements the entrained humidity.[56] Concern about humidity meant increased difficulty in patient management and may have limited early use of HFV technology. With too little fluid or humidity, necrotizing tracheobronchitis might occur, but attempts to supersaturate the inspired gas could lead to "neardrowning" or pulmonary edema.

In response to the potential link between necrotizing tracheobronchitis and humidity, numerous and extensive hardware modifications have been made in all systems. The Bunnell ventilator has incorporated a heated cartridge system that allows for highly sensitive control and measurement of infused fluid. In our experience, a heightened awareness of the problem and improvements in humidification have seemed to reduce the incidence of necrotizing tracheobronchitis.

Direct trauma has also been suggested as a factor for the etiology of necrotizing tracheobronchitis. Wiswell and associates reported severe instances of this disorder in 11 of 17 baboons treated with a high-frequency flow interrupter at 600 breaths/minute in an uninterrupted pattern.[58] It is speculated that the high MAP generated using this strategy contributed to or caused the necrotizing tracheobronchitis. Other investigators using the same machine with a different ventilation strategy reported a much reduced incidence.[28]

The exact incidence of necrotizing tracheobronchitis is not known. The diagnosis initially was made at autopsy because of limitations in technology. In infants who died during clinical trials of the Life Pulse ventilator, the incidence of NTB and erosion of tracheal mucosa at autopsy was 41 percent and 47 percent, respectively.[56]

In a study of 34 infants treated with the Life Pulse HFJV, 9 showed clinical evidence of necrotizing tracheobronchitis, and 1 required intervention for airway obstruction. Bronchoscopic evaluation of 13 infants showed some degree of tracheal inflammation in 9 (71 percent). However, none of the infants who ultimately survived has had airway compromise clearly related to necrotizing tracheobronchitis.[57]

Therapy for this condition depends upon the severity of the clinical presentation. Early recognition is important. Vigorous tracheal toilet can be helpful. Emergency bronchoscopy has been successfully employed to remove debris.[66] Weaning from HFJV may be necessary.

It appears that airway damage may be more frequent with any form of high frequency system than with CMV. While clinically significant necrotizing tracheobronchitis is unusual, its potential must still be considered prior to any application of HFJV.[57]

Reactive airway disease. This disorder has been observed in infants treated with both HFJV and CMV. Characterized by prolonged severe bronchospasm, this process is probably due to irritation of the airways during ventilation—especially in the presence of infection.[67] Because bronchospasms are a known sequela of BPD, reactive airway disease may also be a result of the severity of lung disease and any invasive ventilatory therapy rather than a result of high-frequency ventilation alone.[68] Therapy may include the use of bronchodilators, sedation, and steroids.[67] Bronchoscopy may also be needed to differentiate between true reactive airway disease and airway malacia or necrotizing tracheobronchitis.[69]

Hypotension. An interesting complication or side effect of HFJV is hypotension. This may be due to the extreme effectiveness of this therapy in some patients. High-frequency ventilation can abruptly drop carbon dioxide pressure. Hypocarbia can cause systemic vasodilation, resulting in hypotension.[70,71] Also, rapid and severe hypocarbia can cause cutaneous

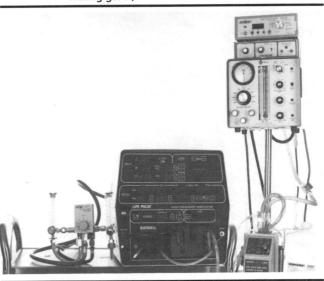

FIGURE 8 ▲ Tandem ventilation. Tandem ventilator setup (note conventional ventilator, high-frequency jet ventilator, airway pressure monitor, and blender for mixing gases).

peripheral vasoconstriction,[70] which may affect transcutaneous monitoring accuracy. Therapy (and prevention) may include close arterial blood gas monitoring, careful ventilator adjustments, volume expansion, and use of vasopressors.

Mechanical Problems

As with all devices, certain mechanical problems or failures can occur. The ventilators used for HFJV have evolved from crude devices to sophisticated, highly technical machines with many built-in safeguards. Proper connection of pressure-monitoring devices as well as an accurate understanding of alarm states are imperative if application of high airway pressure to the patient is to be avoided. Use of HFJV may expose the patient to certain undefined risks. It was recently reported that a part of an HFJV silicone patient-breathing circuit shed debris.[72] Although no malady could be associated with this observation, changes were made in the equipment and operating procedures to eliminate the risk of particle deposition.[56,72]

FIGURE 9 ▲ Life Pulse Ventilator block diagram

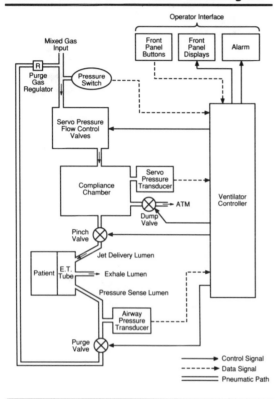

From: Bunnell JB: Life Pulse High Frequency Ventilator Operator's Manual, Salt Lake City, 1987, revision 19, p. IV-3. Reprinted with permission.

Like all methods of mechanical ventilation, HFJV has adverse side effects and complications. As use of the technique increases, these must be closely monitored and reported. Careful analysis of benefits versus risks is required prior to widespread usage of any treatment modality.

THE BUNNELL LIFE PULSE VENTILATOR

The clinical experience and nursing care presented in the remainder of this chapter involve the use of one type of high-frequency jet ventilator—the Bunnell Life Pulse Ventilator. This HFJV device is approved by the Food and Drug Administration for commercial use in the treatment of infants with severe respiratory failure and extraventilatory air. An understanding of the machine itself may help the reader evaluate our experiences.

The Bunnell Life Pulse high-frequency ventilator is a microprocessor controlled, time cycled, pressure limited, constant flow generator, high-frequency jet respirator. The system is capable of delivering and monitoring between 240 and 660 humidified "breaths" per minute. The Life Pulse functions in tandem with a conventional respirator, which supplies entrained gas, controls the PEEP, and provides background conventional mechanical ventilator breaths (Figure 8). Sophisticated microprocessor control systems, utilizing integrated software elements, manipulate gas valves that regulate breath size. The computer also controls the electromagnetic solenoid that activates the pinch valve. Pinch valve movement interrupts a continuous gas flow, creating the jet "breaths" (Figure 9).[56]

On the front of the panel (Figure 10) are ventilator monitoring displays. These include PIP, Delta P, PEEP, Servo pressure (the pressure the machine has to generate internally to meet the desired PIP), and MAP. The PIP is the average peak inspiratory pressure generated with each breath; it is set by the user. The Delta P, the difference between the PIP and the PEEP, is analogous to the tidal volume. The lowest pressure in the cycle, the PEEP is set by the user and controlled by the tandem conventional ventilator. The MAP is the average pressure delivered over the entire respiratory cycle. The pressures are sampled either every inhalation valve cycle or every 2 milliseconds. After start-up, the values displayed are 10-second averages. After regular operations, the pressure samples are averaged over a 20-second period.[56]

Ventilator Performance Indicators

The continuous gas flow that is used to generate the jet "breaths" is varied to meet the required PIP and rate settings. This flow is expressed as the Servo pressure and is the amount of gas pressure needed to keep the system pressurized (compliance chamber) to meet the demand (Figure 9). The Servo pressure ranges from 0–20 cm H_2O. This is servo-controlled by a feedback loop from information obtained from the distal tip of the endotracheal tube. The machine will adjust the Servo pressure to keep the PIP steady. It is affected by factors such as lung compliance or resistance to gas flow. Changes in Servo pressure may indicate improved lung status or acute changes such as atelectasis, tension pneumothorax, or other air leaks (extubation or tracheal air leak). Situations that decrease compliance will result in a low Servo pressure because less gas is needed to meet any given PIP. Situations that increase compliance will increase the Servo pressure needed for any given PIP, and adjusting the PIP itself will directly affect the Servo pressure. The pressure readings are averaged over the last 10–20 seconds with displays updated every 2 seconds.[56]

The jet valve "on/off" light is on when the pinch valve is open and off when closed. During operation, the light flickers on and off at a speed reflecting the ventilator rate. It should flash off whenever an overriding breath is provided. This means the machine is off and not "stacking" breaths.[56]

Ventilator Alarm Displays

The alarm displays are located in the upper right hand corner. High and low alarms are automatically set as follows:
Servo pressure = +1 cm H_2O present value
MAP = +1.5 cm H_2O present value
High = >5 cm H_2O now (current) PIP for
at least 2 seconds
>10 cm H_2O now PIP during a 30-
second period

FIGURE 10 ▲ Life Pulse Ventilator front view

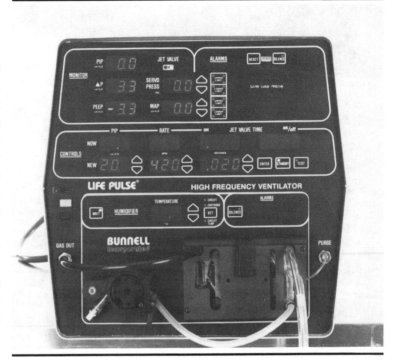

Loss of PIP = <25 percent of now PIP
There are displays and controls for manually adjusting the upper and lower limits for MAP and Servo pressure. The "high PIP," "loss of PIP," "cannot meet PIP," "jet valve fault," "ventilator fault," and "low gas pressure" are backlighted displays. The ready light glows when the alarms are able to work. There are "reset" and "silence" buttons.[56]

Ventilator Controls

There are displays and controls for "PIP," "rate," and "jet on time" (inspiratory time) located on the front panel. These displays show the current or "now" settings. One is able to set different settings without affecting operation by manipulating the "new" control area. These settings can then be entered and acted upon. The PIP can be set between 8 and 50 cm H_2O, the rate from 240 to 660 bpm, and the "jet on time" from 0.02 to 0.034 seconds. These limits were installed to increase machine safety without sacrificing performance.[56]

FIGURE 11 ▲ Patient box

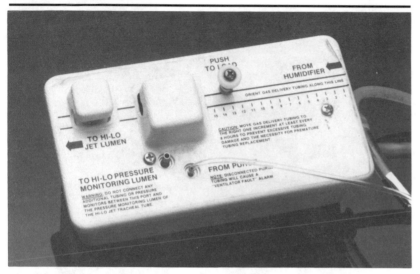

ing the silicone tube of the patient circuit. Silicone tube location is changed every eight hours to prevent premature tube replacement from excessive wear. The purge valve allows a ten-millisecond burst of pressurized dry gas into the pressure monitoring line, helping to keep it free of moisture. The pressure transducer provides the tracheal pressure information used to guide the respirator. These pressures are measured at the distal end of the triple-lumen jet tube and do not reflect alveolar pressures. The patient box must be located as close to the infant as possible to assure accurate pressure data and delivery of crisp jets of gas.[56]

Humidifier Displays and Controls

The humidifier is a heated, low-compliance cartridge system that automatically fills. The circuit temperature is the temperature of the patient breathing circuit measured at the patient box. Both the set and actual temperatures are displayed. The cartridge temperature is the temperature of the cartridge. The amount of humidity in the gas is directly related to this temperature. The range of possible temperatures is 32–42°C. Alarms monitor for system function and for too high or too low temperature or water levels.[56]

The Patient Box

The patient box (Figure 11) is a satellite component that houses the pinch (inhalation) valve, the purge valve, and the pressure transducer. The pinch valves breaks the flow of pressurized gas into small high-energy bursts by alternately pinching and releas-

HI-LO Jet Tracheal Tube

The HI-LO Jet Tracheal Tube (National Catheter Corporation division of Mallinckrodt Co., Argyle, New York) is a triple-lumen

FIGURE 12 ▲ Triple lumen E-T tube. Note pressure line, jet line and ETT adapter.

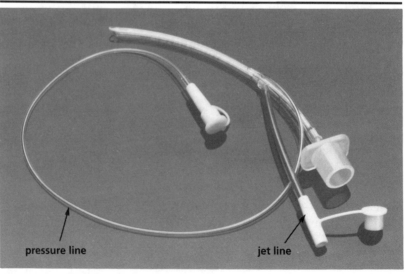

pressure line   jet line

TABLE 1 ▲ HFJV Rescue Therapy Entry Criteria

Severe respiratory disease
  RDS
  Pneumonia
  Persistent pulmonary hypertension of the newborn
    (PPHN)

Significant pulmonary air leak
  Bilateral PIE
  Tension pneumothorax
  Broncho-pleural fistula
  Pneumopericardium
  Pneumomediastinum

Failing conventional ventilation
  PaO_2 <60 mmHg and falling
  $PaCO_2$ >50 mmHg and rising

TABLE 3 ▲ Principal Diagnoses at Initiation of HFJV (N = 100)

	Number (% of total)
Pulmonary air leak	86 (86%)
Prematurity	76 (76%)
Respiratory distress syndrome	75 (75%)
Pneumonia and/or sepsis	30 (30%)
Meconium aspiration syndrome and/or PPHN	26 (26%)
Congenital diaphragmatic hernia/pulmonary hypoplasia	17 (17%)

(Bunnell & Harris: 1987, unpublished data)

1. Changes in airway resistance
2. Tube obstruction or leak
3. Change in lung compliance
4. New pulmonary air leak or resolution of an old leak
5. System leaks or disconnections
6. Patient interaction such as deep, spontaneous breathing

In most alarm situations, the ventilator will continue to operate, but pressure and gas delivery may be held constant. If dangerous situations exist, the ventilator will stop and release patient circuit pressure to the atmosphere to protect the patient.[56] As with all medical devices the user should refer to the latest edition of the operator's manual.

uncuffed endotracheal tube in usual sizes (Figure 12). The external diameter is approximately the size of the next higher regular tube (2.5 jet = 3.0 regular). The main lumen allows for entrained gases and connection to CMV. The insufflation jet lumen is the short green tubing. The long clear tubing is the pressure monitoring line. The pressure line must always be connected during machine start-up or parameter change to protect the patient from potentially excessive airway pressures.[56]

Alarm Systems

The Life Pulse ventilator has many alarm systems to protect the patient and ensure optimal operation. Many of them reflect situations in the patient rather than the ventilator. Changes in the impedance of the patient's respiratory system will cause pressure drops or increases that will initiate alarms. Such situations can include the following:

EIGHT-YEAR CLINICAL EXPERIENCE

Clinical use of HFJV to treat infants with intractable respiratory failure at the Primary Children's Medical Center began in 1982 under the direction of Thomas Harris, MD. The clinical trial was conducted under an investigational device exemption (IDE-G820049) granted to Bunnell, Inc., the Life Pulse developer. Under the research protocol, therapy was limited to infants with severe restrictive pulmonary disease, air leak, or inability to ventilate with conventional therapy. All infants were critically ill and had failed to improve on conventional positive pressure ventilation (Table 1). Many had multisystem failure.

High-frequency jet ventilation was employed as a form of "rescue" ventilation. Its use was

TABLE 2 ▲ Demographic Data for Infants on HFJV (N=100)

		Mean ± SD	(Range)
Birthweight (gm)		1,901 ± 1,025	(600–4,600)
Gestational age (weeks)		32.4 ± 4.9	(24–43)
Age started on HFJV (days)		5.9 ± 4.9	(21–30.4)
Duration on HFJV (days)		6.0 ± 7.1	(0.03–29)
Sex	Females = 39	Males = 61	

(Bunnell, Harris, Karp: 1987, unpublished data)

TABLE 4 ▲ Suggested Physiologic Parameters to be Continuously Monitored

Heart rate and EKG
Arterial blood pressure
Airway pressure
Respiratory rate
Central venous pressure
Ambient oxygen
Blood gas monitoring, both O_2 and CO_2
    (indwelling probes or transcutaneous sensors)
Trending capabilities helpful

approved by the human subjects review committees and parental consent was obtained prior to the initiation of therapy. There have been more than 130 patients treated with HFJV at our institution during the last eight years. Demographics for the first 100 patients are presented in Table 2.

Principal diagnoses were mainly prematurity and pulmonary disease (Table 3). More than 17 infants with congenital diaphragmatic hernia were treated. Excluded from study were infants with severe congenital anomalies or syndromes incompatible with life. All infants were out-born.

Aggressive supportive care was provided before and after the initiation of HFJV. Most infants were paralyzed with pancuronium bromide to facilitate respiratory support and positional therapy.[73,74] Maximal CMV support had been employed with MAP usually greater than 14 cm H_2O. When progressive pulmonary failure or worsening air leak occurred, parents were approached by the attending physician for informed consent to enter the infant into the clinical trial.

Once entered in the study, the infant was reintubated with the HI-LO Jet endotracheal tube, which has lumens for jet gas injection

FIGURE 13 ▲ Tandem ventilation airway pressure wave patterns

Wave Form Method I:

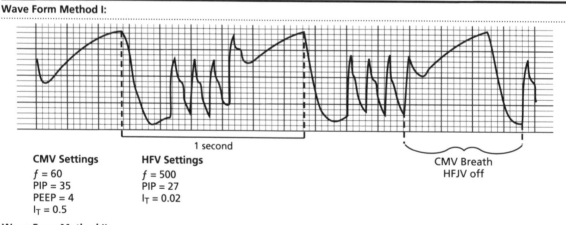

CMV Settings	HFV Settings		CMV Breath
f = 60	f = 500		HFJV off
PIP = 35	PIP = 27		
PEEP = 4	I_T = 0.02		
I_T = 0.5			

1 second

Wave Form Method II:

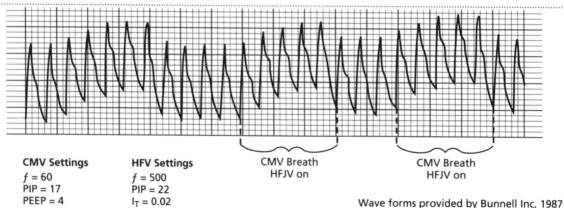

CMV Settings	HFV Settings	CMV Breath	CMV Breath
f = 60	f = 500	HFJV on	HFJV on
PIP = 17	PIP = 22		
PEEP = 4	I_T = 0.02		

Wave forms provided by Bunnell Inc, 1987

and pressure monitoring lines that terminate near the distal end of the tube. A third lumen allows for gas entrainment, exhalation, and suctioning.

After stabilization, baseline blood gases, vital signs, and distal pressure data were collected with the infant still on CMV. Because blood gas values may change rapidly during HFJV, real-time monitoring (with an oximeter or transcutaneous oxygen and carbon dioxide monitors) is a requirement. The suggested physiologic parameters to be continuously monitored are presented in Table 4.

Initial HFJV settings were based upon animal work.[42,44,56,75] The PIP was reduced by 25–33 percent and the PEEP kept constant or increased slightly. The starting rate was usually 450–600 bpm with a 20-millisecond inspiratory time. These settings usually resulted in a decrease in MAP. The pressure values utilized were based upon the in-use CMV settings as measured in the distal trachea and displayed by the HFJV monitor. Provision and regulation of all ventilation parameters except PEEP and oxygen were carried out through the HFJV. The PEEP was provided by a tandem CMV, enriched oxygen by two blenders (Figure 8).

Initiation of HFJV is simultaneous with an attempt to wean the infant from CMV. Early in the study, attempts were made to wean the infant to background CPAP. Later in the study and currently, attempts are made to wean the infant to a low rate (5–10 bpm), intermittent mandatory ventilation. Background CPAP may be used in severe air leak syndrome or lung overdistention (air trapping). The unpredictable blood gas response to HFJV may make many parameter changes necessary. Thus the initiation or trial period of HFJV is often quite time and labor intensive. Carbon dioxide is manipulated by small changes in PIP (1–2 cm H_2O) or large changes in rate (20–50 bpm). Oxygenation still seems dependent upon MAP. PEEP appears to be important: A range of 2–5 has been used in most infants, but higher lev-

FIGURE 14 ▲ Weaning to CMV

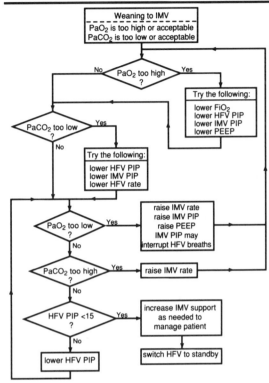

From: Bunnell JB: Life Pulse High Frequency Ventilator Operator's Manual, Salt Lake City, 1987, revision 9, p. VIII-17. Reprinted with permission.

els (up to 10) may be required to stabilize oxygenation even in the face of an air leak. We try to avoid PEEPs less than 2 cm H_2O. In our experience, PEEPs <2 cm can promote air trapping due to airway collapse.

Tandem Ventilation

Progressive atelectasis develops in many infants when they are treated with HFJV alone. Hypoxemia alone or in unison with hypercarbia may ensue. This can be treated with tandem ventilation.

Two methods of providing tandem ventilation have been described.[24,76] One uses CMV PIPs higher than the HFJV. When the distal (CMV) PIP is 5 cm H_2O higher than the set PIP, the HFJV pauses. This method is used to prevent pressure stacking of the HFJV and CMV breaths and movement of the baseline pressure.

The second method of providing tandem

TABLE 5 ▲ Long-Term Therapy (N = 100)

Infants on HFJV	No. (% of total)
0–1 weeks	63 (63%)
1–2 weeks	17 (17%)
2–3 weeks	04 (04%)
3–4 weeks	05 (05%)
4–5 weeks	01 (01%)

(Bunnell, Harris, Karp: 1987, unpublished data)

ventilation utilizes conventional mechanical ventilation of at least a PIP 2–5 cm H_2O less than HFJV.[24,56] The HFJV continues to cycle during the breath. Proponents of this method believe continuation of HFJV at all times enhances its effect without additional risk of barotrauma. There are no studies comparing these two methods. Figure 13 displays an example of the pressure wave patterns that may be seen with the two types of tandem ventilation.

Once the infant has been stabilized, efforts are aimed at reducing MAP. The PIP may be gradually reduced to the low teens and rates to the 250–300 bpm range. Resolution of air leaks may occur in hours to days. We attempt to delay return to full CMV until air leaks are healed for two days so as to decrease the risk of reoccurrence.

Methods of weaning the infant to CMV have not been thoroughly studied. Various techniques have been utilized with the goal of limiting the PIP and MAP as much as possible (Figure 14). Weaning may be hampered by the development of BPD.

Two weaning methods appear to be common. The first involves decreasing PIP while increasing CMV breaths. The HFJV rate remains elevated, usually above 350 bpm. The second method involves lowering the HFJV to 250 bpm while increasing the CMV rate. Pressures remain elevated. The weaning process depends on the presence of air leaks, complications, and degree of improvement. We usually lower support to a baseline level and then over a 12–24 hour period wean the infant to CMV. As one adds background breaths, the

rate may remain elevated. Both HFJV and CMV PIP are adjusted to control ventilation.

During HFJV therapy, aggressive support is provided to all body systems. Nutrition is provided by hyperalimentation, which includes intravenous fat when possible. Cardiac output and circulation are supported with vasoactive agents and volume infusions. Close surveillance for and aggressive therapy of infection are conducted. Bronchodilators may be required in large doses for presumed reactive airway disease. Bronchoscopy may be required as a diagnostic or therapeutic endeavor. Lastly, much parental support is provided by the whole health care team during this crisis situation.

Our present HFJV usage is for short-term "rescue" ventilation. In addition, we have utilized long-term rescue therapy, which has often been required because of an infant's failure to tolerate low-pressure CMV or redevelopment of air leaks (Table 5). Twenty-seven infants received therapy for more than 1 week; our longest usage has been 29 days. During these prolonged therapy periods, the focus of care is shifted from an acute critical orientation to one of more chronic long-term care.

Use of HFJV had at least a short-term positive response on the pulmonary course of more than 80 percent of our patients. Of the infants undergoing therapy, 51 percent survived on a short-term basis and 33 percent on a long-term basis.[75]

The major complications seen in our group were air leak and intraventricular hemorrhage. Some infants also suffered from pneumonia, alone or in combination with bronchospasms and mucus plugging, while receiving HFJV therapy. The bronchospasm and mucus plugging may have been secondary to necrotizing tracheobronchitis.[56]

NURSING CARE

Infants requiring HFJV therapy are critically ill. The clinical course has been one of worsening lung disease reflected by deteriorating blood gases and chest x-rays. Frequently exten-

TABLE 6 ▲ Assessment of Chest Vibrations

Baseline:	Continuous with rapid rise and fall
Lack of vibration:	Plugged or dislodged ET tube, ET tube orientation causing obstruction
	Massive tension pneumothorax
	Machine failure or gas leak
Decreased vibration:	Air trapping
	Worsening lung compliance
	Tube malposition or obstruction
	Worsening air leak
	Excessive weaning of PIP
	Excessive PEEP
Excessive vibration:	Excessive PIP
	Improved pulmonary compliance
	Unconnected pressure monitor

sive air leak syndrome has developed or worsened. These complex patients require the adaptation, revision, and evaluation of various aspects of nursing practice to integrate HFJV technology into bedside care.

Most descriptions of nursing care of patients requiring HFJV are based on the adult population.[77-79] These reports provided the initial framework from which we developed our early care.[76] Recently, Gordin in 1989, and White and associates in 1990, reported their nursing experiences with HFJV therapy. [80,81] These two reports, in addition to our own experiences with 130 infants, represent a compilation of the nursing care provided to over 400 infants. From this perspective, the following section presents a framework of nursing care based upon our eight-year experience; it has allowed for flexibility, adapation, evaluation, and revision.

Assessment

Patient assessment is frequent and extensive, consisting mainly of inspection, auscultation, and palpation. Although the basic nursing methods for gathering data remain unchanged, the interpretation of the information is dramatically affected by HFJV technology. Assessment is also influenced by underlying disease states and drug usage.

Respiratory system. Assessment of the respiratory system is dramatically affected by HFJV. The high breath rates and small pulses of gases cause significant chest vibration. This rapid chest movement makes counting total respiratory rates impractical. During normal ventilator operation, the vibrations are continuous except when the measured distal PIP exceeds the now PIP. This occurs when background CMV PIP or the infant's spontaneous breaths cause the measured PIP to be greater than the now PIP by more than 5 cm H_2O. These pauses are very short and have no obvious adverse effect on the infant. However, it is important to constantly monitor the amount of vibration because it appears related to tidal volume delivery (Table 6). The status of chest vibration is assessed formally every 30 minutes and informally whenever the patient is observed.

Spontaneous respirations can occur provided the infant is not hypocarbic or receiving paralytic agents. These breaths are assessed mostly by inspection for retractions and other signs of distress. Spontaneous aeration is usually not heard until marked improvement in pulmonary compliance occurs. Breaths provided by CMV are assessed in the usual manner. These breaths are often used as the assessment standard.

The breath sounds created by HFJV have a loud "jackhammer" quality with a high-pitched tone. Different than traditional breath sounds, these provide much information, especially when monitored over time. Decreased tone may indicate poor ventilation or pneumothorax. Higher-pitched tones, especially those of musical quality, seem to indicate mucus secretions, plugs, or bronchospasm. Assessment of rales and the "rice crispy" crackles of PIE can be difficult during HFJV. Background CMV breaths can be used for this assessment but may hamper the resolution of air leaks.

Extraventilatory air status should be assessed frequently. Transillumination is performed on each patient during each shift and whenever deteriorations occur.[82] Changes in the air leak rate or occurrence of new leaks will alter therapeutic plans. Constant vigilance for new air leaks, especially pneumopericardium, is vital. Although it is unclear if pneumopericardium is more frequent with HFJV than CMV, it does occur. In situations of acute deterioration, especially with cardiovascular compromise, pneumopericardium must be considered.

Assessment of tracheal secretions is very important during HFJV. Changes in tracheal secretion consistency and color may be the first warning signs of developing necrotizing tracheobronchitis. Nosocomial pneumonia has occurred during HFJV, and the infant must be assessed for this infection.

Cardiovascular system. Most infants requiring HFJV therapy have concomitant cardiovascular compromise. This may be secondary to the underlying disease state or therapeutic maneuvers. Pulmonary hypertension and poor left ventricular output are the most common alterations seen. The high MAP required to support these infants, as well as the accumulation of extraventilatory air, may hamper venous return and subsequent cardiac output. In addition to auscultation, inspection, and palpation, assessment of cardiovascular function requires integration of other information, such as urine output and acid-base balance.

Physical assessment of the cardiovascular system is hampered by the inability to hear the heart sounds during ventilator operation. Murmurs usually cannot be heard unless they are very loud; pulse rate cannot be counted unless the ventilator is on standby. Locating the point of maximal impulse is greatly limited by the chest vibration except in cases of an extremely active precordium. Assessment of peripheral pulses is hampered by the total body vibration. The more peripheral pulses (radial and posterior tibial) are less affected than the central pulses (femoral and brachial) because of the distance from the vibrating thorax.

During HFJV operation, EKG and vascular pressure waveforms can show movement artifact. This appears to depend on the vigor of the body movement, pulmonary compliance, and transducer sensitivity. The CVP waveform is the most affected. Despite the motion artifacts, the pressure value seems valid and useful. Arrythmias and abnormal pressure waveforms have been detected.

Other systems. Assessment of the gastrointestinal tract is influenced by the body vibrations and noise produced during HFJV. Gross assessment can be performed without major impairment, but fine assessments, such as bowel sounds and liver evaluation, can be difficult. Abdominal distention and tenderness can still be determined. Stooling is not impaired.

The genitourinary system is not affected by HFJV. However, the frequent use of paralytics and sedatives in these infants necessitates frequent evaluation for urinary retention.

Assessment for alterations in the integumentary system should be frequent. In our experience, the body vibration does not seem to increase the incidence of skin breakdown. In fact, the movement may help reduce impairment in those infants who are paralyzed.

Assessment of the neurologic status depends more on the severity of the underlying disease state, any specific complications, and pharmacotherapy than on HFJV. Some infants are obtunded; others are active and alert. With adequate ventilation, infants do not appear distressed while on HFJV. Behavioral signs of distress are interpreted in their usual context. Seizure activity can be observed. Fontanel, tone, and basic reflexes can be assessed within limitations of patient status.

Equipment and monitoring needs. Because patients receiving HFJV are critically ill, constant assessment of vital signs and blood gas values is necessary (Table 4). The noise and vibration produced by HFJV precludes many normal assessment activities. Heart sounds cannot be heard, so continuous heart rate moni-

TABLE 7 ▲ Nursing Responsibilities and Interventions for Infants Prior to and During the Application

Responsibilities	Interventions
Obtain and document baseline assessment data.	Perform full system assessment. Draw appropriate blood gases, and correlate results with monitors.
Ensure that appropriate monitoring equipment is available and working.	Gather and apply needed monitoring devices (Table 4) with assistance from other team members. Organize environment to facilitate care.
Orient parents to new bedside environment and patient care status.	Explain new equipment and patient conditions to parents. Allow time for questions, and provide answers or referral.
Ensure that parent consent has been obtained by physician or nurse practitioner.	Act as witness during consent procedure. Assess understanding, and act as advocate as needed.
Assist with needed procedures. Endotracheal tube will be changed to a triple-lumen tube.	Participate with other team members during reintubation procedure or other procedures. Assist with x-ray examinations as needed.
Ensure that patient safety is maintained during transition process from CMV to HFJV.	Prepare for possible patient deterioration necessitating return to CMV and possible drug support.
Provide emotional support for family.	Answer questions as needed. Allow time alone with infant prior to initiation of therapy. Provide anticipatory guidance regarding potential patient instability.
Ensure potential for respiratory gas exchange.	Observe patient for constant chest motion. Maintain ET tube orientation and stability. Suction as needed.
Perform safe and effective suctioning procedure.	If procedure performed while HFJV operates, maintain suction throughout procedure.
Monitor for complications: air leak, NTB, hypotension, etc.	Obtain blood gases as needed. Monitor trends in vital signs. Assess for signs and symptoms of air leak syndrome—especially pneumothorax and pneumomediastinum. Observe quality and quantity of secretions, and listen for musical breath sounds.
Monitor response to therapy.	Document and interpret changes in oxygenation and ventilation status following ventilator manipulations. Frequently assess activity of chest tubes, if present.
Ensure patient safety and comfort.	Administer analgesics, sedatives, and muscle relaxants as needed. Be prepared to return infant to CMV should mechanical failure occur or patient not tolerate therapy.
Continue support of parents.	Provide therapeutic environment at bedside. Allow for physical contact. Allow for expression of feelings. Provide consistent information and education.

toring is vital. We find it useful to employ a monitor that can determine the heart rate from both the QRS complex and the arterial waveform. Chest movement artifact may alter EKG waveform, depending on electrode placement.

Continuous blood gas monitoring is required, as with any critically ill child. Carbon dioxide monitoring is mandatory because HFJV may alter the blood value significantly within a very short time. Oxygen saturation and PaO_2 monitors (internal or surface) can be used to assess the patient's oxygenation status.

Nursing Diagnoses and Goals

Nursing diagnoses are derived from the information obtained during patient assessment. General diagnoses such as altered respiratory gas exchange are adapted to reflect HFJV usage. One example is "potential for airway obstruction." Although airway obstruction can occur with any form of mechanical ventilation, the use of HFJV increases the potential for necrotizing tracheobronchitis. This increases the potential for airway obstruction and air leak syndrome. Nursing care can be focused by the use of adapted nursing diagnoses that reflect the influence of new technology.

Patient care goals are derived from the nursing diagnoses. Both short- and long-term goals are developed, including goals to provide a supportive and safe environment that facilitates recovery.

Interventions

Nursing care interventions are individualized according to the infant's acuity. General nursing interventions are similar to those for infants requiring CMV.

Certain interventions are the result of the HFJV technology (Table 7). The first nursing activity usually is assistance with the procedure to place the special triple-lumen jet endotracheal tube. This procedure can place additional stress on an already compromised patient. Taping the jet tube in place correctly is of greater significance than with conventional tubes. The green jet line is placed facing anterior (the lip). This places the bevel of the jet tube in a left oblique position, which seems to facilitate ventilation. The reintubation procedure often necessitates a chest radiograph to document placement.

The use of HFJV has required modification of our suctioning procedure.[81,83] The most notable changes are the instillation of irrigating fluid in the green jet line and the continuous application of suction during the entire suctioning procedure. When HFJV is operating, continuous suction is required to prevent the buildup of excessive volumes of gas during obstruction of the exhaust port with the catheter.[56, 84] Failure to apply suction may result in significant gas trapping and subsequent air leak. Suctioning may also be performed with the ventilator in standby.[56] When HFJV is not being provided, no suction is applied during the insertion phase.[80,85]

Patient response to ventilator changes on HFJV is somewhat unpredictable, so frequent blood gas analysis is required during periods of instability. Alteration in settings usually takes many factors into consideration. A team approach with frequent consultation is needed. Because much of the care of these infants is still based on anecdote and experience, tremendous flexibility in treatment plans is a necessity.

Evaluation and Revision

Evaluation of nursing care occurs frequently because of the complexity of these patients. The process is an ongoing one providing feedback into the various steps of the nursing process. Most of the evaluation activities occur on an informal level at the bedside between the staff nurse, primary care provider, and attending physician. Evaluation must also occur on a formal level. Two mechanisms are utilized to accomplish this: (1) formal nursing care rounds and (2) the patient care conference. In these conferences, parents and medical, social work, clergy, and nursing staff review the case. The information and decisions from these conferences are then integrated into the daily nursing care plan.

The steps of the nursing process require that information obtained, goals established, interventions performed, and evaluations conducted be analyzed to provide the basis for revision of the care plan. Revision is required as the patient's course progresses or deteriorates. If the infant survives, the degree of residual chronic lung disease will be a prime factor in the planning of future care. If the chronic lung disease is severe or air leaks persist, prolonged HFJV may be required. If improvement does not occur, then plans must be made for care of the infant and family during the terminal portion of hospitalization. Usually death is due to progressive cardiorespiratory failure. The terminal period may be prolonged by the ability of HFJV to support ventilation in very diseased lungs.

Parent Care

Nursing care is given not only to the infant undergoing HFJV, but also to the parent(s). Emotional stress is very great when an infant is sick at birth, and HFJV increases that stress. Not only is their infant extremely ill, but he is receiving experimental therapy to which his responses are unpredictable.

The technology is offered in hopes of rescuing the child but may only delay death. Although survival is important, parents are concerned about outcome. No parent has withdrawn a patient from HFJV without agreement of the care team. Parents have refused entry into the study.

The HFJV technology and stress require additional nursing care time for family education and support. Parents are encouraged to participate in care as much as is feasible. This is especially true with long-term usage. Infants on HFJV can be held, though provisions need to be made for the additional equipment. If the infant is terminally ill, care is provided to support the family through this process. The families of all patients undergoing HFJV therapy are provided with social service support.

Administrative and Professional Issues

The introduction of HFJV technology impacts the management of the intensive care unit. Manpower and capital costs are affected. Staffing requirements are increased to provide adequate patient coverage. Nursing hours per patient day increase as the acuity of the patient population increases. Additional education time is required to orient the staff to HFJV technology. This may increase job stress.

Capital costs may increase. Physical space requirements are increased by the need for two ventilators at the bedside. Additional ventilators and related equipment, such as blenders and carts, must be purchased. The HFJV ventilator may be subject to periods of disuse because of the limited patient base it can be used on. This may prolong the time it takes to recoup the capital cost.

High-frequency jet ventilation technology can also be a revenue source. Our overall patient referral population increased as infants were transferred to our nursery from other Level III units. These were unexpected admissions. The technology can also be a marketing tool for both patient and staff recruitment.

Although HFJV provides an additional means to save infants who would otherwise die, there can be an emotional cost. Certain infants who eventually will die are supported for longer periods than possible with CMV. Ethical issues regarding appropriate patient selection and resource utilization further increase the stress inherent in the care of critically ill infants.

Another source of stress is the use of a machine to which patient response is unpredictable. There is always some degree of mistrust of anything new. The bedside nurse must be prepared to return the infant to CMV at a moment's notice. Improvements in machine reliability have greatly reduced, but not eliminated this source of stress.

HFJV introduction creates further stress on nursing and other personnel by necessitating additional documentation, education, patient assignment changes, and staffing. Even the environment is affected by HFJV: The noise level in the nursery increases from the constant clicking of the patient box valve.

Many of these stresses can be counterbalanced by the positive influences brought about by the introduction and utilization of HFJV. Outcome for some infants appears to be improved. The nurse is given an opportunity to broaden her theoretical basis for care. New concepts of physiology are learned and old ones evaluated. New methods of responding to crisis are available, and the nurse plays an integral role in the therapy. Nursing participation in data collection enables a project to go forward.

Involvement in research seems to foster interest in nursing research in other areas. Experience with HFJV technology also helps pave the way for the introduction of other new care technology. Nursing involvement in this and other new therapies, research, education, and the evolution of nursing practice seems to have a positive impact on job satisfaction.

SUMMARY

High-frequency jet ventilation is a new technology that has been useful for rescue ventilation in infants suffering severe respiratory failure. As with many new technologies, it has had a considerable influence on nursing care. It has required evaluation and adaptation of patient care and unit management practices. Nursing care approaches continue to evolve. However, there is a lack of nursing research to either support or refute many of our assertions. For this we take responsibility and are committed to validate our care through nursing research.

ACKNOWLEDGEMENT

This work was supported in part by Patient Care Services, Primary Children's Medical Center (PCMC) and the Division of Neonatology, University of Utah School of Medicine. The author would like to thank Debbie Wirth, RN, MS; Burt Bunnell, PhD; Tom Harris, MD; and the nursing, respiratory care, and medical staff of the newborn intensive care unit at PCMC.

REFERENCES

1. Bancalari E, and Goldberg RN: High-frequency ventilation in the neonate, Clinics in Perinatology 14(3), 1987, pp. 581–597.

2. Bancalari E, and Eisler E: Neonatal respiratory support, *in* Kirby RR, Smith RA, and Desametels DA, eds., Mechanical Ventilation, New York, 1985, Churchill Livingston, chap. 7.

3. Goldsmith JP, and Karotkin EH, eds., Assisted Ventilation of the Neonate, Philadelphia, 1988, W.B. Saunders.

4. Avery ME, et al.: Is chronic lung disease in low birth weight infants preventable? A survey of eight centers, Pediatrics 79(1), 1987, pp. 26–30.

5. Mandansky DL, et al.: Pneumothorax and other forms of pulmonary air leak in newborns, American Review of Respiratory Disease 120(4), 1979, pp. 729–737.

6. Northway WH, Rosen RC, and Porter DY: Pulmonary disease following respiratory therapy of hyaline membrane disease, New England Journal of Medicine 276, 1967, pp. 357–368.

7. Workshop on bronchopulmonary dysplasia, Journal of Pediatrics 85 (supplement), 1979, pp. 815–819.

8. Slutsky AS, et al.: High-frequency ventilation: A promising new approach to mechanical ventilation, Medical Instrumentation 15(4), 1981, pp. 229–233.

9. Slutsky AS, et al.: Effective pulmonary ventilation with small volume oscillations at high frequency, Science 209(4456), 1980, pp. 609–671.

10. Special Conference Report: High frequency ventilation for immature infants, Pediatrics 71(2), 1983, pp. 280–287.

11. Henderson Y, Chillingworth FP, and Whitney JL: The respiratory dead space, American Journal of Physiology 38(1), 1915, pp. 1–19.

12. Brisco WR, Foster RE, and Comroe J, Jr.: Alveolar ventilation at very low tidal volumes, Pediatric Research 7(7), 1954, pp. 27–30.

13. Sjostrand U: High frequency positive pressure ventilation (HFPPV): A review, Critical Care Medicine 8(6), 1980, pp. 345–364.

14. Klain M, and Smith RB: High frequency percutaneous transtracheal jet ventilation, Critical Care Medicine 5(6), 1977, pp. 280–287.

15. Carlon GC, et al.: Clinical experience with high frequency jet ventilation, Critical Care Medicine 9(1), 1981, pp. 1–6.

16. Marchak BE, et al.: Treatment of RDS by high frequency oscillatory ventilation: A preliminary report, Journal of Pediatrics 99(2), 1981, pp. 282–287.

17. Pokora T, et al.: Neonatal high frequency jet ventilation, Pediatrics 72(1), 1983, pp. 27–32.

18. Harris TR, and Christensen RD: High frequency jet ventilation of pulmonary interstitial emphysema, Pediatric Research 19(4), 1984, p. 326A.

19. Carlo WA, et al.: Decrease in airway pressure during high-frequency jet ventilation in infants with respiratory distress syndrome, Journal of Pediatrics 104, 1984, pp. 101–107.

20. Frantz I, Werthammer J, and Stark A: High frequency ventilation in premature infants with lung disease: Adequate gas exchange at low tracheal pressure, Pediatrics 71(4), 1983, pp. 483–488.

21. Donn SM, et al.: Proximal high frequency jet ventilation of the newborn, Pediatric Pulmonology 1(5), 1985, pp. 267–271.

22. Mammel MC, et al.: High frequency-jet ventilation: The Children's Hospital of St. Paul experience and viewpoint, Ross Special Conference in Neonatology: Two great debates (program syllabus), 1987, pp. 181–182.

23. Boros SJ, et al.: Neonatal high-frequency jet ventilation: Four years experience, Pediatrics 75(4), 1985, pp. 657–663.

24. Spitzer AR, Butler S, and Fox WW: Ventilatory response to combined high frequency jet ventilation and conventional mechanical ventilation for the rescue treatment of severe neonatal lung disease, Pediatric Pulmonary 7(2), 1989, pp. 244–250.

25. Pauly TH, et al.: Predictability of success of high-frequency jet ventilation in infants with persistent pulmonary hypertension, Ross Special Conference in Neonatology: Two great debates (program syllabus), 1987, p. 172A.

26. Gonzalez F, et al.: Decreased gas flow through pneumothoraces in neonates receiving high-frequency jet ventilation versus conventional ventilation, Journal of Pediatrics 110(3), 1986, pp. 464–466.

27. Keszler M, Donn SM, and Bucciarelli RL: Controlled multicenter trial of high-frequency vs conventional ventilation, Pediatric Research 27(2), 1990, p. 309A.

28. Bodenstein CJ, et al.: VDR-1 programmable high-frequency ventilation in severe neonatal respiratory failure, Ross Special Conference in Neonatology: Two great debates (program syllabus), 1987, pp. 181–182.

29. Pfenninger J, and Gerber AC: High-frequency ventilation in hyaline membrane disease: A preliminary report, Intensive Care Medicine 13(1), 1987, pp. 71–75.

30. Gaylord MS, Quissell BJ, and Lair ME: High frequency ventilation in the treatment of infants weighing less than 1,500 grams with pulmonary interstitial emphysema: A pilot study, Pediatrics 79(6), 1987, pp. 915–921.

31. Gaylord MS, et al.: Predicting mortality in low-birth-weight infants with pulmonary interstitial emphysema, Pediatrics 76(2), 1985, pp. 219–224.

32. Schur MS, et al.: High-frequency jet ventilation in the management of congenital tracheal stenosis, Anesthesiology 68(6), 1988, pp. 952–955.

33. Carlo WA, et al.: Early randomized intervention with high-frequency jet ventilation in respiratory distress syndrome, Journal of Pediatrics 117(5), 1990, pp. 765–770.

34. Mammel MC, et al.: Comparison of high frequency jet ventilation and conventional mechanical ventilation in meconium aspiration syndrome, Journal of Pediatrics 103(4), 1983, pp. 630–634.

35. Trindale O, et al.: Conventional versus high frequency jet ventilation in a piglet model of meconium aspiration: Comparison of pulmonary and hemodynamic effects, Journal of Pediatrics 107(1), 1985, pp. 115–120.

36. Keszler M, et al.: Combined high frequency jet ventilation in a meconium aspiration model, Critical Care Medicine 14(1), 1986, pp. 34–38.

37. Carlo WA, and Martin RJ: Principles of neonatal assisted ventilation, Pediatric Clinics of North America 33(1), 1986, pp. 221–237.

38. Jacob J, et al.: The contribution of PDA in the neonate with severe RDS, Journal of Pediatrics 96(1), 1980, pp. 79–87.

39. Cartwright DW, Willis MM, and Gregory GA: Functional residual capacity and lung mechanics at different levels of mechanical ventilation, Critical Care Medicine 12(5), 1984, pp. 422–427.

40. Frantz I, and Close RH: Elevated lung volumes and alveolar pressure during jet ventilation of rabbits, American Review of Respiratory Disease 131(1), 1985, pp. 134–138.

41. Wetzel RC, and Gioia FR: High frequency ventilation, Pediatric Clinics of North America 34(1), 1987, pp. 15–38.

42. Bunnell JB, Karlson KH, and Shannon DC: High frequency positive pressure ventilation in dogs and rabbits, American Review of Respiratory Diseases 117 (supplement), 1978, pp. 289–294.

43. Johnston J, et al.: Exhalation time effects on arterial and venous blood oxygen content and arterial pCO_2 during high frequency jet ventilation of surfactant depleted cats, Pediatric Pulmonology 3(1), 1987, pp. 19–23.

44. Smith DW, Frankel LR, and Ariagno RL: Influences of ventilator rate and inspiratory time (T_I) on tidal volume (V_T), rate of CO_2 elimination (V_ECO_2) and lung (LV) using the Bunnell Life Pulse high frequency ventilator, Pediatric Pulmonology 3(10), 1987, p. 377A.

45. Korventranta H, et al.: Carbon dioxide elimination during high frequency jet ventilation, Journal of Pediatrics 111(1), 1987, pp. 107–113.

46. Bancalari A, et al.: Gas trapping with high frequency ventilation: Jet versus oscillatory ventilation, Journal of Pediatrics 110(4), 1987, pp. 617–622.

47. Weisberger SA, et al.: Effects of varying inspiratory and expiratory times during high frequency jet ventilation, Journal of Pediatrics 108(4), 1986, pp. 596–600.

48. Chang HK: Mechanisms of gas transport during high frequency ventilation, Journal of Applied Physiology 56(3), 1984, pp. 553–563.

49. Permutt S, Mitzner W, and Weinmonn G: Model of gas transport during high-frequency ventilation, Journal of Applied Physiology 58(6), 1985, pp. 1956–1970.

50. Slutsky AS: Mechanisms affecting gas transport during high frequency oscillation, Critical Care Medicine 12(9), 1984, pp. 713–717.

51. Allen JL, et al.: Alevolar pressure magnitude and a synchrony during high-frequency oscillation of excised rabbit lungs, American Review of Respiratory Diseases 132(2), 1985, pp. 343–349.

52. Haselton FR, and Scherer PW: Bronchial bifurcation of respiratory mass transport, Science 208(4), 1980, pp. 69–71.

53. Scherer PW, and Haselton FR: Convective exchange in oscillatory flow through bronchial-tree models, Journal of Applied Physiology 53(4), 1982, pp. 1023–1033.

54. Taylor GI: Dispersion of matter in turbulent flow through a pipe, Proceeding of the Royal Society of London A, 223, 1954, pp. 446–468.

55. Jaegar MJ, Kursweg UH, and Banner MJ: Transport of gases in high frequency ventilation, Critical Care Medicine 12(9), 1984, pp. 708–710.

56. Bunnell JB: Life Pulse High Frequency Ventilator Operator's Manual, Salt Lake City, 1987, Bunnell, Inc., revision 9.

57. Mammel MC, and Boros SJ: Airway damage and mechanical ventilation: A review and commentary, Pediatric Pulmonology 3(6), 1987, pp. 443–447.

58. Wiswell TE, et al.: Tracheal and bronchial injury in high-frequency oscillatory ventilation and high-frequency flow interruption compared with conventional positive-pressure ventilation, Pediatrics 112(2), 1988, pp. 249–256.

59. Clark RH, et al.: Tracheal and bronchial injury in high-frequency oscillatory ventilation compared with conventional positive pressure ventilation, Journal of Pediatrics 111(1), 1987, pp. 114–118.

60. Kirpalani H, et al.: Diagnosis and therapy of necrotizing tracheobronchitis in ventilated neonates, Critical Care Medicine 13(10), 1985, pp. 792–797.

61. Ophoven JP, et al.: Tracheobronchial histopathology associated with high frequency jet ventilation, Critical Care Medicine 1(9), 1984, pp. 829–832.

62. Boros SJ, et al.: Necrotizing tracheobronchitis: A complication of high-frequency ventilation, Journal of Pediatrics 109(1), 1986, pp. 95–100.

63. Cohen DJ, Baumgart S, and Stephenson LW: Pneumopericardium in neonates: Is it PEEP or is it PIP? Annals of Thoracic Surgery 35(2), 1983, pp. 179–183.

64. Pramanik A, Romero M, and Wissing D: Inadvertent positive end expiratory pressure (PEEP): A complication of high frequency jet ventilation, Pediatric Pulmonology 3(10), 1987, p. 376A.

65. Harris TR, Gooch WM, and Wilson JF: Necrotizing tracheobronchitis associated with high frequency jet ventilation, Clinical Research 32(2), 1984, p. 132A.

66. Pietsch JB, et al.: Necrotizing tracheobronchitis: A new indication for emergency bronchoscopy in the neonate, Journal of Pediatric Surgery 20(4), 1985, pp. 391–393.

67. Karp TB, and Harris TR: Neonatal bronchospasm and its complications, Perinatology-Neonatology 9, 1985, pp. 35–37.

68. Koops BL, Abman SH, and Accurso FJ: Outpatient management and follow-up of bronchopulmonary dysplasia, Clinics in Perinatology 11(1), 1984, pp. 101–122.

69. Bhuntani VK, et al.: Effect of high-frequency jet ventilation on preterm and rabbit tracheal mechanics, Pediatric Pulmonology 2(5), 1986, pp. 327–331.

70. McDowall RJS: The effect of CO_2 on the circulation, part I, Journal of Physiology 70(3), 1930, pp. 301–315.

71. Peckham GJ, and Fox WW: Physiologic factors affecting pulmonary artery pressure in infants with persistent pulmonary hypertension, Pediatrics 93(6), 1978, pp. 1005–1010.

72. Minton S, et al.: Silicone particulate debris in the Life Pulse high frequency jet ventilator, Pediatric Pulmonology 3(10), 1987, p. 375A.

73. Nugent SK, Laravuso R, and Rogers MC: Pharmacology and use of muscle relaxants in infants and children, Journal of Pediatrics 94(3), 1979, pp. 481–487.

74. Swingle HM, Eggert LD, and Bucciarelli RL: New approach to the management of unilateral tension pulmonary interstitial emphysema in premature infants, Pediatrics 74(2), 1984, pp. 354–357.

75. Bunnell JB: Personal communication, Salt Lake City, March 1988.

76. Karp TB, et al.: High frequency jet ventilation: A neonatal nursing perspective, Neonatal Network 4(5), 1986, pp. 42–50.

77. Griffin JP, and Carlon GC: Pulmonary aspects of critical care and rehabilitation, Heart and Lung 13(3), 1984, pp. 250–254.

78. Loder BJ, Guy Y, and Carlon GC: Critical care nurses and high-frequency ventilation, Critical Care Medicine 12(9), 1984, pp. 798–799.

79. Warren TE, and Howell C: High-frequency jet ventilation: A nursing perspective, Heart and Lung 12(4), 1983, pp. 432–437.

80. Gordin P: High-frequency jet ventilation for severe respiratory failure, Pediatric Nursing 15(6), 1989, pp. 625–629.

81. White C, Richardson C, and Rabstein L: High-frequency ventilation and extracorporeal membrane oxygenation, AACN Clinical Issues in Critical Care Nursing 1(2), 1990, pp. 427–444.

82. Kuhns LR, et al.: Diagnosis of pneumothorax or pneumomediastinum in the neonate by transillumination, Pediatrics 56(3), 1975, pp. 354–359.

83. Olson DK, et al.: High frequency jet ventilation: Endotracheal suction procedure, Neonatal Network 4(5), 1986, pp. 66–68.

84. Guntupalli K, Sladen A, and Klain M: High-frequency jet ventilation and tracheobronchial suctioning, Critical Care Medicine 12(9), 1984, pp. 791–792.

85. Kuzenski BM: Effect of negative pressure on tracheobronchial trauma, Nursing Research 27(4), 1978, pp. 260–263.

8 High-Frequency Oscillation

M. Susan Inwood, RN
Mount Sinai Hospital
Toronto, Ontario, Canada

High-frequency oscillation (HFO) is a form of mechanical ventilation still in the experimental stages. Its value as a "rescue" treatment to reduce hypercarbia is well documented, but its use as a primary mode of ventilation has not been completely investigated.

This chapter presents an overview of high-frequency oscillation, including its historical background, the laboratory and clinical experience, and the theories of gas transport. The nursing responsibilities for the oscillated infant are also discussed.

Slutsky and associates first defined high-frequency ventilation (HFV) as any form of mechanical ventilation operating at least four times the normal respiratory rate for that person.[1] This definition was difficult for clinicians because adults, children, and infants all breathe at different rates. The problem is compounded by the variety of mechanisms used to deliver HFV, the most common being high-frequency positive pressure ventilation, high-frequency jet ventilation, and high-frequency oscillation. The complexity increases even more with the combined use of high-frequency and conventional ventilation.

Fortunately, Froese has suggested a sensible solution to the problem of nomenclature based on the single aspect of differentiation between all methods of high-frequency ventilation—the nature of expiration.[2] Only with oscillation is the gas actively pulled out during expiration. All other forms of HFV allow for the passive recoil of the lungs and chest wall to expel the gas. Froese suggests that HFV be divided into two classifications: HFV-A for those systems using active expiratory flow and HFV-P for those with passive expiratory flow.[2]

HISTORICAL PERSPECTIVE

Mechanical ventilation for the neonate suffering from respiratory distress, although common today, has been in clinical use for only the past 20 years.[3] Prior to this, many scientists had attempted to develop devices to assist infants with breathing. The first such instrument for use in resuscitation and short-term ventilation of neonates was developed in France in 1879. A tube with a rubber bulb attached was inserted into the infant's upper airway. Compressions of the bulb produced inspirations and expirations.[4] Shortly after this, Alexander Graham Bell designed and built a body-enclosing machine for negative/positive pressure resuscitation of newborns.[5]

Progress was slow because of an incomplete knowledge of pulmonary physiology and available technology, and this was reflected in the high mortality rate. Swyer, in 1969, reported a mortality rate of greater than 60 percent for infants with respiratory distress syndrome (RDS).[6]

With the introduction of continuous positive airway pressure (CPAP) by Gregory in the early 1970s, positive end-expiratory pressure (PEEP), and improved respiratory technology, the mortality rate decreased.[7] However, many survivors of severe respiratory distress suffered from lung injury associated with mechanical ventilation. Northway and colleagues were the first to describe this lung injury in 1967, naming it bronchopulmonary dysplasia (BPD).[8] The introduction of high-frequency, low-volume ventilation provided neonatologists with an alternative to conventional ventilation and the opportunity to attempt to reduce the serious complications that can occur with this form of treatment.

As early as 1915, Henderson and colleagues had suggested that, contrary to the opinion of physiologists, ventilation could be adequate using tidal volumes less than dead space. Their very simple experiment consisted of blowing smoke through a thin glass tube (Chapter 7, Figure 3). The smoke formed a thin spike rather than filling the tube from side to side in a cylindrical fashion: "The quicker the puff, the thinner the spike." Once the puff stops, "the spike breaks instantly everywhere; and the tube is seen to be filled from side to side with a mixture of smoke and air." They concluded that "a tidal volume even smaller than the volume of dead space may thus afford a very considerable gaseous exchange."[9]

The first person to experiment with high frequencies was John H. Emmerson. In 1959, he invented and patented a device he called an "apparatus for vibrating a patient's airway." He speculated, in his patent application, that "vibrating the column of gas doubtless causes the gas to diffuse more rapidly within the airway and therefore aids in the breathing function by circulating the gas more thoroughly to and from the walls of the lungs." Emmerson even offered a clinical application for his device

when he stated, "another object is to provide an apparatus and method which may be used to expand the lungs of newborn babies when their lungs are initially stuck together."[10] Unfortunately, this line of thinking was not pursued at the time, the equipment was never built, and the patent expired.

As reported in 1980 in an experiment that was not directly related to ventilation, Sjostrand was able to verify Emmerson's claims. During an investigation of the carotid sinus reflex, he encountered problems with artifacts in the recordings of blood pressures and decided that these could be eliminated by increasing the ventilatory rate to 60–100 breaths per minute and by decreasing the tidal volume. He found that gas exchange could be well supported using this system, which was called HFPPV. It has been successfully used in adult and neonatal intensive care as well as during laryngoscopy, bronchoscopy, and general surgery.[11]

Actual experimentation with HFO first started in Germany in 1972. Lunkenheimer and colleagues proposed to study the myocardial response to pericardial pressure oscillations by using a loudspeaker to produce the oscillations, which were then directed down the trachea. It was deemed necessary to render the dogs apneic in order to avoid the interface produced by the respirations on the pericardial pressure. Measurements would therefore be kept brief to avoid carbon dioxide retention. Very much to the surprise of the investigators, carbon dioxide retention did not become a problem, even though the oscillations were delivered for several hours. Because of difficulties encountered with metabolic acidosis and depressed cardiac output, however, further investigations were not pursued by this group.[12]

THEORIES OF GAS TRANSPORT MECHANISMS

Although the theory of Henderson and associates has been amply demonstrated using HFV, understanding of the mechanisms of gas trans-

FIGURE 1 ▲ **Direct ventilation occurs in a fraction of alveoli even if inspired volume is smaller than total anatomical dead space**

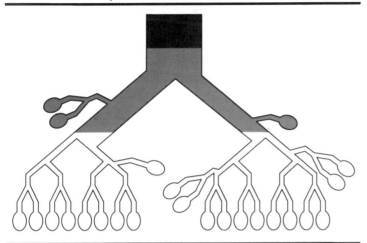

From: Chang HK: Mechanisms of gas transport during ventilation by high-frequency oscillation, Journal of Applied Physiology 56, 1984, pp. 553–563. Reprinted with permission.

port is still not complete. Six different mechanisms appear to contribute to the transportation of gases.[13]

1. Bulk convection. Because the physiology of the human bronchial tree exhibits considerable variation, inspiration of fresh gas will reach only a portion of the total alveoli.[14] The number of alveoli affected will depend on the tidal volume inspired and on the distance from the mouth to the alveoli (Figure 1). Thus HFO, even while using small tidal volumes, can provide some amount of direct alveolar ventilation.

2. "Penduluft" or out-of-phase HFO. The rate of filling and emptying of a particular alveolus depends on two mechanical properties.[13] Compliance describes the elasticity or the ability of the lung to distend. Resistance is the property of the lungs to resist airflow. Both compliance and resistance are used to calculate the time necessary to equalize pressure in the lung unit. The following equation is used to calculate this time constant:[15]

$$Time\ constant\ (seconds) = Resistance\ (cm\ H_2O/liter/second) \times Compliance\ (liter/cm/H_2O)$$

Individual lung units can have different time constants, according to Otis and associates. In 1956, they showed that this would produce disparities between the time it took to fill one alveolus and empty another, resulting in an exchange of gases between neighboring alveoli known as "penduluft."[16] This mechanism may also explain how ventilation occurs in those alveoli not reached by the initial tidal volume.

3. Asymmetric velocity profiles. Based on studies done by Schroter and Sudlow that showed more skewing of the velocity profile in the inspiratory than in the expiratory flow, Hazelton and Scherer

FIGURE 2 ▲ **Illustration of convective exchange mechanism due to asymmetric oscillatory velocity profiles in a tube.**
A uniform bolus (top) is dispersed (middle) because of parabolic velocity profile to the right. On reverse stroke with flat velocity profile, marker material will be transported uniformly to the left (bottom). A net dispersion of initial bolus has occurred as a result of to-and-fro motion with marker particles near center of tube displaced to right and those near wall displaced to left.

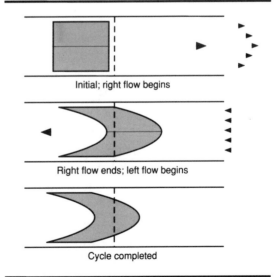

From: Chang HK: Mechanisms of gas transport during ventilation by high-frequency oscillation, Journal of Applied Physiology 56, 1984, pp. 553–563. Reprinted with permission.

FIGURE 3 ▲ Modes of gas transport during high-frequency oscillation and tentative sketch of their zones of dominance. These modes are not mutually exclusive and may interact to achieve efficiency observed in animal or patient studies.

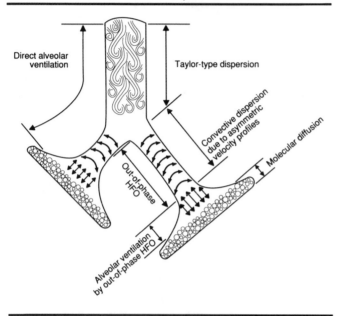

From: Chang HK: Mechanisms of gas transport during ventilation by high-frequency oscillation, Journal of Applied Physiology 56, 1984, pp. 553–563. Reprinted with permission.

proposed that there would be net convective transport of material during oscillation.[17,18] This mechanism is illustrated in Figure 2. Initially, the marker material forms a uniform block. When flow to the right is introduced, there is dispersal to the right, and the velocity profile is parabolic. Reversal of the flow to the left produces a flat velocity profile. The new result is transportation of the marker material at the center of the tube to the right while the material near the wall is displaced to the left. Chang and El Masry found that the peak velocities occurred near the inner wall of the bifurcations, suggesting that the mechanism is most effective at this location.[19]

4. Taylor dispersion. Based on Henderson and coworkers' experiment that showed gas forming a parabolic velocity profile in a straight tube, Taylor described, in 1953, the concept of gas dispersion resulting from the interaction of the axial velocity profile and radial diffusion of gases in motion.[9,20] He showed that, in addition to the forward motion of gas, molecular diffusion along concentration gradients occurs laterally through radial diffusion. This increases gas mixing.[20]

Fredberg was the first to suggest that gas transport during HFV is based on Taylor dispersion.[21] His theory suggests that carbon dioxide elimination depends upon the product of tidal volume and frequency but not on each individually. Later studies showed that tidal volume is more influential than frequency regarding gas exchange.[22,23] Taylor dispersion thus appears to play a role during HFV, but further studies are required to determine the other factors involved.

5. Cardiogenic mixing. Froese and Bryan propose that the lung is constantly subjected to a natural oscillation produced by the action of the pounding of the heart on the lung.[24] Fukuchi and associates showed that the transport of gases in the lung periphery is increased five times during cardiogenic mixing.[25]

6. Molecular diffusion. The gas transport mechanism of molecular diffusion results from the random movement of gas molecules. Creation of a diffusion gradient causes both oxygen and carbon dioxide to be transported across the alveolar capillary membrane. Chang states that "during ventilation by HFO there is no reason to doubt that this role of molecular diffusion is altered."[13]

The mechanisms discussed all appear to play a role in the transport of gas during HFO. None of these is mutually exclusive, and all interact in order to increase gas exchange. The importance of each is not yet fully understood but may well vary in different areas of the lung as shown in Figure 3.

THE MECHANICS OF OSCILLATION

Whenever artificial ventilation is being used, whether conventional or high-frequency, there

FIGURE 4 ▲ **Schematic pressure-volume (P-V) curve of surfactant deficient lung (solid line) bounded by zones of opening (OP) and closing pressure (CP).** Dotted line represents a lung with hyaline membranes showing loss of hysteresis and rise in both opening and closing pressures.

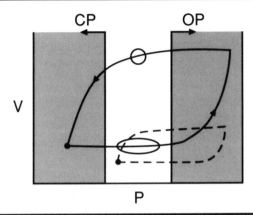

From: Bryan AC: Mechanical ventilation: The role of high-frequency ventilation, *in* Walters DV, and Strang LB, eds., Proceedings of the International Symposium on Physiology and Pathophysiology of the Fetal and Neonatal Lung, Brussels, 1985. Reprinted with permission.

are two basic critical mechanisms at work: oxygenation and carbon dioxide clearance. With conventional mechanical ventilation (CMV), it is difficult to distinguish between oxygen and carbon dioxide regulatory mechanisms. In the presence of hypercarbia, it is necessary to move the gas mechanically in and out of the lungs. With hypoxia as the presenting problem, treatment requires the recruitment of additional lung volume. This calls for adjustments in the CPAP, the PEEP, or the mean airway pressure (MAP, a measure of the average pressure to which the lungs are exposed during the respiratory cycle).

The dilemma with CMV is that making an adjustment in one of these settings can easily alter another. In contrast, HFO provides independent control over the mechanisms that affect oxygen and carbon dioxide.

LUNG VOLUME AND OXYGENATION

In order for a lung to provide adequate gas exchange, there must be good perfusion, a large number of open alveoli, and the presence of gas from the airways. The number of open alveoli is in direct relationship to the MAP. It takes a large amount of pressure, occurring during the late phase of inspiration, to open the diseased lung being ventilated by CMV (Figure 4), and during the expiratory phase, the alveoli will collapse unless PEEP is maintained. Even with PEEP, some loss of open alveoli occurs. Of course, the PEEP can be increased, but the higher pressures can damage tissues and impair circulation.

Because of the rapid delivery of breaths characteristic of oscillation, these continual swings in pressure are not encountered. Therefore, the alveoli remain open continuously as long as the infant receives the oscillations at the set MAP. However, if the infant is disconnected from the circuit (for instance, to be suctioned), then the pressure drops, and the alveoli will collapse. Recruitment of the alveoli can be achieved through a sustained inflation (SI or sigh). The sigh is delivered at a pressure 8–10 cm H_2O higher than the MAP and held for ten seconds before returning to the set MAP.

In order to assess the desired effect of maintaining pressure above the closing or collapsing pressure of the alveoli, a transcutaneous oxygen pressure ($TcPO_2$) monitor is used. A sustained rise in transcutaneous PaO_2 indicates that the pressure is indeed above the closing pressure, alveoli are open, adequate gas exchange is occurring, and the inspired oxygen can be reduced.

However, if the rise in PaO_2 is only transitory, then the MAP must be increased by a small amount and the sigh repeated until a sustained rise in transcutaneous PaO_2 is achieved. Hamilton and colleagues effectively demonstrated this maneuver on adult rabbits following lung lavage (Figure 5).[26]

Froese and Bryan point out that this form of alveolar recruitment is not effective if there is already hyaline membrane disease formation, which may occur after even a few hours of mechanical ventilation.[24]

FIGURE 5 ▲ Plot of arterial oxygen tension (PaO₂) against time for five-hour experiments. Values appearing immediately before and after wide cross-hatched areas represent control values before and after pulmonary lavage. Values appearing before and after narrow cross-hatched area represent presigh and postsigh values. Vertical bars denote standard error (SE).

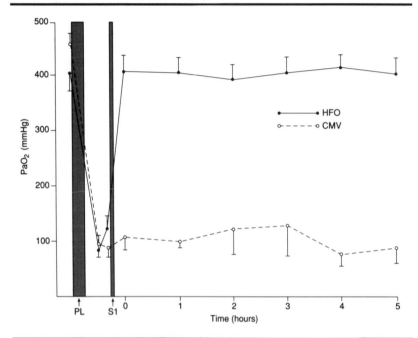

From: Hamilton PP, et al.: Comparison of conventional and high-frequency ventilation: Oxygenation and lung pathology, Journal of Applied Physiology 55, 1983, pp. 131–138. Reprinted with permission.

CARBON DIOXIDE ELIMINATION

Tidal volume and frequency are the two factors controlling the elimination of carbon dioxide during HFO, as they are with CMV. Difficulties in altering these parameters without changing the pressures are encountered with conventional ventilation. This is not a problem with HFO. The tidal volume is adjusted with changes to the amplitude or peak-to-peak pressure that has been generated by the stroke volume of the piston. Monitoring of the infant's carbon dioxide either by transcutaneous monitor or blood gases will provide the best information as to what setting is required for the amplitude. The measurement of the amplitude is taken at the endotracheal tube connector, which will provide a much higher reading than that in the lower respiratory tract.

The frequency used during HFO is 15 Hertz (1 Hz = 1 cycle/second), which delivers 900 breaths per minute. Bohn and associates describe this as the ideal frequency because carbon dioxide elimination reaches a plateau at higher frequencies.[27]

THE HFO CIRCUIT

The delivery of fresh gas is from a wall source through a blender and is controlled by a flow meter. This gas is directed through a heating and humidification system, then through the inspiratory tubing to the endotracheal tube. The oscillator creates the high-frequency oscillations at a preselected rate or frequency of 15 Hz by means of a piston pump. The oscillations are directed along a second tubing to the endotracheal tube and are there superimposed on the fresh gas flow.

The expiratory tubing connected to the endotracheal tube provides for the exit of the expired gases. A low-pass filter on the expiratory circuit provides a low resistance to the oscilations, thus directing them to the baby, the path of least resistance. In some systems, a Venturi jet provides further resistance (Figure 6).

The ratio between the fresh gas flow entering the circuit and the resistance provided by the expiratory line and the low-pass filter determines the MAP. Leaks in the system will cause a decrease in MAP. The sigh is delivered by stopping the oscillation motor and increasing the expiratory resistance until the desired pressure is attained.

Because oxygenation is controlled by the MAP and carbon dioxide elimination by the amplitude, weaning is accomplished by independently reducing these settings on the oscillator, as indicated by the $PaCO_2$ and PaO_2, until CPAP has been achieved.

EXPERIENCE WITH HFO

As was previously mentioned, Lunkenheimer and his coworkers abandoned their work with HFO after their unsatisfactory experiences with acidosis, but others have reopened this area of investigation.[12] In 1980, Bohn and associates published data demonstrating that HFO can support both carbon dioxide elimination and oxygenation without incurring problems of cardiac dysfunction or acidosis. They applied high-frequency oscillation to anesthetized dogs with normal lung function. A piston pump, which allowed for altering both amplitude and frequency, was used to provide oscillations. It was found that the optimal frequency for carbon dioxide elimination was 15 Hz. The arterial oxygen and carbon dioxide tensions remained normal throughout five hours of uninterrupted oscillations.[27]

Butler and coworkers then went one step further by investigating the use of HFO in the presence of lung disease. In 1980, they reported the successful use of HFO with a group of patients ranging in age from 3 days to 74 years. The patients required ventilation for a variety of reasons, including support following vascular surgery, respiratory disease due to RDS or chronic obstructive pulmonary disease, and septic shock. Each received up to one hour of HFO using a piston pump at frequencies of 15 Hz. Excellent gas exchange without cardiac impairment was achieved in all patients. The investigators also concluded that HFO may reduce barotrauma because it causes little distension of the lung.[28]

FIGURE 6 ▲ Breathing circuit for the high-frequency oscillator

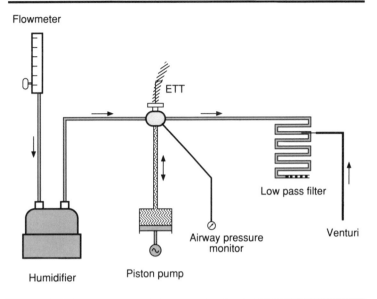

From: Inwood S, Finley GA, and Fitzhardinge PM: High-frequency oscillation: A new mode of ventilation for the neonate, Neonatal Network 4(5), 1986, pp. 53–58. Reprinted with permission.

Further research involving the diseased lung was reported by Marchak and associates in 1981. They studied eight neonates with severe RDS ranging in age from 12 to 60 hours. A piston pump was used to deliver oscillations with frequencies ranging from 8 to 20 Hz. The study time ranged from 67 to 233 minutes. Prior to oscillation, while receiving CMV, an FiO_2 of 0.66 ± 0.15 achieved a PaO_2 of 59.6 ± 17 mmHg. With HFO, a mean FiO_2 of only 0.41 ± 0.11 was required to provide similar oxygenation. However, they concluded that "a higher mean airway pressure need not mean greater distension of the lung."[29] This study showed that HFO is effective in promoting gas exchange in infants with RDS. It also clarified the relationship between mean airway pressure and oxygenation.

Kolton and his group used rabbits to compare oxygenation during CMV and HFO. They induced two different pulmonary injuries in the animals: one using oleic acid, the other by lung lavage with physiologic saline. Each animal was ventilated with HFO, then with CMV, using the same MAP.[30] The importance of the sustained inflation maneuver during HFO, in order to achieve larger lung volume and better oxygenation, was clearly demonstrated in this experiment.

With the realization that HFO could provide adequate gas exchange, studies progressed from patients with RDS to those with pulmonary interstitial emphysema (PIE), a respiratory condition in which gas is trapped throughout the interstitium, with dissection into the perivascular, peribronchial, and bronchial spaces.[31,32] This trapping decreases lung compliance, requiring higher pressures to achieve adequate ventilation.

Clark and coworkers reported the use of HFO on 27 infants who developed PIE while receiving CMV. Although 10 patients died (6 with documented sepsis), all showed initial improvement in oxygenation, with decreasing MAP. These researchers concluded that HFO was an effective mode of ventilation in treating PIE and hypothesized that the interstitial air leaks decrease during HFO because of lower peak distal airway pressures.[32]

In a study addressing the issue of the safety and efficacy of HFO when used as the primary method of ventilation, Froese and colleagues compared infants who were randomized to either HFO or CMV. The MAPs used in HFO was greater than those used in CMV, with an aggressive protocol designed for rapid FiO_2 reduction. For those infants treated with HFO, a sustained inflation (SI) was delivered after each disconnection when there was a demonstrated decrease in transcutaneous oxygenation. This was delivered at a MAP of 5–10 cm/H_2O above the maintenance MAP for 15–20 seconds. The efficacy of this form of treatment was based on adequate gas exchange, which was easily achieved. The issue of safety was judged on the incidence of pulmonary complications. The authors concluded that the experimental ventilator is safe because no infant treated solely with HFO developed BPD. In addition, no

new hazards were noted (i.e., adequate humidification was maintained, and there were no incidences of necrotizing tracheitis). The importance of the SI was also commented upon; it was noted to reverse early atelectasis and allow for rapid, early reduction of oxygen if adequate MAP was used to keep the lungs expanded.[33]

Cortambert and his colleagues compared 17 premature infants born in 1986 who had RDS and were treated with HFO with retrospective data compiled on 16 prematures born in 1985 with a similar degree of RDS who had been treated with CMV. The results showed a significant difference in mortality rates between the two groups. Ten (62.5 percent) of the infants treated with CMV died—6 from pulmonary and 4 from neurological causes (Grade 4 intraventricular hemorrhage and/or periventricular leukomalacia). Six (35.3 percent) of those ventilated with HFO died—2 from pulmonary and 4 from neurological causes. During the course of ventilation, there was no difference in the incidence of complications, either pulmonary or neurological, between the two groups. There were 2 cases of BPD in the 6 survivors who had been ventilated with CMV but none in those treated with HFO.[34]

The most recent clinical study is a multicenter, randomized trial conducted by the HIFI Study Group and sponsored by the National Heart, Lung, and Blood Institute of Bethseda, Maryland. In order to test the hypothesis that HFO is the better form of treatment for respiratory failure, 673 premature babies, weighing between 750 and 2,000 gm, were randomized to either CMV or HFO as the primary means of ventilation. High-frequency oscillation was provided by a piston-driven oscillator, Hummingbird model 20N, Senko Medical Instruments Manufacturing Co., Ltd., Tokyo, Japan, as shown in Figure 7.[35]

Results indicated no significant difference in the incidence of BPD: Thirty-nine percent in the HFO group were diagnosed with BPD as compared to 41 percent in the CMV group.

FIGURE 7 ▲ The Hummingbird Oscillator, Model 20N from Senko Medical Instruments Manufacturing Company, Limited, Tokyo, Japan

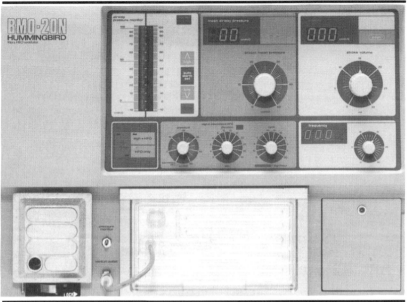

Reprinted with permission of Senko Medical Instrument Mfg. Co. Ltd.

This diagnosis was based on the need for oxygen for more than 28 days and radiological evidence of chronic lung changes. Other parameters—days on oxygen, mortality, pneumothoraces, and length of hospital stay—were also not statistically significant. There was, however, an increase in incidence of Grade 3 or 4 hemorrhage in the HFO group, 26 percent against 18 percent in the control group ($p = .02$), as well as an increase in periventricular leukomalasia in the HFO group, 12 percent versus 7 percent ($p = .02$). The investigators concluded that HFO "as used in this trial, offers no significant advantage over CMV in the treatment of respiratory failure in preterm infants and may be associated with undesirable side effects."[35]

However, there has been some controversy over these conclusions. Froese, in a letter to the editor of the *New England Journal of Medicine*, indicated that the use of the "lowest possible peak and mean airway pressures" was not the best method to achieve lung reexpansion. She also felt that the SI was not fully understood at the time of the study design, and had its use been built into the study, the

outcome could have been different.[36]

The HIFI Study Group responded by stating that the protocol called for a sigh following suctioning but, due to concerns about air leaks and intracranial hemorrhage, additional sighs were optional.[36]

Further analysis of the data from the HIFI Study Group was offered by I. D. Franz, one of the study investigators. He observed that the study allowed for crossover from the randomized form of treatment to the other mode. This could occur if there was treatment failure, based on strict criteria. A total of 25 percent of all infants entered into the study were crossed over, but data analysis maintained the infants in their assigned groups. If the data were analyzed without these infants, the results regarding the Grade 3 or 4 hemorrhage becomes smaller and no longer statistically significant. Again, by addressing the data in a different manner, the rates of hemorrhage between study centers were vastly different, ranging from 6 percent to 48 percent.[37]

The studies described here have certainly demonstrated the effectiveness of HFO in providing adequate gas exchange, but they do not completely address the issue of whether HFO is more effective in reducing damage to the lungs. Nor do they provide adequate follow-up data on these infants. The HIFI Study Group is following their patients to 18 months corrected age but has yet to publish its results.

CRITERIA FOR HFO USE IN RESCUE THERAPY

Because HFO is still deemed an experimental form of ventilation, it is not used as the primary method of treatment but solely for "rescue" ventilation. There have been no set criteria for HFO use among neonatal patients. Essentially, infants presenting with severe respiratory distress due to RDS, PIE, persistent pulmonary hypertension of the newborn, or pneumonia in whom hypercarbia and hypoxia persist regardless of numerous adjustments to conventional ventilation, are candidates for HFO.

TABLE 1 ▲ Nursing Responsibilities and Interventions for Oscillated Infants Prior to HFO

Responsibility	Intervention
Obtain and record baseline physiological data.	Record temperature, heart rate, respiratory rate, systolic and diastolic blood pressure, $TcPO_2$ and $TcPCO_2$.
Obtain and record baseline biochemical data.	Draw blood samples for arterial gases.
Maintain current ventilation.	Record ventilator parameters: rate, peak inspiratory pressure (PIP), positive end expiratory pressure (PEEP), mean airway pressure (MAP), inspiratory-expiratory ratio, FiO_2.
Assemble and prepare equipment.	Ensure that infant is attached to monitoring devices for heart rate, intra-arterial blood pressure, transcutaneous oxygen and carbon dioxide.
	Check alarms on all monitors.
	Assist with arterial line insertion.

High-frequency oscillation has also been used in treating patients with congenital diaphragmatic hernia for its effectiveness in lowering $PaCO_2$ and raising the pH while using minimal peak pressures and MAP.[38,39] Several centers have reported success in utilizing HFO as an alternative to extracorporeal membrane oxygenation, particularly in infants presenting with severe RDS and pneumonia.[40,41].

The use of HFO is contraindicated for patients with meconium aspiration because the thick meconium in the airways acts as a high resistance to the oscillated gas flow, thus directing the flow away from the baby and out the expiratory tubing.

IMPLICATIONS FOR NURSING

The clinical use of HFO is still experimental, so there is little literature available regarding nursing care.[42] Other forms of HFV, specifically HFJV, have well-documented nursing care plans.[43–45] Development of nursing care plans for patients on HFO have evolved from those in use for conventionally ventilated patients, incorporating specifics for HFO patients. As clinical experience increases, so will our knowledge regarding nursing care.

Providing care for the critically ill infant requiring HFO necessitates a multidisci-

plinary approach. Physicians, nurses, and respiratory therapists combine their expertise in managing these patients. One-to-one nursing is usually the ratio for the infant being oscillated as a rescue treatment. However, in a recent study being conducted in our hospital where HFO was used as the primary ventilation, a two-to-one infant-nurse ratio was used quite successfully.[35]

Although nursing care is similar to that given to infants being ventilated with CMV, the nurse must be aware of the differences in theory regarding HFO and its implications for nursing care (Tables 1 and 2). Baseline measurements must be taken while the infant is receiving CMV. These measurements of heart rate, respiratory rate, blood pressure, arterial blood values, transcutaneous oxygen and carbon dioxide, and FiO_2 will provide data regarding the effectiveness of HFO once the switch to oscillation has occurred. An arterial line allows easy access for gas sampling as well as arterial systemic pressure.

The nurse must be aware that because HFO is still an experimental form of therapy; the physician must obtain informed consent from the parents or legal guardian for its use. The parents are already stressed by the premature delivery and the serious illness affecting their baby. They may be over-whelmed by these circum-stances and by the technology being used on their tiny infant. Reactions will vary from grief and anger to euphoria.

Communication be-tween parents and staff is an important aspect of parental care during this time of crisis. The nurse must be available to inter-pret information, ensuring that parents understand the medical terminology, and to offer continuing sup-port. It is not unusual for parents to repeatedly ask the same questions. The nurse must be prepared for this behavior and be patient while the parents work through this period. Par-ents should be encouraged to interact with their baby; stroking or holding hands will not interfere with oscil-lation. In addition to the support offered by the bedside nurse, the parents should be encouraged to attend parent support groups or be referred to the services of a clinical nurse special-ist or a social worker.

The most striking fea-ture of HFO treatment is the shaking of the infant.

TABLE 2 ▲ Nursing Responsibilities and Interventions for Oscillated Infants During Oscillation

Responsibility	Intervention
Monitor and document physiological parameters.	Record hourly—temperature, heart rate, spontaneous respirations, systolic and diastolic blood pressure.
	Measure and record accurate intake and output of fluids every 8 hours.
Monitor and document biochemical parameters.	Draw arterial blood gases as ordered.
Maintain patent airway.	Monitor for continuous vibration of chest.
	Assess $TcPO_2$ and $TcPCO_2$ hourly.
	Perform endotracheal suctioning every 2 hours and prn.
	Record amount, color, and consistency of secretions.
	Assess bilateral air entry while hand bagging at sigh pressures, pre- and post-suctioning.
	Ensure adequate humidification of gas flow.
Prevent pneumothorax.	Maintain ordered MAP.
	Observe for decreased vibrations of the chest.
	Assess infant for signs of respiratory difficulty: increased spontaneous respirations, increased chest retractions, diminished air entry, increased FiO_2 requirements, increased $TcPCO_2$ readings.
	Obtain chest x-ray film as required, ensuring that oscillator is stopped during filming.
Provide pulmonary support.	Monitor and record MAP, amplitude, frequency, and FiO_2 hourly.
	Perform a sustained inflation after endotracheal suctioning and disconnection at ordered pressure and duration.
	Record infant's response to sigh.
Provide physical care.	Reposition infant from side to side, or prone to supine every 2 hours.
Provide emotional support to the family.	Provide accurate, consistent information.
	Promote bonding by encouraging nurse specialist or social worker for assistance with coping skills.
	Encourage parents to attend parents' support group.

This is most visible in the thorax and the abdomen; however, it can extend to the hands and feet, depending on the amplitude and the weight of the baby. Assessing the motion is very subjective, but the nurse must note this movement because a decrease without an amplitude change indicates that oscillated gas flow is not reaching the baby. A blocked or displaced tube, machine failure, or a pneumothorax may be the reason for this change.

The oscillated infant's breathing pattern is radically different from that of one receiving

CMV. Researchers have noted that apnea occurs at normocarbia during HFO.[28,29] Apnea is most prevalent during the immediate postnatal period when only brief periods of spontaneous respiration occur during rapid eye movement (REM) sleep. As the infant gets older, REM sleep is the more common state, so the nurse will see an increase in the amount of spontaneous breathing and decrease in apnea.

Because of the amount of noise produced in the chest with HFO, the nurse must disconnect the baby from the oscillator and hand bag him to assess air entry. In our nursery, we bag at the pressures used to deliver a sustained inflation and observe for chest movement. Once air entry has been assessed, oscillations are restarted, and a sigh is delivered if ordered.

The nurse should pay careful attention to the carbon dioxide measurements, either $TcPCO_2$ or $PaCO_2$, especially when the baby is first placed on the oscillator. Infants requiring the rescue treatment of oscillation generally are hypercarbic. High-frequency oscillation is quite effective at decreasing carbon dioxide, but careful adjustment of the amplitude is required so that the reverse trend of hypocarbia is avoided. Constant transcutaneous carbon dioxide monitoring is recommended for the first 36 hours of HFO treatment.

Suctioning the oscillated infant requires the same sterile technique as that for babies receiving CMV. However, a sustained inflation may be delivered to the baby once suctioning is completed in order to reexpand the lungs and allow for adequate gas exchange. Following suctioning, the amount, color, and consistency of secretions are recorded. The nurse will also note the sigh pressure delivered, the duration of the sigh, the number of times the sigh was performed, and the baby's response to the sigh as indicated by the $TcPO_2$ monitor.

Chest x-ray examinations are done as clinically indicated. The nurse should turn the oscillator off during the moment of filming because its vibrations create motion artifact on the film, making it unreadable and requiring a repeat x-ray.

Although there is no literature available regarding feeding the oscillated infant, it has been our experience that institution of feedings on our regular schedule for ventilated infants has not been detrimental. Intermittent gavage feedings are usually started 48 hours after delivery, beginning with one feed of dextrose and then changing to breast milk or formula. The volume is gradually increased as the intravenous volume is decreased.

The oscillated baby can be placed in an incubator and may be repositioned as needed. The prone position somewhat limits the assessment of shaking, but careful attention to other assessment tools ($TcPO_2$ and $TcPCO_2$ probes) will make the nurse aware of potential problems. Sedation is not generally necessary because these infants do not fight the oscillator. Other areas of concern, such as fluid management and treatment of hyperbilirubinemia, are managed following usual procedures.

COMPLICATIONS

In caring for the oscillated baby, the nurse must be aware of the complications that may arise from this mode of ventilation, including presentation, possible causes, and treatment. The two complications discussed here—a blocked or displaced endotracheal tube and pneumothorax—relate directly to the respiratory system. No other complications have yet been identified in the literature.

As with the conventionally ventilated infant, the endotracheal tube in the oscillated infant may become blocked or displaced. Blocking due to decreased humidification is not a major problem, as it can be with HFJV. However, a blocked tube can be caused by increased secretions or inadequate suctioning. The nurse will observe that chest vibrations will lessen, the $TcPCO_2$ will gradually climb, the required FiO_2 will increase, and the infant may either start to have spontaneous respirations or the rate of spontaneous respirations already present will increase.

Physiologically, gas exchange is not occurring: The blockage in the tube creates an impedance to the oscillations, which then take the path of least resistance and exit via the expiratory tubing. Assessment of air entry is required to differentiate between a blocked and a displaced tube. The treatment calls for suctioning and/or replacing the blocked or displaced tube.

When a pneumothorax occurs in an oscillated baby, it does not present in the sudden, life-threatening manner as with a baby receiving CMV. The gradual increase in carbon dioxide and the slow but steady fall in $TcPO_2$ are subtle signs that will alert the nurse. This allows for a controlled situation whereby the necessary equipment and personnel can be mobilized to take the appropriate action. Transillumination and/or a chest x-ray may be required to confirm the diagnosis. Physiologically, the loss of available alveoli for adequate gas exchange accounts for the increased need for oxygen and the increasing carbon dioxide. As with a CMV patient, standard treatment is chest tube insertion.

FUTURE DIRECTIONS

Though its value as a "rescue" treatment is well documented scientifically, high-frequency oscillation as a primary method of ventilation still needs to be investigated. Also, the timing and the technique of the recruitment of lung volume by means of the sustained inflation must be researched further. It is still not known whether oscillation reduces the amount of barotrauma as compared to conventional ventilation. Follow-up data are as yet nonexistent, leaving a large gap in our knowledge of these infants.

Research is continuing worldwide. In Japan, a large trial is being conducted using an updated model of the Hummingbird, which can provide both HFO and CMV and is being used for both rescue and primary ventilation. Further investigations are being conducted in France using a different machine. And in many research centers throughout the United States and Canada, high-frequency oscillation is attracting scientists' attention.

High-frequency oscillation will continue to be the focus of research for many years, and the day may come when it will be used frequently in neonatal intensive care nurseries.

REFERENCES

1. Slutsky AS, et al.: High-frequency ventilation: A promising new approach to mechanical ventilation, Medical Instrumentation 15, 1981, pp. 229–233.
2. Froese AB: High-frequency ventilation: Current status, Canadian Anaesthetist's Society Journal 31(supplement), 1984, pp. 9–12.
3. Silverman WA, et al.: A controlled trial of management of respiratory distress syndrome in a body-enclosing respirator: Evaluation of safety, Pediatrics 39, 1967, pp. 740–748.
4. Daily WJR, and Smith PC: Mechanical ventilation of the newborn infant I, Current Problems in Pediatrics 1, June 1971, pp. 1–37.
5. Stern L, et al.: Negative pressure artificial respiration: Use in treatment of respiratory failure of the newborn, Canadian Medical Association Journal 182, 1970, pp. 595–601.
6. Swyer PR: An assessment of artificial respiration in the newborn, *in* Problems of Neonatal Care Unit, Report of the 59th Ross Conference on Pediatric Research, Columbus, Ohio, 1969, pp. 25–35.
7. Gregory GA, et al.: Treatment of the idiopathic respiratory distress syndrome with continuous positive airway pressure, New England Journal of Medicine 284, 1971, pp. 1333–1340.
8. Northway WH, Jr, Rosen RC, and Porter DY: Pulmonary disease following respirator therapy of hyaline-membrane disease, New England Journal of Medicine 276, 1967, pp. 357–368.
9. Henderson Y, Chillingworth FP, and Whitney JL: The respiratory dead space, American Journal of Physiology 38, 1915, pp. 1–19.
10. Emmerson J: Apparatus for vibrating portions of a patient's airway, U.S. Patent #2,918,917, December 1959.
11. Sjostrand U: High-frequency positive-pressure ventilation (HFPPV): A review, Critical Care Medicine 8, 1980, pp. 345–364.
12. Lunkenheimer PP, et al.: Experimental studies with high-frequency oscillation, International Anesthesiology Clinics 21, 1983, pp. 51–62.
13. Chang HK: Mechanism of gas transport during ventilation by high-frequency oscillation, Journal of Applied Physiology 56, 1984, pp. 553–563.
14. Horsfield K, et al.: Models of the human bronchial tree, Journal of Applied Physiology 31, 1971, pp. 202–217.
15. Carlo WA, and Martin RJ: Principles of neonatal assisted ventilation, Pediatric Clinics of North America 33, 1986, pp. 221–237.

16. Otis AB, et al.: Mechanical factors in distribution of pulmonary ventilation, Journal of Applied Physiology 8, 1956, pp. 427–443.

17. Schroter RC, and Sudlow MF: Flow patterns in models of the human bronchial airways, Respiratory Physiology 7, 1981, pp. 341–355.

18. Hazelton FR, and Scherer PW: Flow visualization of steady streaming in oscillatory flow through a bifurcating tube, Journal of Fluid Mechanics 123, 1982, pp. 315–373.

19. Chang HK, and El Masry OA: A model study of flow dynamics in human central airways I: Axial velocity profiles, Respiratory Physiology 49, 1982, pp. 75–95.

20. Taylor G: The dispersion of matter in turbulent flow through a pipe, Proceedings of the Royal Society: Series A (London) 56, 1954, pp. 553–563.

21. Fredberg JJ: Augmented diffusion in the airways can support pulmonary gas exchange, Journal of Applied Physiology: Respiratory Environmental Exercise Physiology 49, 1980, pp. 232–238.

22. Brusasco V, Knopp TJ, and Rehder K: Gas transport during high-frequency ventilation, Journal of Applied Physiology: Respiratory Environmental Exercise Physiology 55, 1983, pp. 472–478.

23. Fletcher PR, and Epstein RA: Constancy of physiological dead space during high frequency ventilation, Respiratory Physiology 47, 1986, pp. 39–49.

24. Froese AB, and Bryan AC: High frequency ventilation, American Review of Respiratory Diseases 135, 1987, pp. 1363–1374.

25. Fukuchi Y, et al.: Convection, diffusion and cardiogenic mixing of inspired gas in the lung: An experimental approach, Respiratory Physiology 26, 1976, pp. 77–90.

26. Hamilton PP, et al.: Comparison of conventional and high-frequency ventilation: Oxygenation and lung pathology, Journal of Applied Physiology 55, 1983, pp. 131–138.

27. Bohn DJ, et al.: Ventilation by high-frequency oscillation, Journal of Applied Physiology 48, 1980, pp. 710–716.

28. Butler WJ, et al.: Ventilation by high-frequency oscillation in humans, Anesthesia and Analgesia 59, 1980, pp. 577–584.

29. Marchak BE, et al.: Treatment of RDS by high-frequency oscillatory ventilation: A preliminary report, Journal of Pediatrics 99, 1981, pp. 287–292.

30. Kolton M, et al.: Oxygenation during high-frequency ventilation compared with conventional mechanical ventilation in two models of lung injury, Anesthesia and Analgesia 61, 1982, pp. 323–332.

31. Franz ID, Werthammer J, and Stark AR: High-frequency ventilation in premature infants with lung disease: Adequate gas exchange at low tracheal pressure, Pediatrics 71, 1983, pp. 483–488.

32. Clark RH, et al.: Pulmonary interstitial emphysema treated by high-frequency oscillatory ventilation, Critical Care Medicine 14, 1986, pp. 926–930.

33. Froese AB, et al.: High-frequency oscillatory ventilation in premature infants with respiratory failure: A preliminary report, Anesthesia and Analgesia 66, 1987, pp. 814–824.

34. Cortambert F, et al.: Ventilation a haute frequence par oscillation dans le traitement de la maladie des membranes hyalines de forme severe, Resultats preliminaires, unpublished data.

35. The HIFI Study Group: High frequency oscillatory ventilation compared with conventional mechanical ventilation in the treatment of respiratory failure in preterm infants, New England Journal of Medicine 320, 1989, pp. 88–93.

36. Froese AB: Letter to the editor, New England Journal of Medicine 320, 1989, pp. 1694–1695.

37. Franz ID: Newer methods for treatment of respiratory distress, Ross Conference on Pediatric Research, Carefree, Arizona, May 1989.

38. Karl SR, Ballantyne TVN, and Snider MT: High-frequency ventilation at rates of 375 to 1800 cycles per minute in four neonates with congenital diaphragmatic hernia, Journal of Pediatric Surgery 18, 1983, pp. 822–828.

39. Boynton BR, et al.: Combined high-frequency oscillatory ventilation and intermittent mandatory ventilation in critically ill neonates, Journal of Pediatrics 105, 1984, pp. 297–302.

40. Rosenberg R, et al.: High frequency ventilation for acute respiratory failure, an alternative to ECMO, (abstract) 7th Annual Children's National Medical Center ECMO Symposium, Feb. 1991.

41. Null D: Alternative therapies: high frequency ventilation, (proceedings) 7th Annual Children's National Medical Center ECMO Symposium, Feb. 1991.

42. Inwood S, Finley GA, and Fitzhardinge PM: High-frequency oscillation: A new mode of ventilation for the neonate, Neonatal Network 4, 1986, pp. 53–58.

43. Karp TB, et al.: High frequency jet ventilation: A neonatal nursing perspective, Neonatal Network 4, 1986, pp. 42–50.

44. Kaplow R, and Fromme LR: Nursing care plan for the patient receiving high-frequency jet ventilation, Critical Care Nursing 5, 1985, pp. 25–27.

45. Warren TE, and Howell C: High-frequency jet ventilation: A nursing perspective, Heart and Lung 12, 1983, pp. 432–437.

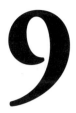

9 Surfactant Replacement

Louis Gluck, MD
University of California
Irvine, California

Jan Nugent, RNC, MSN
Ochsner Foundation Hospital
New Orleans, Louisiana

Successful surfactant replacement is a new and exciting therapy—one which has been considered and trailed since surfactant deficiency in neonatal respiratory distress syndrome (RDS) was initially implicated. The earliest surfactant replacement experiments, first attempted around 25 years ago, met with little success. However, recent clinical trials have demonstrated that surfactant replacement therapy can reverse the pulmonary insufficiency of RDS. It must be cautioned that confounding factors, most of which stem from a poor understanding of the pathophysiology of RDS, may hamper its effectiveness. Specifically, there is an inadequate appreciation of the role of the patent ductus arteriosus (PDA) in RDS. Until it is understood how to manage the PDA in infants with RDS, only partially effective or even poor results from surfactant replacement can be predicted.

This chapter discusses lung development; surfactant function, development, and chemistry; the relationship of RDS and PDA; and the experience with surfactant replacement to date. It highlights the fallacies in the understanding of the etiology and course of RDS, a number of which have become widely accepted in neonatal/perinatal medicine. The effect of these, unfortunately, has been to encourage widespread inappropriate therapy and to engender more and more chronic lung disease.

LUNG DEVELOPMENT

The lung develops very early, arising at about 25 days of embryonic life from an outpouching of the primitive gut that branches and sub-branches. After 17 subdivisions, at about 26 weeks gestation, the alveolar ducts and the beginnings of the alveoli are formed. The alveoli are complex structures requiring about 7 more divisions, to a total of approximately 24 divisions, maturing at about 31–32 weeks gestation. Twenty-six weeks gestation is crucial because this marks the time of viability for the fetus.

The basic alveolus consists of a capillary mesh overlaid with two types of cells:

▶ Type I cells are the major cells for oxygenation and carbon dioxide diffusion. They are extremely thin, flattened, and attenuated—much like large sheets. These cells are thus adapted to provide a huge surface area for oxygen and carbon dioxide exchange. They occupy the major part of the alveolus and cover the capillaries.

▶ Type II cells manufacture, store, and secrete surfactant into the alveoli. They are large, cuboidal, and arranged in no discernible pattern. They contain intracellular lamellar inclusion bodies, which progressively fill these cells during gestation. These lamellar bodies are the sites of synthesis and storage of surfactant and are ejected whole into alveoli as the means of releasing surfactant.

Fetal alveoli are not empty. They contain fluid secreted under pressure into which the lamellar bodies are excreted. The fluid with its lamellar bodies is carried into the amniotic fluid, partly with the help of cilia farther up in the respiratory tract.

The unique alveolar structure with its complex subdivisions forming a single alveolus also forms a huge cross-sectional area. If the cross-sectional area of the tubular airways is measured against the velocity of air traveling in the respiratory tract, it is found that *the flow of tidal volume stops at the level of the respiratory bronchioles*—that is, tidal volume with each breath normally does not extend into the alveoli. *The exchange of gases in the alveoli occurs purely by diffusion.*

Clinically, this is a major consideration in the problem of the wet alveolus in the infant with RDS. When such an infant is managed with extensive mechanical ventilation, the tidal volume is pounded by the ventilator into the alveoli, which normally receive none. This is almost a guarantee that this ventilation, together with high concentrations of oxygen, will result in significant and sometimes extensive lung damage.

Eventually, the fetus is born and becomes an air breather. The alveolar fluid is replaced by air, although a layer of water remains on top of the alveolar lining cells. Careful studies have demonstrated that there is a layer of surfactant on the surface of the water layer on top of the Type I cells.[1] The surfactant thus sits at the interface between the air and water in the alveolus. In so doing, it acts in its absolutely essential role as a biological detergent to lower the surface tension at this air/water interface.

SURFACTANT

As a biological detergent whose primary function is to lower the surface tension of the water surface, surfactant opposes the collapsing effect of the extreme intermolecular attraction among the water molecules of the surface layer. In the clinical setting, the effect of surface tension is to make the water layer as small an area as possible. The water tension is so high that, if unopposed, it will collapse the tiny 50 μm diameter alveoli of the premature infant. Because of surfactant's reduction of this surface tension, the alveoli stay open and do not collapse on expiration.

Surfactant thus functions to *stabilize alveoli at low lung volumes on exhalation*. Clinically, the *initiation of RDS* occurs with expiratory instability: The baby, who lacks adequate surfactant, breathes out and begins the progressive collapse of lung—the hallmark of RDS.

Surfactant is a mixture of about 90 percent lipid and 10 percent protein. The lipid is composed of about 90 percent phospholipids and 10 percent cholesterol, cholesterol esters, free fatty acids, and mono-, di-, and triglycerides. The proteins are a confusing assortment of various molecular weights. Many claims for functions of these proteins have been made, but none has been clearly demonstrated. Some of the proteins even have been cloned at a tremendous effort and expense. However, the clinical necessity for the proteins remains unknown.

The surfactant phospholipids include two major classes. First, the glycerophospholipids are derivatives of the three-carbon alcohol, glycerol, to which two fatty acids are esterified on the first and second carbons. A phosphate is esterified on the third carbon, giving the basic prefix "phosphatidyl-" for this group of compounds. Attached to the phosphate molecule is another compound that gives the phospholipid both its name and its chemical characteristics; for example, choline plus phosphate would produce the compound, phosphatidylcholine.

The major glycerophospholipids in surfactant include *phosphatidylcholine,* better known as *lecithin, phosphatidylinositol,* and *phosphatidylglycerol.* Lecithin is the major component, accounting for 50–70 percent of the total phospholipids in surfactant. As the lung matures, lecithin concentration increases. Its fatty acids (principally palmitic acid) become progressively more saturated and consequently more active. Phosphatidylinositol and phosphatidylglycerol are synthesized by a different reaction than that of lecithin, but they compete with each other for their synthesis.

The second class, the sphingolipids, represented by sphingomyelin, contain a long-chain sphingosine (rather than glycerol) backbone with one fatty acid amide (instead of two fatty acid esters). The sphingolipids, like phosphatidylcholine, also contain phosphate and choline. Though sphingomyelin is a minor component, it does lower surface tension, as do the other components.

Developmental Sequence of Phospholipids

There is a regular developmental sequence for phospholipids, different for each, which governs the timing of their appearance in the alveolar effluent and in the amniotic fluid. The observation that the lamellar bodies containing surfactant are dumped into amniotic fluid is therefore clinically useful: If we know the composition of the lamellar bodies (their qualitative phospholipid composition) at any point in gestation, we can determine the maturation of the fetal lung. This is the basis for our L/S ratio and lung profile. We then can know when the baby may be delivered safely without fear of RDS.

In the developmental sequence, lecithin, the major component, slowly increases in content until about 34 or 35 weeks gestation, when it jumps abruptly and rises to high levels. Sphingomyelin has an almost inverse relationship to lecithin, starting out at around the same concentration, then dropping while lecithin

rises at about 34 or 35 weeks. The ratio of these two compounds to each other is called the L/S ratio, and it has an accuracy of about 98 percent for predicting lung maturity.

Phosphatidylinositol and phosphatidylglycerol, the acidic phospholipids, are especially unique compounds. Their importance lies in the fact that lecithin *by itself* is not a surfactant. It will wet easily with water and become inactive. In the presence of phosphatidylglycerol, however, lecithin forms a stable surfactant. Therefore, lung maturity is assured with the appearance of phosphatidylglycerol. (In fact, the compositions of effective totally synthetic surfactant are between 6:1 and 8:3 ratios of lecithin to phosphatidylglycerol.)

Thus, phosphatidylglycerol—the last of the surfactant phospholipids to appear in amniotic fluid—marks the absolute maturation of fetal lung surfactant. In some women with high-risk pregnancies, notably gestational or Class A or B diabetics, it is the standard of care not to deliver unless phosphatidylglycerol is found in the amniotic fluid.

The appearance of the mature L/S ratio (2:1) and of phosphatidylglycerol (at about 35–36 weeks gestation) as heralds of fetal lung maturity is amazingly constant in normal gestation. However, there are notable exceptions. Those of the greatest clinical importance involve accelerated maturation of the lung associated with some kinds of intrauterine stresses. Usually, these are maternal conditions such as hypertensive disorders, prolonged rupture of membranes, infection, retroplacental separation with scarring, and degenerative diabetes mellitus. Delayed maturation of the lung may occur in the gestational diabetic or the diabetic who is out of control. In such cases, the production of phosphatidylglycerol is delayed from 1 to 3 weeks, and the fetal lung remains immature.

WHAT IS RDS?

The concept is widespread that the only pathology contributing to respiratory distress syndrome is a surfactant inadequacy. Therefore, it is argued, all one needs to do to "cure" these babies is to replace the surfactant. This is a bold and naive oversimplification. It is important to understand and define RDS rigorously and, in fact, quite rigidly.

The most widely accepted description of RDS takes into account only the surfactant deficiency and therefore is not complete. RDS is a progressive, collapsing, expiratory atelectasis, confined almost entirely to low-birthweight infants owing to a surfactant deficiency, with consolidation of the lung, progressive damage of the alveoli, and production of hyaline membranes. This clinical picture is limited because it does not take into account the contribution of a patent ductus arteriosis to the pathophysiology of RDS.

Clinically, the typical patient with RDS is a low-birthweight, prematurely born baby who from birth breathes fast and with difficulty; shows significant substernal, suprasternal, and intercostal retractions; uses the accessory muscles, including tensing of the sternocleidomastoids; has an open mouth; flares the alae nasi in an attempt to lower airway resistance, which begins at the nose; develops paradoxical breathing in which the abdomen balloons up and the chest caves in with each inspiration; grunts at the end of each expiration; requires obligatory oxygen; continues to worsen; and lies rather limply in what the British call "a position of surrender."

At play in the production of these signs and symptoms is a tremendous mismatch: A noncompliant lung is mismatched with an overly compliant chest wall, and the downward pull of the strong diaphragm causes the chest to cave in with each inspiration. These infants, by virtue of the lack of surfactant, have a noncompliant lung, which resists expansion on inspiration and tends to collapse on expiration. They are, in addition, born with weak thoracic muscles, soft ribs, and poor muscle fixation. At the same time, a very strong diaphragm, developed by about 3 months gestation, causes the whole chest to cave in on descent. This is the basis for the paradoxical breathing and the difficulty in oxygenating which is characteristic of RDS.

The amounts of inspired and expired air from the first breaths in these babies are almost of the same volume. Unless some kind of assisted ventilation is given beyond oxygen, which helps only temporarily, they will die.

Except for the external signs described, the x-ray examination is the most helpful in revealing the features of RDS. It shows a widespread bilateral reticulogranular pattern, which extends all the way out to the periphery of the lung. The reticulogranular pattern is produced by the collapse of alveoli and the overdistension of the respiratory bronchioles. The baby has air bronchograms which are indicative of collapsing lung around tubular airways.

Overall, the chest shows a decreased volume. That, plus the reticulogranular pattern and air bronchograms, results from lack of surfactant. The x-ray films demonstrate why the lung is not compliant and why the baby has difficulty oxygenating.

But the x-ray films reveal much more. The heart is enlarged. There are left-to-right shunt vessels, evident particularly in the right hilum. The right side of the chest is used for diagnosis in a nonrotated film, particularly the right hilum. The lower right lung is most useful for the evaluation of air bronchograms. The combination of enlarged heart, left-to-right shunt vessels, and frequent haziness (that may progress all the way to a "white out" after asphyxiation) represents the effect of the patent ductus arteriosus.

There is a regular progression to the course of RDS. Initially, there is a problem with oxygen that requires assisted ventilation and results directly from a lack of surfactant.

Relatively soon after the onset of RDS, metabolic acidosis develops—even in the baby who was in good condition at birth and did not start life with acidosis. This is due to the left-to-right PDA shunt, which depletes the peripheral circulation and results in shock from inadequate blood flow.

Soon after this, respiratory acidosis is indicated by an elevated carbon dioxide pressure. This also results from the left-to-right PDA shunt, which causes filling of the interstitial lung space between the alveolar capillary wall and the Type I cells. This is the major effect of the shunt because it causes a decrease in alveolar gas diffusion and the retention of carbon dioxide.

On top of the problems with oxygenation and acidosis is the ever more irreversible complication of damage to the lung from the mechanical ventilation. This results in leaky lungs and a further decrease in compliance, further burdening the lung that is already noncompliant because of the initial surfactant lack as well as the added accumulation of fluid from the PDA. These all add up to problems in later oxygenation and contribute further to the accumulation of carbon dioxide.

The Patent Ductus Arteriosus

In the very low-birthweight infant with RDS, the PDA usually either is not diagnosed or the signs and symptoms are misinterpreted as being caused by surfactant lack and lung collapse. There are several reasons for the confusion.

Echocardiograms performed on very low-birthweight infants requiring ventilatory support may not be sensitive enough to detect blood flow through the PDA. Furthermore, very small infants have murmurs only infrequently. The reason for this is that, in these infants, the PDA is equal to or larger than the aorta. Without turbulence, owing to a mismatch of sizes, there are no murmurs. Also, because the heart is already dilated and is operating at maximum stroke volume, there is neither bounding pulses nor a precordial thrust. Consequently, all the presenting signs and symptoms are attributed to the lack of surfactant and the PDA is not treated effectively. Indomethacin may not work or may work only

partially. Mechanical ventilation is clearly inadequate, and the same may be said for any nonsurgical intervention for the PDA.

At birth, all infants, preterm or term, have a patent ductus arteriosus. *In utero,* the pulmonary vessels are constricted, and every fetus has natural physiological pulmonary hypertension. After birth, in the normal term baby, the foramen ovale closes, the left side of the heart develops systemic blood pressure, and the pulmonary artery pressure falls as the lungs are expanded. This baby is able to control pulmonary blood flow through an extensive system of miles of arterioles, which also have thick arteriolar walls. The pulmonary and systemic blood flow pressures are equal to each other after 6 to 18 hours, and there is no net flow into the pulmonary system. The PDA at this point becomes functionally closed, although it will take about 14 to 21 days for true anatomical closure and fibrosis.

By contrast, the premature infant has fewer and shorter pulmonary arterioles and is unable to use these as resistance vessels. In addition, the arteriolar walls are much thinner in the premature because there is an increase in arteriolar thickness with gestation. Thus, the premature infant is unable to control or equalize the left-to-right shunt. The interstitial space between the capillary and the Type I cells fills with fluid, primarily plasma.

Developmentally, the PDA derives from the embryonic left sixth aortic arch. From autopsy material, we have observed that the PDA is as large or larger than the aorta until 32 weeks gestation! The most important clinical aspect to remember, therefore, is that *every case of RDS actually is respiratory distress/PDA syndrome.* Effective management dictates that both the surfactant deficiency and PDA be treated concurrently.

EXPERIENCE WITH SURFACTANT REPLACEMENT

Surfactant replacement/replenishment was attempted as early as 1964. That attempt and at least three other acknowledged failed attempts all tried the replacement therapy using synthetic dipalmitic lecithin aerosols to deliver the surfactant.[2-5] Today we know that the primary reason for failure was the substance. Lecithin by itself is not effective as a surfactant because it is so easily wetted. It depends upon phosphatidylinositol and phosphatidylglycerol for its stability.

The largest study of attempted replacement therapy that failed was reported in 1967 in Singapore. Owing to a series of miscalculations, however, the report added a serious measure of confusion to the understanding of RDS. The investigators advocated that RDS should properly be considered "hypoperfusion syndrome."[3] Actually, RDS is associated with serious overperfusion of the lung. Unfortunately, this association of hypoperfusion with RDS, despite its fallacy, still finds its way into medical publications.

In 1972, the problem of how to replace surfactant was solved by Enhorning and Robertson. They dripped surfactant prepared from adult rabbits into the tracheae of prematurely delivered rabbit fetuses. This restored lung compliance and pulmonary function.[6] All subsequent experimental and clinical studies with surfactant have used the same techniques.

Enhorning and Robertson's work was verified in sheep by Adams and associates at UCLA. They reported on the successful instillation of adult sheep surfactant into the tracheae of prematurely delivered lambs with subsequent normal compliance and lung function.[7] One of the members of the team was Tetsuro Fujiwara, later to be part of the first team to instill artificial surfactant successfully into human infants.

One of the more important studies, which, unfortunately, has received inadequate recognition, was published in 1973 by McAdams and colleagues. They showed that hyaline membranes appeared in the lungs of monkeys and humans about *5 minutes after the initiation of*

mechanical ventilation. This is a devastating finding. After about 30 minutes, the lesions had become extensive and widespread. Although the infants studied were terminally ill (having such conditions as previability or absent kidneys), none had instrinsic lung disease.[8]

In 1978, in conjunction with another study, Nilsson and associates, including Enhorning, verified the work of the McAdams team. They found that barotrauma lesions appeared in rabbits about 7 minutes after the beginning of mechanical ventilation; after 27 minutes, the lesions had become extensive. The purpose of this study was to evaluate possible protective effects from surfactant instilled into the lungs of premature rabbits *prior* to their being ventilated mechanically. The control animals showed evidence of extensive damage compared to those that had received surfactant or had never been ventilated.[9]

An earlier landmark study in surfactant replacement was published in 1974 by Enhorning and coworkers showing the protective effects of surfactant instilled into premature rabbits before their first breaths—before they required assisted ventilation. These studies with rabbits established the significant efficacy of surfactant instilled before the first breath.

Another landmark study was published in 1980 by Fujiwara and associates, who instilled artificial surfactant into the tracheae of human infants with RDS for the first time and with some success. The surfactant used by this group was an extract of beef lung with added lecithin and phosphatidylglycerol. The number of survivors was greater in the surfactant-treated group than among the controls. However, the proportion of deaths in the treated group was still quite high, and there were cases of bronchopulmonary dysplasia. These investigators also noted the worsening of the PDA in the treated babies.[10]

In publications in 1983 and 1985, Hallman and associates in San Diego described the first use of human surfactant as replacement therapy. The surfactant was harvested and purified from human term amniotic fluid. Initially, as in the studies by Fujiwara's group, the surfactant was used for salvage in infants with already established RDS. All were babies who already had been ventilated for an average of about 15 hours before surfactant was instilled.[11,12]

Dramatic results were seen—for example, an oxygen pressure reading (PaO$_2$) of 30 jumped almost immediately upon surfactant instillation up to 300! However, 1 or 2 hours after this initial dramatic improvement, after ventilator settings and oxygen requirements had been reduced rapidly, these babies became much worse. Their settings on ventilators and their oxygen requirements then had to be increased to levels higher than they had been before surfactant instillation.[11]

Part of the reason for this failure of salvage therapy, in which surfactant is given after RDS has been under way for a number of hours, was shown by Ikegami and associates. They demonstrated that, during mechanical ventilation in lambs, a protein that inhibits surfactant activity is secreted into the airway.[13]

In 1985, three separate groups (Enhorning and associates in Toronto, Kwong and associates in Buffalo, and Shapiro and associates in Rochester) in a general collaboration but publishing independently, all gave surfactant from calf lung extract before the first breath to infants with RDS and reported consistently fair to good results. There still were problems with babies who did not achieve 100 percent efficacy. However, the group showed that artificial surfactant given with or before the first breaths is of benefit to humans.[14–16]

In reports published in 1986 and 1987, Hallman and associates again documented the value of instilled human surfactant. This time the surfactant was instilled with or before the first breaths at the time of birth. They achieved fairly good results, with lower requirements for oxygen and ventilation and fewer infants with bronchopulmonary dysplasia than in their control group.[17,18]

In 1987 also, Gitlin and colleagues published results of a three-center trial of beef extract surfactant and reported fairly good results demonstrating that surfactant replacement reduces the severity of RDS in the premature infant.[19]

There are currently three major types of surfactant available for commercial or clinical trial use: natural, semisynthetic, and synthetic. Natural preparations are isolated from human amniotic fluid, or harvested cow (Infasurf) or pig lungs (Curosurf).[20–23] One semisynthetic preparation (Survanta) consists of a natural bovine preparation that is supplemented with dipalmitoylphosphatidylcholine (DPPC), the active lipid component of natural surfactant, and with palmitate.[24] Synthetic preparations consist of mixtures of DPPC and chemical spreading agents. Exosurf Neonatal, for example, uses tyloxapol and cetyl alcohol as spreading agents.[28] The synthetic preparations have the advantages of being protein-free, thereby avoiding the risk of antigenisity; carrying no known risks of infectious transmission (eg., HIV, herpes virus, CMV); and presumably can be made available in large quantities.

Clinical trials are currently underway with the surfactant preparations mentioned above. Exosurf Neonatal is the only preparation to date to receive FDA approval for marketing.

Exosurf Neonatal has been approved for the following indications:[26]

1. Prophylactic treatment of infants with birth weights of less than 1350 grams who are at risk of developing RDS
2. Prophylactic treatment of infants with birth weights greater than 1350 grams who have evidence of pulmonary immaturity
3. Rescue treatment of infants who have developed RDS.

Exosurf Neonatal is available as a sterile, lyophilized powder that is reconstituted with preservative-free sterile water for injection. Exosurf Neonatal is stable at room temperature for up to 24 months as a dry powder and for up to 12 hours after reconstitution.[26]

The dosage of Exosurf Neonatal is based upon the infant's birthweight. Three 5 ml/kg doses administered 12 hours apart are recommended for prophylactic treatment.[27] Two 5 ml/kg doses administered 12 hours apart are recommended for rescue treatment. The first dose should be administered as soon as possible after birth for prophylaxis, and between 2 and 24 hours of age for rescue treatment.[26,28–31] Infants must be intubated and on mechanical ventilation for dosing. Each dose is administered, without interrupting ventilation, in two 2.5 ml/kg aliquots through a luer-lock sideport on special endotracheal tube adapters that are supplied with Exosurf Neonatal.

Of all surfactants, Exosurf Neonatal has the most extensive clinical experience to date. Over 4,400 patients were entered into 11 randomized, placebo-controlled, double-blind trials conducted in the United States and Canada. More than 3,000 infants have been randomized in European trials to date. Over 11,000 additional patients at over 450 North American hospitals were treated with Exosurf Neonatal under a separate treatment IND.[32] Since the commercial release in the U.S.A. on August 2, 1990, more than 15,000 patients have received Exosurf Neonatal.

Because mortality and morbidity vary with birth weight, the Exosurf Neonatal clinical trials divided the premature newborn population into three distinct subpopulations (tiny, middle-sized, and large). Tiny infants weighed between 501–699 grams or 500–749 grams, depending on the protocol; middle-sized infants weighed between 700–1,100 grams, 750–1,250 grams, or 700–1,350 depending on the protocol; large infants weighed ≥1,250 grams or >1,350 grams, depending on the protocol. Single-dose prophylaxis, one versus three dose prophylaxis, and two-dose rescue treatments were studied. Improvements in severity of RDS were apparent in all weight classes: significantly less supplemental oxygen and respiratory support were required in

the Exosurf Neonatal group.[28–31,33] In tiny infants, a single prophylactic dose of Exosurf Neonatal resulted in a 50 percent reduction in death from RDS and in the incidence of pneumothorax.[33]

In 700–1,100 gram infants, a single prophylactic dose resulted in a (a) 50 percent reduction in death from RDS, (b) 33 percent reduction in one-year mortality from any cause, and (c) 44 percent reduction in the incidence of pneumothorax.[29] An additional 44 percent reduction in mortality from any cause was seen at 28 days and at one year of life with three prophylactic doses in 700–1,100 gram infants.[27] In 700–1,350 gram infants, a single prophylactic dose showed a 29 percent decrease in death or bronchopulmonary dysplasia (BPD).[28] A two-dose rescue study in middle-sized infants resulted in (a) 50 percent reduction in mortality from any cause at 28 days and at one year of life, (b) 66 percent reduction in death from RDS, (c) 21 percent increase in intact cardiopulmonary survival (defined as survival at 28 days without BPD), (d) 31 percent reduction in the incidence of pneumothorax, and (e) 48 percent reduction in the incidence of pulmonary interstitial emphysema.[30]

Large infants who received two rescue doses of Exosurf Neonatal had (a) 40 percent reduction in mortality from any cause at 28 days, (b) 68 percent reduction in death from RDS, (c) 51 percent reduction in the incidence of pneumothorax, (d) 47 percent reduction in the incidence of pulmonary interstitial emphysema, and (e) a 44 percent reduction in the incidence of death or bronchopulmonary dysplasia. In addition, large infants had a 51 percent reduction in the incidence of BPD, two day reduction in the number of days on mechanical ventilation, and a 17 percent reduction in patent ductus arteriosus.[31]

One year follow-up evaluation of 1,450 infants (tiny, middle-sized, large infants) in the controlled clinical trials showed slightly fewer visual and motor handicaps for infants who received Exosurf Neonatal despite an increase in the number of survivors. In addition, Bayley mental (MDI) and motor (FDI) scores appeared to be improved in tiny infants who received Exosurf Neonatal.[34]

Exosurf Neonatal did not affect the incidence of nosocomial infections, sepsis or death from sepsis in any of the clinical trials. An increase in the incidence of apnea was seen with both prophylactic and rescue treatment.[29–31] The increase in the incidence of apnea was associated with a reduction in the length of time on mechanical ventilation in one study.[31] Indeed, infants who lived to develop apnea had better survival, fewer air leaks, and fewer intraventricular hemorrhages.[30]

A cross-study analysis of six controlled trials showed an increased incidence of pulmonary hemorrhage in the Exosurf Neonatal group (2 percent) versus the placebo group (1 percent).[35] A four percent incidence of pulmonary hemorrhage was seen in the more than 11,000 infants who received Exosurf Neonatal under the treatment IND.[32] Pulmonary hemorrhage was associated with younger gestational age, male gender, lower birthweight (<700 grams), ductal patency, and non-Caucasian race.[35] This complication appears to be related to improvement in pulmonary function and subsequent increased left to right shunting through the ductus arteriosus. Aggressive diagnosis and treatment of the PDA during the first 24 hours of life, as well as preferential weaning of the FiO₂ rather than ventilator pressure 24–26 hours after dosing, may minimize this risk.[28,29]

Survanta, a semisynthetic surfactant preparation currently in clinical development, is an organic solvent extract of mined cow lung that has been supplemented with DPPC, palmitic acid, and tripalmitin. It is supplied as a liquid which is warmed prior to use. Each 4 ml/kg dose is administered in four equal aliquots through a 5-French feeding tube that is inserted into the infant's endotracheal tube. The ventilator must be briefly disconnected during dosing.[36]

Both prophylactic and rescue treatments with Survanta have been studied using single-dose and multiple-dose treatment regimens. A single-dose, randomized, placebo-controlled, prophylactic trial has been completed in which Survanta was administered within 15 minutes of birth to infants between 24 and 30 weeks gestation and with birthweights between 750 and 1,250 grams.[36] Two single-dose, randomized, placebo-controlled rescue trials in which Survanta was administered within 8 hours of birth to infants with birth weights between 750 and 1,750 grams and who had RDS severe enough to require assisted ventilation with at least 40 percent oxygen also have been completed.[37,38] The single prophylactic dose resulted in a decrease in severity of respiratory distress syndrome as indicated by chest radiographic findings 24 hours after treatment and an improvement in oxygenation during 72 hours after treatment.[36] A single rescue dose resulted in a reduction in RDS severity 48 hours and 72 hours after treatment.[37,38] No reductions in mortality or long-term morbidity were reported with either prophylactic or rescue treatment.[36–38] One single-dose multicenter rescue study conducted in Europe was prematurely discontinued due to an increase in the incidence of periventricular-intraventricular hemorrhage in infants receiving Survanta.[39] Apparently multiple-dose clinical trials are also complete but little published information is available.

Infasurf (calf lung surfactant extract) is one of the natural surfactants currently in clinical development.[39–41] It consists of surfactant that has been isolated after lavage of calf lungs, and suspended in saline. It is then frozen and must be thawed to a liquid state prior to use. Unlike some of the other surfactants, the dosage is fixed at 3 ml regardless of the infant's birth weight. The infant must be intubated prior to dosing. Each 3 ml dose is administered in four equal aliquots through a 5-French feeding tube that is inserted into the infant's endotracheal tube. Infants are then hand-ventilated for two minutes after each dose. Dosing necessitates brief disconnection of the ventilator.

Early trials with Infasurf were randomized, placebo-controlled, single-dose prophylactic trials in which viable infants at less than 30 weeks gestational age were dosed before their first breath.[39,40] A reduction in RDS severity was seen during the first 24 hours with one prophylactic dose but the benefit was not sustained past 24 hours. No placebo-controlled data indicating benefits after 24 hours have been published. A later randomized trial comparing multiple-dose prophylaxis with multiple-dose rescue treatment of CLSE (calf lung surfactant extract) prepared in Rochester, New York showed a reduction in mortality with prophylactic treatment.[41]

Shapiro and coworkers demonstrated that significantly improved results could be obtained if multiple doses of CLSE were given to infants who met specific clinical respiratory criteria. This multiple dose study demonstrated an improvement in survival from 71–94 percent in infants between 24 and 29 weeks gestation when compared to a previous one dose study.[42] A recently published study of bovine surfactant comparing placebo administration at birth, prophylactic administration (surfactant given at birth) and late administration (surfactant given <6 hours of age) demonstrated significant improvement in gas exchange during the first week of life in the surfactant treated groups. Surfactant therapy also resulted in lower incidence of pulmonary air leak and severe chronic lung disease.[42] There was no difference between the prophylactic and late surfactant groups in any of these parameters. However, the group treated prophylactically demonstrated a higher incidence of mild chronic lung disease than the late treatment group, i.e., 29 percent of survivors in late treatment group compared with 58 percent in the early group required supplemental oxygen beyond 28 days of life.[43] This suggests that there may be no clinical justification for using a prophylactic approach to surfactant replacement therapy in infants less than 30 weeks gestation.[43]

Surfactant replacement therapy is not without significant risks and hazards. The infant's clinical condition must be evaluated prior to, during, and for at least 30 minutes after each dose by a clinician skilled in ventilatory management and endotracheal intubation. Clinical trials have demonstrated that lung compliance may increase rapidly following administration, and that peak inspiratory pressure should be decreased as indicated to avoid pneumothorax. Hyperoxia and hypocarbia may occur requiring reduction of FiO_2 and ventilatory rate. Mucus plugging, which can obstruct the endotracheal tube, has been reported. To minimize this hazard suction the infant prior to dosing or if an obstruction is suspected. Reintubate if an obstruction persists.

In summary, decreased morbidity and increased survival rates have been demonstrated after administration of surfactant preparations. Although there are some problems associated with surfactant replacement therapy, available long-term follow-up data indicate that the benefits of surfactant replacement therapy clearly outweigh the risks. Indeed, surfactant therapy for RDS has become the standard of care in the United States.

REFERENCES

1. Kikkawa Y, Motoyama EK, and Gluck L: Study of the lungs of fetal and newborn rabbits morphological biochemical and surface-physical development, American Journal of Pathology 52, 1968, pp. 177–209.

2. Robillard E, et al.: Microaerosol administration of synthetic ß-γ-Dipalmitoyl-Γ–α-Lecithin in the respiratory distress syndrome: A preliminary report, Canadian Medical Association Journal 90, 1964, pp. 55–57.

3. Chu J, et al.: Neonatal pulmonary ischemia: Clinical and physiologic studies, Pediatrics 40, 1987, pp. 709–782.

4. Shannon DC, and Bunnell JB: Dipalmitoyl lecithin aerosol in RDS, Pediatric Research 10, 1976, pp. 467–470.

5. Ivey H, Roth S, and Kattwinkel J: Nebulization of sonicated phospholipids (PL) for treatment of respiratory distress syndrome (RDS) of infancy, Pediatric Research 11, 1978, pp. 178–182.

6. Enhorning G, and Robertson B: Lung expansion in the premature rabbit fetus after tracheal depositions of surfactant, Pediatrics 50, 1972, pp. 58–66.

7. Adams FH, et al.: Effect of tracheal instillation of natural surfactant in premature lambs: Clinical and autopsy findings, Pediatric Research 12, 1978, pp. 841–848.

8. McAdams AJ, et al.: The experimental production of hyaline membranes in premature rhesus monkeys, American Journal of Pathology 70, 1973, pp. 277–290.

9. Nilsson R, Grossmann G, and Robertson B: Lung surfactant and the pathogenesis of neonatal bronchiolar lesions induced by artificial ventilation, Pediatric Research 12, 1978, pp. 249–255.

10. Fujiwara T, et al.: Artificial surfactant therapy in hyaline membrane disease, Lancet 1, 1980, pp. 55–59.

11. Hallman M, et al.: Isolation of human surfactant from amniotic fluid and a pilot study of its efficacy in respiratory distress syndrome, Pediatrics 71, 1983, pp. 473–482.

12. Hallman M, et al.: Exogenous human surfactant for treatment of severe respiratory distress syndrome: A randomized prospective clinical trial, Journal of Pediatrics 106, 1985, pp. 963–969.

13. Ikegami M, et al.: A protein from the airway of premature lambs that inhibits surfactant function, Journal of Applied Physiology 57, 1984, pp. 1134–1142.

14. Enhorning GE, et al.: Prevention of neonatal respiratory distress syndrome by tracheal instillation of surfactant: A randomized clinical trial, Pediatrics 76, 1985, pp. 145–153.

15. Kwong MS, et al.: Double-blind clinical trial of calf lung surfactant extract for the prevention of hyaline membrane disease in extremely premature infants, Pediatrics 76, 1985, pp. 585–592.

16. Shapiro DL, et al.: Double-blind, randomized trial of a calf lung surfactant extract administered at birth to very premature infants for prevention of respiratory distress syndrome, Pediatrics 76, 1985, pp. 593–599.

17. Hallman M, et al.: Effect of surfactant substitution on lung effluent phospholipids in respiratory distress syndrome: Evaluation of surfactant phospholipid turnover, pool size, and the relationship to severity of respiratory failure, Pediatric Research 20(12), December 1986, pp. 1228–1235.

18. Merritt TA, et al.: Prophylactic treatment of very premature infants with human surfactant, New England Journal of Medicine 15(13), September 25, 1986, pp. 785–790.

19. Gitlin JD, et al.: Randomized controlled trial of exogenous surfactant for the treatment of hyaline membrane disease, Pediatrics 79, 1987, pp. 31–37.

20. Hallman M, et al.: Isolation of human surfactant from amniotic fluid and a pilot study of its efficacy in respiratory distress syndrome, Pediatrics 71(4), 1983, pp. 473–482.

21. Wallman M, et al.: Exogenous human surfactant for treatment of severe respiratory distress syndrome: A randomized prospective clinical trial, Journal of Pediatrics 106(6), 1985, pp. 963–969.

22. Egan EA, et al.: Natural and artificial surfactant replacement in premature lambs, Journal of Applied Physiology 55, 1983, pp. 676–883.

23. Collaborative European Multicenter Study Group: Surfactant replacement therapy in severe neonatal respiratory distress syndrome, an international randomized clinical trial, Pediatrics 82, 1988, pp. 683–691.

24. Fujiwara T: Surfactant replacement in neonatal RDS *in* Robertson B, Van Golde LNG, Bratenburg JJ, eds., Pulmonary surfactant, Amsterdam, The Netherlands, Elsevier, 1984, pp. 479–804.

25. Durand DJ, et al.: Effects of a protein-free synthetic surfactant on survival and pulmonary function in preterm lambs, Journal of Pediatrics 107, 1988, pp. 775–780.

26. EXOSURF Neonatal Product Insert, Burroughs Wellcome Co., Research Triangle Park, North Carolina, 1990.

27. Gerdes J, et al., and the EXOSURF Neonatal Study Groups I & II: Effects of three vs one prophylactic doses of EXOSURF Neonatal in 700–1,100 gram Neonates, Pediatric Research 29, 1991, p. 214A.

28. Rose C, et al.: Improved outcome at 28 days of very low birth weight infants treated with a single dose of synthetic surfactant, Journal Pediatrics 117, 1990, pp. 947–953.

29. Corbet AJ, et al.: Decreased mortality in small premature infants treated at birth with a single dose of synthetic surfactant: A multicenter trial, Journal of Pediatrics 118( ), 1991, pp. 277–284.

30. Long WA, et al.: Effects of two rescue doses of a synthetic surfactant on mortality in 700–1,300 gram infants with RDS, Journal of Pediatrics 118, 1991, pp. 595–605.

31. U.S. and Canadian EXOSURF Pediatric Study Groups: Effects of two rescue doses of EXOSURF Pediatric in 1,232 infants ≥1,250 grams, Pediatric Research 27, 1990, p. 320A.

32. Burroughs Wellcome Co. EXOSURF Neonatal Treatment IND Newsletter, 3(4), March 1991.

33. Long W, et al., and the American EXOSURF Neonatal Study Group I, Effects of a single prophylactic dose of EXOSURF Neonatal in 215 500–700 gram infants, Pediatric Research 29, 1991, p. 223A.

34. Walter D, et al., the American EXOSURF Neonatal Study Group I, and the Canadian EXOSURF Neonatal Study Group, Double blind one year follow up in 1,480 infants randomized to EXOSURF Neonatal or air, Pediatric Research 29, 1991, p. 270A.

35. Pramanik AK: New synthetic surfactant helps infants breathe more easily, Neonatal Intensive Care, Jan/Feb. 1991, pp. 32–46.

36. Soll RP, et al.: Multicenter trial of single-dose modified bovine surfactant extract (Survanta) for prevention of respiratory distress syndrome, Ross Collaborative Surfactant

Prevention Study Group, Pediatrics 55(6), June 1990, pp. 1092–1102.

37. Horbar JD, et al.: A European multicenter randomized controlled trial of single dose surfactant therapy for idiopathic respiratory distress syndrome, European Journal of Pediatrics 149(6), March 1990, pp. 416–423.

38. Horbar JD, et al.: A multicenter randomized placebo-controlled trial of surfactant therapy for respiratory distress syndrome, New England Journal of Medicine 320(15), April 13, 1989, pp. 959–965.

39. Shapiro DK, et al.: Double-blind, randomized trial of a calf lung surfactant extract administered at birth to very premature infants for prevention of respiratory distress syndrome, Pediatrics 76(4), October 1985, pp. 593–599.

40. Kendig JW, et al.: Surfactant replacement therapy at birth: final analysis of a clinical trial and comparisons with similar trials, Pediatrics 82(5), November 1988, pp. 756–762.

41. Kendig JW, et al.: A comparison of surfactant as immediate prophylaxis and as rescue therapy in newborns of less than 30 weeks gestation, New England of Medicine 324(13), March 28, 1991, pp. 865–871.

42. Shapiro D: Surfactant Replacement Therapy *in* Nelson N, ed., Current Therapy in Neonatal-Perinatal Medicine-2, BC Decker, Philadelphia, 1990, pp. 477–480.

43. Dunn MS, et al.: Bovine surfactant replacement therapy in neonates of less than 30 weeks' gestation: A randomized controlled trial of prophylaxis versus treatment, Pediatrics 87(30), 1991, pp. 377–386.

BIBLIOGRAPHY

▶ Enhorning G, Grossmann G, and Robertson B: Tracheal deposition of surfactant before the first breath, American Review of Respiratory Diseases 107, 1973, pp. 921–927.

▶ Jacob J, et al.: The contribution of PDA in the neonate with severe RDS, Journal of Pediatrics 96(79), 1980, pp. 79–87.

▶ Metcalfe IL, Burgoyne R, and Enhorning G: Surfactant supplementation in the preterm rabbit: Effects of applied volume on compliance and survival, Pediatric Research 16(10), October 1982, pp. 834–839.

▶ Robertson B, and Enhorning G: The alveolar lining of the premature newborn rabbit after pharyngeal deposition of surfactant, Laboratory Investigation 31(54), 1974, pp. 54–59.

10 Extracorporeal Membrane Oxygenation in the Newborn

Jan Nugent, RNC, MSN
Ochsner Foundation Hospital
New Orleans, Louisiana

Respiratory failure is a serious medical problem that has significant impact on neonatal mortality and morbidity. Recent advances in technology have challenged clinicians to consider alternative therapies for the 5–10 percent of infants with severe pulmonary dysfunction who respond poorly to maximal conventional ventilatory, medical, and surgical treatment.[1] The past decade has witnessed intense research in the field of high-frequency ventilation and extracorporeal membrane oxygenation (ECMO).[2] In the clinical arena, these new techniques have found application in the care of neonatal respiratory distress.

After current standard therapy has been exhausted, ECMO can provide life-saving cardiopulmonary support in some neonates with predictably fatal pulmonary failure. Nurses caring for these infants need a basic understanding of the principles of ECMO perfusion as well as excellent physical assessment and psychosocial skills. The nurse's ability to provide this sophisticated level of care will have direct and significant impact on the outcome of this mode of therapy.

CONVENTIONAL VENTILATORY THERAPY

Despite significant advances in the care of infants with severe pulmonary dysfunction, respiratory failure remains the most frequent cause of neonatal death. Failure of conventional ventilatory therapy accounts for an estimated 15,000 neonatal deaths annually.[3] Contributing respiratory pathology includes respiratory distress syndrome, meconium aspiration syndrome; persistent pulmonary hypertension of the newborn (PPHN), which may occur as a primary entity or as a secondary complication of respiratory distress syndrome; and pulmonary hypoplasia associated with congenital diaphragmatic hernia.

Conventional ventilatory therapy includes use of 100 percent oxygen, positive pressures, and rapid ventilator rates via a pressure-limited, time-cycled, continuous flow mechanical ventilator. Frequent adjuncts to this therapy are use of inotropic agents (dopamine, dobutamine) to augment systemic circulation, pulmonary vasodilators (tolazoline, prostaglandin E_1) to reduce pulmonary vascular resistance, and sodium bicarbonate to induce alkalosis and dilate pulmonary vasculature.[4–7]

Unfortunately, the aggressive management required to treat severe pulmonary parenchymal dysfunction and PPHN can contribute significantly to acute parenchymal damage. This can lead to therapeutic failure and death or chronic respiratory disease. An estimated 10 percent of infants who survive the acute stages of their disease may be chronically crippled by bronchopulmonary dysplasia from barotrauma and oxygen toxicity.[8]

ECMO: A HISTORICAL PERSPECTIVE

ECMO, "the process of prolonged extracorporeal circulation (cardiopulmonary bypass) achieved by extrathoracic vascular cannulation," provides cardiorespiratory support for infants in reversible, profound respiratory or cardiac failure.[8]

Rashkind and associates were the first to report use of neonatal extracorporeal oxygenation via femoral arteriovenous shunt through a bulb oxygenator in 1965.[9] Initial work with a membrane oxygenator was reported by other investigators during the late 1960s and early 1970s.[10–12] There were no survivors reported in these early trials, but the work of these clinicians established the feasibility of ECMO as a treatment modality and demonstrated the need for further refinements in apparatus and technique.

The chief problems the early investigators encountered were fairly daunting. The heart-lung machine required a large blood reservoir, which necessitated complete suppression of coagulation and a large priming volume. The oxygenator, which functioned by direct exposure of blood to oxygen, damaged blood cells and proteins if operated for more than a few hours. The blood pump hemolyzed red cells and caused significant leukopenia. Vascular access was a problem: Umbilical vessels or vessels in the leg were used to gain access to the infant's circulation, but these proved too small to provide extracorporeal flow sufficient for adequate respiratory support.

The final concern was that of coagulation control since extracorporeal therapy required that the patient be heparinized until coagulation ceased. This practice was safe for only a limited period of time because of the real potential of producing life-threatening hemorrhage when extended over a period of days. No simple laboratory procedure for instantaneous evaluation of clotting time existed. This made accurate titration of systemic anticoagulants impossible.[13]

Medical researchers, lured by the prospect of developing a clinical revolution in cardiopulmonary support, began extensive clinical trials supported by grants from the National Institutes of Health. Kolobow and coworkers began work on the roller pump and membrane lung in 1969, demonstrated the superior blood compatibility of silicone in a membrane lung in 1974, and published data on long-term survivability of lambs perfused up to ten days in 1976.[14–16]

Concurrent clinical work on the technique of extracorporeal circulation via extrathoracic vascular cannulation was begun by Bartlett and coworkers in 1971. They managed their first newborn patient in 1973 and to date have performed more than 100 neonatal ECMO procedures. Of these infants, 45 were reported in the literature in 1982—with a 55 percent survival rate.[17] The years of painstaking research had led to dramatic improvements in machinery and patient management.

Since that time, the survival rate has improved because of extensive experience with the technique, case selection, and earlier intervention. Bartlett and associates determined that ECMO was safe (the risks of the treatment itself were less than the risks of the disease) and effective in a study that included 55 moribund patients treated in three centers over a nine-year period. Of the 40 infants with birthweights of more than 2 kg, 28 (70 percent) survived. Of the 15 infants with birthweights of less than 2 kg, 3 (20 percent) survived.[18]

Encouraged by the reported overall survival rate of 56 percent, groups in several major medical centers began to evaluate the use of ECMO in neonates.[3,19] During this phase of clinical research, ECMO was used when all other therapy had failed and the infant was considered moribund. The moribund condition was quantified by objective criteria predictive of high mortality (more than 80 percent), chief of which were the newborn pulmonary insufficiency index and the alveolar-arterial gradient (Table 1).[20–22]

Prompted by the successful outcome of this phase of research, Bartlett and associates designed and conducted a prospective controlled randomized study. From October 1982 until April 1984, a group of 12 infants with birthweights greater than 2 kg who met 80 percent mortality risk criteria entered the study. One patient was randomly assigned to conventional therapy and died. The 11 patients randomly assigned to ECMO survived.[18]

This study used the "randomized play-the-winner" technique, which assigns an infant to treatment based on the outcome of each previous patient in the study—that is, if one treatment is more successful, more patients are randomly assigned to it. This randomly assigned pattern was to continue until ten patients had been treated with ECMO or ten control patients died. The researchers utilized this methodology to address the scientific/ethical issue of withholding an unproven but potentially life-saving treatment. Thus some patients were saved from exposure to an inferior treatment. The research of this phase documented that survival is better with ECMO (90 percent) than with conventional ventilation.[18] These results, the small study size, and the statistical method used generated significant controversy.[23,24]

This controversy compelled O'Rourke and associates to design a prospective clinical trial comparing ECMO with conventional mechanical therapy (CMT). To limit the number of infants assigned to what might ultimately be a less effective therapy, they used an adaptive design with both a randomized and nonrandomized phase. If the therapies were proven to be of equal efficiency, all patients would have been ran-

TABLE 1 ▲ Criteria Predictive of Potential Mortality

1. Newborn Pulmonary Insufficiency Index (NPII)
The NPII score is a single-number cumulation of oxygen requirement, acidosis, and time. This score assesses the severity of an infant's respiratory distress in the first day of life. It is calculated by plotting the newborn's FiO_2 and pH on a graph over the first 24 hours of life. The NPII graph has 10 percent FiO_2 increments and one-tenth pH increments on the vertical axis and hourly time increments on the horizontal axis. The score is determined by the number of boxes outlined between the FiO_2 and pH lines when the plotted FiO_2 is greater than the plotted pH on the graph.[30,52] In the past, the NPII was used effectively as a measure of high mortality risk (greater than 80 percent). Since the advent of induced alkalosis as a treatment for PPHN, the NPII has not been applicable.[18,54]

2. Alveolar-arterial gradient >620 mmHg for 12 hours
Alveolar-arterial oxygen difference ($AaDO_2$) is a measure of alveolar efficiency in transporting oxygen to pulmonary capillaries. Use of this criterion assumes that the baby is ventilated with 1.0 FiO_2 and that the $P_ACO_2 = PaCO_2$. The following calculation is used:
$$AaDO_2 = (FiO_2)(713) - PaO_2 - PaCO_2$$
The numerical value 713 assumes an atmospheric pressure of 760 mmHg minus vapor pressure (47 mmHg); PaO_2 and $PaCO_2$ are measured by assaying arterial blood gases. Retrospective reviews demonstrate that an $AaDO_2$ >620 for 12 consecutive hours correlates with greater than 80 percent mortality.[21,22,55]

3. Acute deterioration despite optimal therapy: either a PaO_2 <40 mmHg or a pH ≤7.15 for two hours

4. Lack of response to treatment of PPHN. [Two of the following indications for three hours]: PaO_2 <55 mmHg; pH <7.4; hypotension

5. Severe barotrauma, with four of the following indications:
   Interstitial emphysema
   Pneumothorax
   Pneumopericardium
   Pneumoperitoneum
   Subcutaneous emphysema
   Persistent air leak for 24 hours
   Mean airway pressure of ≥15 cm H_2O

6. Congenital diaphragmatic hernia with respiratory failure:[18,30,56]
PaO_2 <80 mmHg on FiO_2 >0.8/24 hours after surgery
$PaCO_2$ >40 mmHg (2 hours after surgery) with ventilation index (mean airway pressure × respiratory rate) >1,000 [56]

7. The oxidation index
The oxidation index can be utilized to predict mortality and incidence of bronchopulmonary dysplasia. The oxygenation index is calculated by dividing the product of the FiO_2 (times 100) and the mean airway pressure by the postductal PaO_2:
$$\frac{Mean\ Airway\ Pressure \times FiO_2 \times 100}{Postductal\ PaO_2}$$
Retrospective data demonstrates that an oxidation index ≥40 correlates with a predicted mortality risk of 80–90 percent; an index ≥25–40 correlates with a 50–60 percent mortality.[8]

Adapted from: Nugent J: Extracorporeal membrane oxygenation in the neonate, Neonatal Network 4(5), 1986, p. 29. Reprinted with permission.

domized. The mortality rates did differ significantly, and the assignment of patients to CMT was halted after the tenth patient. Enrolled in the study were 39 newborn infants (weight >3 kg, 39–40 weeks gestation) with severe PPHN and respiratory failure who met 85 percent mortality criteria. The overall survival of ECMO treated infants was 99 percent (28 of 29), compared with 60 percent (6 of 10) in the CMT group.[25]

To date, the ECMO registry, which includes international data from institutions in the United States and abroad, lists more than 4,400 infants treated with ECMO since 1975 and documents an overall survival rate of 83 percent. These statistics include all the early cases at participating medical institutions.[26] Bartlett and colleagues, in a published summary of their group's first 100 cases, validate an overall survival rate of 72 percent.[27] In infants weighing more than 2 kg, the survival rate is 83 percent.[8] In experienced hands, this treatment modality has proven itself to be an effective life-support system for the very critically ill infant who is greater than 34 weeks gestation.

In the current phase of this research, Bartlett is addressing the need for additional data to support the use of ECMO. The present research protocol requires patients who meet specific criteria to be randomized to ECMO or to continue ventilator management when the risk of mortality is 50 percent. The morbidity and cost of the medical treatment of these two groups will be studied and compared.[27]

CRITERIA FOR USE OF ECMO

Extracorporeal membrane oxygenation is an extreme life-support procedure with significant inherent risks. Presently, neonates are considered candidates only if their risk of mortality is estimated at 80 percent or more despite use of 100 percent oxygen, high-pressure ventilation, and vasoactive drug therapy.

The ECMO procedure acts as a temporary heart-lung substitute. A neonate's pulmonary or cardiac pathology must be acute and reversible within the one- or two-week period that it is feasible for ECMO to safely support the infant.[28] Neonatal respiratory disorders that may fit this criteria are respiratory distress syndrome, meconium aspiration syndrome, PPHN, congenital diaphragmatic hernia with respiratory failure, and pneumonia.

Utilizing ECMO as a mode of therapy subjects the neonate to risks of serious complications and requires sacrificing the right common carotid artery. Selection criteria must identify infants destined to die using conventional care while excluding the hypoxic neonate who would survive without ECMO.

To detect high-risk patients and exclude those with poor prognosis, the patient selection process must have a high degree of predictability and specificity. To achieve this specificity, each neonatal ECMO center must determine its own mortality indicators and criteria.[8]

Final selection is based on objective criteria predictive of greater than 80 percent mortality (see Table 1). Currently, the most frequently used criteria are nonresponse to treatment and the alveolar-arterial oxygen gradient.[26] In certain situations, use of $AaDO_2$ results in either false-negative or false-positive results. The potential for this error lies in the $AaDO_2$ equation: The arterial carbon dioxide pressure ($PaCO_2$) and the arterial oxygen pressure (PaO_2) are weighted equally; hence it is the sum of these values that is important and not the individual numbers. If the sum is high, the patient does not qualify; if it is low, the patient does qualify. Infants with a high $PaCO_2$ and low PaO_2 may not qualify, or infants with an artificially low $PaCO_2$ may qualify despite acceptable PaO_2 levels. Further research is required to enhance specificity. At present, criteria based specifically on PaO_2 may decrease false-negative and false-positive results.[28]

In the early stages of the development of such an invasive and inherently risky technique as ECMO, it was appropriate to begin with patients who had failed conventional therapy and were moribund. As more patients survive and the efficacy of this treatment modality is validated, the selection criteria has and will continue to undergo a natural metamorphosis toward earlier intervention.

Contraindications to ECMO include the following:
1. Cyanotic congenital heart disease
2. Irreversible pulmonary damage
3. Any nonreversible condition incompatible with normal quality of life (such as bilateral pulmonary hypoplasia, certain chromosomal abnormalities, or severe neurological damage)
4. Intracranial hemorrhage
5. A birthweight of less than 2 kg
6. Gestation age of less than 35 weeks

Before ECMO is initiated, each candidate has a pediatric cardiology evaluation, cranial ultrasound, and electroencephalogram.

In the infant with congenital heart disease (which can mimic PPHN), the treatment of choice would be palliative surgery. An exception would be the infant who requires stabilization and life-support prior to or post cardiac surgery.[29]

An abnormal electroencephalogram, although not in itself a contraindication, will help the pediatric neurologist determine whether there is irreversible neurological damage. An electroencephalogram is of particular importance if neurological assessment is hindered by chemical paralysis.

Intracranial hemorrhage is a contraindication because the systemic heparinization of ECMO patients significantly increases the risk of extension of the hemorrhage. A birthweight of less than 2 kg or a gestational age of less than 35 weeks is considered a contraindication because the incidence of intracranial hemorrhage occurring during ECMO in this group is significant; consequently, the survival rate of these infants is discouragingly low.[18,27]

FIGURE 1 ▲ Anterioposterior chest film demonstrates correct placement of (1) venous cannula (left arrow) in the right atrium via the right interal jugular vein and (2) the arterial cannula (right arrow) in the aortic arch via the right common carotid artery.

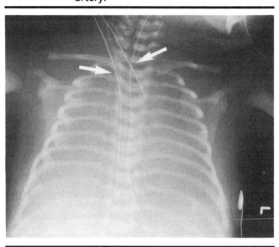

From: Nugent J: Extracorporeal membrane oxygenation in the neonate, Neonatal Network 4(5), 1986, p. 30. Reprinted with permission.

ROUTES OF PERFUSION

In the ECMO circuit, blood is drained from the venous system and diverted outside the body, where oxygen is added and carbon dioxide removed by the membrane oxygenator; this oxygenated blood is then returned to the patient. This support achieves adequate gas exchange and permits ventilator settings to be reduced to low parameters, minimizing barotrauma and oxygen toxicity. The two most common methods of perfusing infants on ECMO are venoarterial bypass and venovenous bypass.

The venoarterial (VA) route drains blood from the right side of the heart through a catheter placed in the right atrium via the right internal jugular vein. Oxygenated blood is returned through the right common carotid artery into the ascending aorta (Figure 1).[30] The carotid artery is the arterial vessel of choice because it is the largest vessel able to provide adequate blood flow to the aortic arch. If the patient demonstrates any degree of cardiac failure, venoarterial bypass must be used. This is presently the preferred—and most common—method of bypass.

The venoarterial route provides excellent support for the heart and lungs by (1) decompressing the pulmonary circulation, which decreases pulmonary artery pressure and pulmonary capillary filtration pressure, (2) supporting the pumping action of the heart and systemic circulation, and (3) perfusing coronary arteries with oxygenated blood. There are several technical advantages of this route: The lungs can be lavaged and suctioned without hazarding hypoxia, positive pressure ventilation can be reduced to minimal parameters, less surgical time is required to initiate VA bypass, and stabilization and total respiratory support can be achieved in less time and at lower pump flow rates than with the venovenous (VV) route.[30]

There are two major risks inherent in venoarterial bypass: Emboli (air or particulate) could be infused directly into the arterial circulation, and the obligatory ligation of the carotid artery may adversely affect cerebral perfusion.[30]

The venovenous route has been used successfully to support neonates in respiratory failure.[31,32] This route drains blood from the right atrium via a right internal jugular cannula and returns the oxygenated blood to the systemic circulation through a femoral vein.

Theoretically, this route is advantageous because it spares the common carotid artery and perfuses oxygenated blood into a vein.[31] This mode does not decompress the right atrium and ventricle and hence has no overall effect on cardiac output or pulmonary artery pressure. Venovenous bypass provides no cardiac support. Oxygenated blood returns to the right side of the heart and lungs, minimizing the danger of arterial embolization and perfusing the pulmonary artery. Perfusion of the pulmonary arterial system with well-oxygenated blood was thought possibly to reduce pulmonary vascular resistance and help resolve PPHN. In practice, studies have shown that there is no difference between VA and VV ECMO in this regard.[32]

Technically, venovenous bypass is more difficult to manage because two surgical incisions and dissections are needed and stabilization on ECMO requires more time. The problem of "pump recirculation" of oxygenated blood from the femoral vein cannula into the internal jugular cannula necessitates 20 percent greater pump flows to achieve total respiratory support. Consequently, less oxygenated blood is available for the patient's circulation because a portion of oxygenated circulating blood volume goes into the drainage cannula.

Patients on VV bypass require more ventilator support (higher FiO_2 and mean airway pressures) and must have good cardiac function. These patients are also at risk for groin wound infections and serious venous insufficiency in the leg with femoral vein ligation.[31] Additionally, VV ECMO has not always been successful in the best of candidates and has required conversion to VA for subsequent survival.[32]

The research documenting the efficacy of venovenous bypass has prompted the development of a double-lumen venovenous catheter. This 14 Fr catheter provides a route for ECMO support via single site cannulation of the internal jugular vein. This catheter has been used successfully in laboratory and clinical trials[33,34] and has been released for limited use in designated ECMO centers. When this catheter becomes readily available for clinical use, infants may well be treated earlier in the course of respiratory failure. Hence, the need for total support will lessen, and venovenous bypass may become the route of choice for neonatal ECMO.[27]

THE ECMO CIRCUIT

Components of the ECMO circuit include cannulas; a system of polyvinylchloride (PVC) tubing with luer lock connectors, stopcocks, and silicone rubber bladder with infusion sites; bladder box assembly; roller pump; membrane oxygenator; and heat exchanger. An activated clotting time machine completes the system (Figure 2). A detailed description of the development of the ECMO circuit is available in the literature.[35]

The cannulas are for removing deoxygenated venous blood and returning oxygenated blood to the infant's arterial circulation. ECMO bypass flow and the ability to deliver oxygen are limited by the amount of venous drainage blood. This volume is limited by the size and position of the venous drainage catheter. The venous cannula must be capable of delivering the total cardiac output (120–150 ml/kg/minute) and should be positioned to drain blood from the superior and inferior vena cava.[8]

The internal diameter of the cannulas has the greatest impact on resistance to flow. Because the ECMO system must be capable of providing total heart-lung support, cannulas of the largest possible internal diameter are inserted. This assures adequate venous drainage to support the required bypass flow rates. Argyle chest tubes ranging in size from 8 to 16 French have been the most widely used because they are thin walled and offer low resistance to flow.[35] However, specifically designed ECMO cannulae (Biomedicus, Elecath) are now available and demonstrate superior flow characteristics when compared to the Argyle chest tubes.[36]

After the patient has received local anesthesia and morphine, the surgeon carefully isolates and dissects the right internal jugular vein and carotid artery. Extensive manipulation can produce vasospasm, particularly of the internal jugular vein, making cannulation with an adequate sized cannula almost impossible.[37] Lidocaine hydrochloride 1 percent may be infiltrated into the surgery site to relieve vasospasms.

The patient is systemically heparinized just before introducing the cannulas. Before administering a heparin loading dose of 100–200 units/kg, the nurse assesses all invasive sites for adequate hemostasis.[38] Once the patient's acti-

FIGURE 2 ▲ Components of the ECMO circuit: (a) PVC tubing with stopcocks, (b) silicone rubber bladder with infusion sites, (c) bladder box assembly, (d) roller pump, (e & f) membrane oxygenator and gas sources, (g & h) heat exchanger and water bath, (j) ACT machine, and (k) heparin infusion.

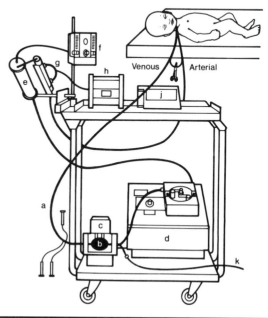

From: Nugent J: Extracorporeal membrane oxygenation in the neonate, Neonatal Network 4(5), 1986, p. 31. Reprinted with permission.

vated clotting time (ACT) has reached 250 seconds, the artery and then the vein are cannulated with saline-filled cannulas. Before the internal jugular vein catheter is introduced, succinylcholine or pancuronium bromide (Pavulon) is given systemically to prevent respiratory movement and air embolism. These medications may be given via the existing arterial lines because peripheral venous infusion sites may have been discontinued.

Preceding the introduction of each cannula, the carotid artery and the internal jugular vein are ligated distally. Perfusion of the brain is maintained by collateral circulation through the external carotid artery, the circle of Willis, and the ophthalmic artery.[39] The arterial cannula is advanced so that the catheter tip reaches just to the aortic arch. The venous cannula is positioned so that the tip lies in the right atrium with the side holes draining the right atrium and the superior vena cava.[37] The cannulas are flushed with a retrograde blood flow from the right atrium and aortic arch, sutured to the skin of the upper neck, and connected to the ECMO circuit tubing. The position of the cannulas is immediately determined by chest x-ray examination.

The PVC tubing with its system of connectors, stopcocks, and silicone bladder provides for circulation of blood from the infant through the components of the circuit as well as for removal of blood and administration of fluids, medications, and blood products. This system has a volume of approximately 350–400 ml.

Prior to cannulation, the circuit is primed: It is flushed with carbon dioxide, which aids in the removal of microbubbles by making them more soluble, and filled with a crystalloid solution. Albumin 25 percent is added to precondition and coat the circuit surface area, minimizing fibrinogen surface area adherence and platelet destruction. This solution is displaced with citrated packed red blood cells to which calcium and heparin have been added. The pH of the blood is corrected with THAM, and 25 percent albumin is added to equalize oncotic pressure. It is essential to determine that the electrolytes, blood gases, and acid-base balance are physiologic prior to instituting bypass. Concentrated platelets are added to the prime solution once bypass is begun and the ACT is within the desired range.

The system of stopcocks on the PVC tubing and the infusion sites on the bladder provide access to the venous side of the circuit. Each of the ports is designed for a singular purpose. The stopcock closest to the patient is used to remove blood samples; the second, third, and fourth ports are for administering blood products, medications, and alimentation solutions. The number and position of stopcocks will vary with each institution's protocols.

Because fluid can stagnate in the bladder, infusing heparin, alimentation solutions, and medications through the stopcocks is preferable to using the infusion sites on the bladder. These sites are suitable for administering blood products and, in emergencies, for removing air. To avoid contamination, sampling sites should be used for blood withdrawal only and infusion sites for infusion only.

Because all ECMO patients are heparinized, all intravenous infusion sites may be discontinued prior to cannulation. This reduces the possibility of bleeding from puncture sites. All medications, fluids, and blood products except platelets are given through the venous side of the ECMO circuit. The only exceptions are fluids infused via the umbilical or peripheral arterial lines. Care is taken to aspirate each syringe gently for air bubbles because there is no in-line air filter.

The same precautions and guidelines for safe administration of medications and blood directly into patients are used when medications and blood are infused into the ECMO circuit. Platelets are infused on the arterial side of the circuit between the membrane oxygenator and the heat exchanger. This prevents inadvertent filtration of platelets by the membrane oxygenator.

The bladder box assembly is a fail-safe alarm system. The collapsible silicone bladder distends with returning venous blood. If the flow into the ECMO circuit is not adequate, the bladder will collapse, causing a microswitch to sound an audible alarm and stop the roller pump. Upon reexpansion of the bladder, the microswitch reengages the pump, and normal pump operation continues.[30] This servo-regulation feature prevents the pump flow rate from exceeding venous return.

Transducer-based technology which allows for servoregulation of extracorporeal flow, independent of bladder volume, is now available (Polystan). Transducers placed in-line in the circuit monitor premembrane (venous) and postmembrane (arterial) pressures. This advance in servoregulation technique allows for early detection of flow problems and timely intervention.

A rise in premembrane pressure signals decreased venous return prior to the collapse of the silicone bladder. Causes of decreased and inadequate venous return are: hypovolemia, kinked venous catheter, incorrect position of the venous catheter in the right atrium, inadequate catheter diameter, or pneumothorax. Adequate venous return is critical to achieving pump flows needed for cardiorespiratory support. Persistent decreased venous return promotes a hemodynamically unstable patient. Hence, the cause for decreased return must be recognized and corrected immediately. A rise in postmembrane pressure could indicate: kinking of the arterial catheter, accidental clamping of the catheter, clot in the membrane oxygenator or heat exchange, or impending oxygenator failure.

The ECMO blood pump is a simple roller device that compresses and displaces the blood in the PVC tubing that is positioned in the pump raceway. The action of the pump pushes fluid forward, creating a suction within the venous catheter. The pumping action will assist left ventricular function when on VA bypass. The pump is electrically powered and can be hand cranked or attached to a battery power source if a power failure occurs. A digital display indicating the circuit flow in cubic centimeters per minute appears on the face of the pump.

The membrane oxygenator or lung (Sci-Med/Kolobow) is a solid silicone polymer membrane envelope with a plastic space screen. This is spirally wound around a spool and encased in a silicone rubber sleeve.[30] In the lung, oxygen is added, and carbon dioxide and water vapor are removed. Membrane oxygenators are the oxygenators of choice. They have the advantages of eliminating the blood gas interface effects (damaging plasma proteins, lipoproteins, red cells), assuring constant blood volume, and providing ease of operation.[40]

A heat exchanger is located downstream from the oxygenator and provides for warming of the blood, which is kept normothermic.[30] Heat loss from the blood occurs during ECMO from the cooling effect of ventilating gases inside the oxygenator and circuit exposure to ambient air temperature. It has been our experience that the infant also requires heat from a radiant heat source to maintain normal body temperature during the ECMO procedure.

A bubble detector (Polystan, Cobe, Shiley) can be placed distal to (patient side) the heat exchanger. These devices are capable of detecting air bubbles as small as 600 microns. If a bubble is detected, the roller head pump is immediately shut off and flow to the patient ceases.

Fiberoptic technology which provides continuous monitoring of arterial and venous blood gases is now available. These monitoring devices (Cardiovascular Devices, Inc.), which are clamped around an arterial and venous site of the PVC circuit, provide digital readouts of arterial pH, PaO_2, $PaCO_2$, base excess/bicarbonate (BE/HCO_3^-) and venous pH, PvO_2, $PvCO_2$ and saturation. The arterial monitoring allows for assessment of membrane oxygenator function. Venous monitoring assists in assessing the adequacy of extracorporeal perfusion and the efficiency of the extracorporeal circulation in meeting the infant's metabolic needs.

An ACT machine and an infusion pump are used intermittently to monitor the patient's ACT and continuously infuse a heparin solution into the ECMO circuit. Heparin must be given to prevent clotting in the extracorporeal circuit. Once the loading dose of heparin is given at the time of cannulation, the ACT is maintained at 180–250 seconds. Low-dose heparin of approximately 40–50 units/kg/hour is continuously infused into the circuit.

Heparin activity is monitored by whole blood activated clotting time. It is essential to use whole blood ACT, rather than plasma partial thromboplastin time (PTT), because of the interactions between platelets, white cells, and heparin.[40] Activated clotting time is checked every 30–60 minutes, and the heparin infusion is titrated to keep the ACT within the desired range. To control the amount of heparin administered, none is added to any other medications or fluids. An exception may be fluids infusing through umbilical or peripheral arterial lines. Factors that will influence heparin requirements are thrombocytopenia, abnormal coagulation studies, and urinary output.[30]

PHYSIOLOGY OF EXTRACORPOREAL CIRCULATION

Physiologic function during prolonged cardiopulmonary bypass differs considerably from normal physiology. The normal functions of blood flow, gas exchange, blood surface interface effects, and reticuloendothelial functions are replaced in various degrees by the extracorporeal device.[40]

Venoarterial bypass is instituted by draining venous blood by siphon into the extracorporeal circuit; a like amount of arterialized blood is returned to arterial circulation. As bypass flow is gradually increased, flow through the pulmonary artery decreases at a faster rate than bypass flow, reducing total flow in the systemic circulation. Peripheral and pulmonary hypotension occur. Though the exact mechanisms causing hypotension are not well understood, reduction in blood viscosity and the release of vasoactive substances may contribute to this phenomenon.[40] Blood volume replacement is required for optimal tissue perfusion and prevention of metabolic acidosis.

Extracorporeal membrane oxygenation perfusion is nonpulsatile, meaning that pulse contour decreases as venoarterial flow rate increases. The precise nature of the physiologic effects of nonpulsatile flow during extracorporeal circulation has been the subject of controversy. Experts agree, however, that the kidney interprets the nonpulsatile flow as inadequate, resulting in renin and aldosterone production and antidiuresis.[40]

The total flow to the patient during ECMO is a function of blood volume and the diameter of the venous catheter. An increase in blood volume at a stable ECMO flow will increase pulmonary-artery-to-left-atrial flow, decreasing the relative percentage of cardiopulmonary bypass. Conversely, a reduction in patient blood volume can inadvertently increase extracorporeal flow and decrease pulmonary-artery-to-left-atrial flow.

Total patient flow is the sum of extracorporeal flow plus pulmonary blood flow. Adequate flow is reached when oxygen delivery and tissue perfusion result in normoxia, normal pH, normal venous oxygen saturation (SvO_2), and normal organ function. Normal cardiac output in an infant is 120–150 ml/kg/minute. Total gas exchange and support are usually achieved at this flow rate.

Gas exchange is accomplished via the membrane lung. The lung consists of two compartments divided by a semipermeable membrane: Ventilating gas is on one side, and blood is on the other. As the blood flows past the membrane, oxygen diffuses into the blood because of a pressure gradient between the 100 percent oxygen in the ventilating gas in the gas phase and the low oxygen pressure in mixed venous blood. The chemical binding of oxygen to hemoglobin proceeds very rapidly.

The limiting factor in oxygenation of flowing blood is the rate of oxygen diffusion through plasma. Therefore, the thickness of the blood film between the gas exchange membranes becomes the rate-limiting factor in oxygen transfer.

Simultaneously, carbon dioxide diffuses from the blood compartment, responding to a pressure gradient between the venous carbon dioxide pressure and the ventilating gas. The rate of carbon dioxide transfer is greater than that of oxygen; hence a carbon dioxide enriched mixture is usually necessary for ventilating the oxygenator. This prevents inadvertent hypocapnea, respiratory alkalosis, and cessation of the infant's spontaneous respirations.

The carbon dioxide pressure is controlled by gas flow through the membrane oxygenator. To remove excessive carbon dioxide, the sweep flow (the total liter flow of oxygen, carbon dioxide, and compressed air to the oxygenator) may be increased. The manufacturer's recommended limit for sweep flow should not be exceeded. If the pressure on the gas side of the membrane exceeds that on the blood side, gas embolization could occur.

Oxygen transfer capacity of a membrane oxygenator is related to the rate of blood flow through the membrane and the degree of oxyhemoglobin desaturation of the blood entering the oxygenator. The flow rate at which venous blood leaves the oxygenator at 95 percent saturation is referred to as "rated flow." As blood flow through the membrane oxygenator is increased, a point is reached when the thickness of the blood film limits the rate that oxygen can diffuse into blood. At this point, the outflow blood will exit at less than 95 percent saturation. The rated flow for a membrane oxygenator is that at which this limitation is reached.

The rated oxygen delivery is the amount of oxygen that can be taken up by the blood at the rated flow. Oxygen delivery is related to flow and to the amount of unsaturated hemoglobin presented to the oxygenator per minute. Oxygen delivery depends entirely on flow; decreasing flow decreases delivery.[40]

In selecting an oxygenator, one should be sure that the "rated flow" is greater than cardiac output—that is, the infant's oxygen requirement should not exceed the oxygenating performance of the membrane lung. The Sci-Med 0.4 m² membrane lung has a rated flow of 40 ml/minute/m² with a recommended blood flow rate of 350 ml/minute; the 0.8 m² size has a rated flow of 60 ml/minute/m² with a recommended blood flow rate of 1,400 ml/minute. Either can be used effectively in the neonate whose usual maximal flow rate requirement is 120–150 ml/kg/minute.

There are other factors that control systemic oxygenation during ECMO. Total oxygen delivery to tissues is equal to extracorporeal oxygen plus pulmonary oxygen. Increasing extracorporeal flow and decreasing patient lung flow will increase the infant's PaO_2. Decreasing extracorporeal flow and increasing patient lung flow will decrease the infant's PaO_2 as long as the infant's lung function is not adequate.

A less than optimal hematocrit (less than 45 percent) will decrease oxygenation. Rapid or overinfusion of blood products will decrease oxygenation because a larger percentage of blood flow will be shifted to the pulmonary-artery-to-left-atrial flow, decreasing the relative percentage of cardiopulmonary bypass. As the infant's lung function improves, more oxygen diffuses into the blood perfusing the infant's lung. This increases the infant's systemic PaO_2, and extracorporeal flow can then be gradually decreased and the infant weaned from ECMO.[30]

During ECMO, at least 80 percent of the cardiac output is exposed to a large artificial surface each minute. All blood cellular components and protein molecules come into contact with a foreign surface hourly. Flow patterns in the circuit include areas of stagnation and turbulence.[30] All these factors stimulate both the protein and the platelet arms of the clotting system.

Within seconds of blood exposure to a foreign surface, a molecular layer of protein adheres to that surface. One of these proteins is fibrinogen, which is converted into fibrin, and subsequent clot formation occurs within a few minutes. Other protein clotting factors are absorbed to some extent by foreign surface exposure, resulting in a decrease of clotting factors at the initiation of bypass. Concurrently, the liver and spleen increase synthesis of fibrinogen and other clotting factors, returning their serum concentration to prebypass levels within a period of hours.[40] Preexposure of the circuit's inner surface to albumin appears to minimize fibrin surface adherence and platelet destruction.[30] In the presence of heparin, fibrinogen is not converted to fibrin, and clotting does not occur.

Platelets show the greatest effect of exposure to a foreign surface, as evidenced by continuous platelet aggregate formation and decreasing platelet count and function. The concentration of platelets drops abruptly with onset of extracorporeal circulation and continues to fall as long as bypass continues. The thrombocytopenia is due in part to platelets adhering directly to the foreign surface but to a greater extent to platelets adhering to each other and to white cells, forming platelet aggregates of 2–200 micron units, which are infused into the patient. These aggregates are picked up by the liver, spleen, and to a lesser extent by the lung, where they are bound or phagocytized. Platelet aggregate formation is not detrimental to microcirculation, as evidenced by lack of microembolic tissue damage even in prolonged bypass (16 days).[30,40]

Because a large number of platelet aggregates is generated continuously, it can be estimated that all circulating platelets are incorporated into aggregates every few hours. These platelets disaggregate and recirculate. The platelet count plateaus at 30,000–60,000 when a balance between aggregation, regeneration from bone marrow, disaggregation, and recirculation is achieved.[30] This chronic thrombocytopenia requires frequent platelet transfusions.

Platelet transfusions are necessary when the platelet level drops below 70,000/mm³. If the patient is experiencing abnormal amounts of bleeding, the platelet count is maintained at 100,000/mm³, and the ACT is restricted to 180–200 seconds. Platelet transfusions do increase heparin consumption, and to compensate, the heparin infusion may need to be increased. Transfusion of a whole unit of adult platelets (rather than platelet concentrate) may be preferable because platelets are very sensitive to contact and temperature.[8]

After cessation of extracorporeal circulation,

clotting factors and platelets return to normal or above normal levels.[40] However, thrombocytopenia can occur up to four days after the cessation of ECMO. Platelet counts must be monitored during this critical period. Infants at highest risk for prolonged thrombocytopenia are those with meconium aspiration syndrome or sepsis and those whose ECMO course was marked by technical complications.[42]

Physiologic changes occur as a result of systemic heparinization. Several of the steps between activation of the surface factor (factor XII) and fibrin formation are inhibited by heparin.[40] This action results in prolonged clotting times. Heparin has an almost immediate onset of action following intravenous administration. It is inactivated by the liver and excreted by the kidney. Clotting times return to normal within two to six hours after the drug is discontinued.

The effects of prolonged extracorporeal circulation on blood cell survival and function demonstrate that hemolysis is negligible and the survival of red blood cells is not altered by continuous exposure to the ECMO circuit. All the various types of white cells decrease in concentration because of the combined effects of dilution and aggregation. Studies of phagocytosis and bacterial killing of circulating leukocytes during extracorporeal circulation demonstrate significantly decreased phagocytic activity in the circulating white cells. It is postulated that these effects are due to the mechanical or chemical effects of the ECMO circuit on blood. It is thought that the phagocytes may become saturated with platelet aggregates, which reduces their ability to further phagocytize bacteria.[38] White cell concentration rebounds after cessation of ECMO.[32]

Fluid and electrolyte changes occur frequently during extracorporeal circulation. Sodium retention, expanded extracellular fluid, and decreased total body potassium are characteristic changes. These conditions are thought to be attributable to third spacing of albumin the source of which is the circuit priming fluid, as well as the action of aldosterone, which causes sodium retention, increased extracellular fluid, and kaliuresis. Potassium replacement is required, and excessive extracellular fluid can be removed via continuous hemofiltration or use of furosemide.[27] Calcium and magnesium levels can remain low throughout the ECMO run; correction is achieved with moderate supplementation via parenteral fluids.[40]

CARE OF THE INFANT UNDERGOING ECMO

Cannulation and the initiation of bypass usually occur in the NICU under local anesthesia and with an operating room staff member in attendance. This avoids the formidable risks inherent in moving a critically ill newborn to and from the operating room with bypass in progress. The operating room team provides an ECMO surgical case cart, an electrocautery unit, and a fiberoptic headlight. While the team is readying the surgical equipment, the ECMO specialist assembles and primes the circuit.

It is essential that the infant have an indwelling arterial line for arterial sampling as well as for continuous blood pressure monitoring. The site of choice is the umbilical artery; if this is not feasible, a postductal site such as the left radial artery will be utilized. A peripheral venous line may also be inserted in an extremity or in a scalp vein for infusion of parenteral fluids and medications during the surgical procedure. All necessary lines are kept to a minimum and are inserted prior to heparinization.

During the surgical procedure, the NICU nursing personnel constantly monitor the infant's cardiopulmonary status and administer the necessary medications. Blood products and emergency drugs are drawn up and are avail-

FIGURE 3 ▲ Arterial pressure waveform and bypass flow rates. On venoarterial bypass, conduction and contraction continue even though little blood is flowing through the heart. The EKG pattern will remain normal. The normal peaked pattern of the arterial pressure waveform will flatten as bypass flow increases. Total bypass (70–80 percent of cardiac output) is reached when the arterial pressure tracing flattens and no peaked contours are evident during positive pressure inflation.

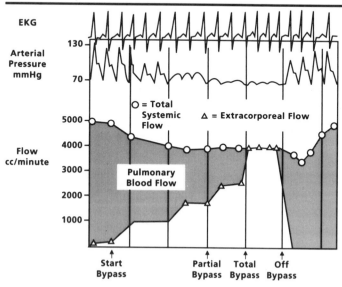

From: Chapman R, Toomasian J, and Bartlett R: Extracorporeal Membrane Oxygenation Technical Specialist Manual, 9th ed., Ann Arbor, Michigan, 1988, University of Michigan Press, p. 8. Reprinted with permission.

able. Initiation of bypass frequently causes hypotension, which is generally corrected with volume replacement. Care must be taken not to dislodge the infant's endotracheal tube and arterial or venous lines during the procedure.

Following cannulation, bypass is gradually instituted until approximately 80 percent of the infant's cardiac output is extracorporeally diverted through the ECMO circuit. This usually requires flow rates of 120–150 cc/kg/minute (Figure 3). At maximum flow, hypoxia, hypercarbia, and acidosis will be reversed. The infant will become normotensive, and vasoactive drugs and muscle relaxants can be discontinued.

Ventilator parameters are reduced to minimal settings to "rest" the lungs. The extracorporeal flow is adjusted to maintain systemic arterial PaO_2 at 60–80 torr, $PaCO_2$ at 35–45

TABLE 2 ▲ ECMO Complications

Physiological	Rationale and Treatment
Electrolyte/glucose/fluid imbalance	Sodium requirements decrease to 1–2 mEq/kg/day. Potassium requirements increase to 4 mEq/kg/day secondary to action of aldosterone. Calcium replacement may be required if citrate is a component of prime blood anticoagulant. Hyperglycemia may occur if citrate-phosphate-dextrose anticoagulated blood is used: Reduce dextrose concentration of maintenance and heparin infusions. Maintain total fluid intake 100–150 ml/kg/day. Fluid intake should balance output; furosemide may be required if positive fluid balance occurs.[39]
Central nervous system deterioration: cerebral edema, intracranial hemorrhage, seizures	This significant complication of ECMO can be related to pre-ECMO hypoxia, acidosis, hypercapnea, or vessel ligation. Drug of choice for seizures is phenobarbital. Serial EEGs and cranial ultrasounds may be required.
Generalized edema	Extracellular space is enlarged by distribution of crystalloid solution from the prime fluid and action of aldosterone and antidiuretic hormone. Furosemide or hemofiltration may be indicated if edema causes brain or lung dysfunction.
Renal failure	Acute tubular necrosis results from pre-ECMO hypotension and hypoxia. Monitor output and indicators of renal failure: blood urea nitrogen (BUN), creatinine. Increase renal perfusion by increasing pump flow and use of dopamine (5 µg/kg/minute). Hemodialysis may be added to the circuit if necessary.
Bleeding/thrombocytopenia	This is the most frequent cause of death. Large foreign surface of ECMO circuit lowers platelet function and count. This is most common in infants requiring surgery or chest tubes. Minimize with good control of ACT (180–200 seconds) and judicious use of platelets and fresh frozen plasma. All surgical procedures must be done with electrocautery.
Decreased venous return/hypovolemia	Infant must have adequate circulating volume to obtain adequate flow rates. This is manifested by collapsing silicone bladder triggering bladder box alarm, decrease in extracorporeal flow rate, arterial pressure, and arterial pulse amplitude. Blood sampling, wound drainage, or peripheral dilatation may account for hypovolemia. Check for pneumothorax, partial venous catheter occlusion, or malposition, which may decrease venous drainage and return. Replace volume with packed cells, fresh frozen plasma. Treat pneumothorax with chest tube placement. Raise level of bed to enhance gravity drainage of venous blood.
Hypervolemia	This is caused by overinfusion of blood products, which causes a larger percentage of blood to flow through malfunctioning lungs. It can also be caused by renal ischemia and excretion of renin/angiotension. It is manifested by widening pulse amplitude and decreasing systemic oxygenation at a fixed extracorporeal flow rate. Treat overinfusion by removing blood from the circuit. Renal hypertension may dictate use of captopril or labetalol.
Patent ductus arteriosus	Left-to-right shunting may occur, causing increased blood flow to the lungs, necessitating high pump flows without expected increase in PaO_2. Ligation may be indicated because weaning will not be successful.

Mechanical	Rationale and Treatment
Tubing rupture, Air in circuit, Oxygenator malfunction	Increase ventilator to pre-ECMO parameters. Take patient off bypass. [Repair circuit, aspirate air, replace oxygenator.] Be prepared to resuscitate infant.
Power failure	Always plug pump into hospital's emergency power supply. Hand crank until emergency power is available.
Decannulation	Apply firm pressure. Come off bypass; increase ventilator parameters. Repair vessel; replace blood volume. Be prepared to resuscitate infant.

Adapted from: Nugent J: Extracorporeal membrane oxygenation in the neonate, Neonatal Network 4(5), 1986, p. 33. Reprinted with permission.

torr, pH at 7.35–7.45, SvO_2 at more than 70 percent, and arterial saturation at more than 90 percent. Extracorporeal flow is considered adequate when oxygen delivery and perfusion of body tissues results in normoxia, normal pH, normal SvO_2, and normal organ function. SvO_2 is considered an excellent indicator of adequate flow because it is a measure of tissue perfusion. A decrease in SvO_2 indicates tissue hypoxia. Continuous monitoring of venous and arterial oxyhemoglobin saturation via fiberoptic technology allows for optimal management of bypass flow.

Total blood flow to the infant on bypass is the sum of extracorporeal flow and pulmonary blood flow. Total oxygen delivery is the combination of extracorporeal oxygen delivery and pulmonary oxygen delivery. The resultant systemic arterial blood gases reflect the sum of these relative oxygen contents.

Oxygen delivery is maximized by maintaining the hematocrit at 45–50 percent. Blood products are also given to correct hypovolemia, excessive bleeding, and thrombocytopenia. Maintenance and alimentation fluids are administered at 100–150 cc/kg/day. Usual sodium requirements are 1–2 mEq/kg/day, and potassium requirements are 4 mEq/kg/day. Gastric feedings are withheld. Significant insensible water loss can occur secondary to radiant warmer and membrane lung. Daily weights are the best indicator of fluid balance. A weight gain will occur the first 24–48 hours, followed by diuresis and weight loss. Antibiotics are ordered routinely, as well as daily blood cultures and chest films.

The infant should receive endotracheal suctioning based on individual assessment and need. Hourly recording of vital signs, intake and output, neurological checks, and arterial blood gases are mandatory. Oozing at the cannulation site may require frequent dressing changes. The amount of blood loss must be quantified and replaced. The infant's position should be changed every one to two hours.

TABLE 3 ▲ Circuit Emergency Procedures

Circuit Emergencies	
Air embolism (arterial)	Power failure
Tubing rupture	Gas source failure
Oxygenator malfunction	
Decannulation	
Pump failure	
↓	
Come off bypass	

Circuit Emergency Procedures	
Nurse	*ECMO specialist*
Ventilation	Clamp catheters
Anticoagulation	Open bridge
Chemical resuscitation	Remove gas source
Replace blood loss	Repair circuit

Catheter dislodgment is a fatal complication; caution must be taken at all times to avoid inadvertent decannulation. The ECMO specialist should assist the nurse in all position changes.

Complications associated with ECMO are both physiological and mechanical. Mechanical problems frequently create emergency situations that require immediate recognition and resolution. Tables 2 and 3 outline these complications with their rationale and corrective actions.

The ECMO Team

The complex and challenging care of infants on ECMO requires a highly trained and skilled team of professionals, including a physician, perfusionist, neonatal intensive care nurse, and ECMO specialist. The most important factor in maintaining ECMO for days or weeks is the team. Maintaining the procedure without mistakes requires constant, diligent concentration. Providing this mode of care is not feasible for many hospitals because of the expense and commitment involved in training personnel. In our institution, the training of an ECMO specialist alone requires a minimum of 80 hours of class and laboratory work.

Both a nurse and an ECMO specialist are assigned to care for the ECMO patient each shift. The nurse is responsible for ongoing assessment, hemodynamic monitoring, data

TABLE 4 ▲ Nursing Responsibilities and Interventions for ECMO

Prior to Cannulation

Responsibility	Intervention
Obtain and document base-line physiological data.	Record weight, length, head circumference.
	Draw blood samples for complete blood count (CBC), electrolytes, calcium, glucose, BUN, creatinine, PT/PTT, platelets, arterial blood gases.
	Record vital signs: heart rate, respiratory rate, systolic, diastolic, mean blood pressure, temperature.
Assure adequate supply of blood products for replacement.	Draw type-and-cross match samples for two units of packed red cells, fresh frozen plasma.
	Keep one unit of packed cells and fresh frozen plasma always available in the blood bank.
Maintain prescribed pulmonary support.	Maintain ventilator parameters.
	Administer muscle relaxants if indicated.
Assemble and prepare equipment.	Prepare infusion pumps to maintain arterial lines and infusion of parenteral fluids and medications into the ECMO circuit.
	Place the infant on a radiant warmer with the head positioned at the foot of the bed to provide thermoregulation and access for cannulation.
	Attach infant to physiological monitoring devices for heart rate, intra-arterial blood pressure, transcutaneous oxygen, etc.
	Insert urinary catheter and nasogastric tube; place to gravity drainage.
	Remove intravenous lines just prior to heparinization (optional).
	Prepare loading dose of heparin (100 u/kg).
	Prepare heparin solution for continuous infusion (100 u/cc/D$_5$W).
	Prepare paralyzing drug (pancuronium bromide, 0.1 mg/kg or succinylcholine 1–4 mg/kg).
	Assist in insertion of arterial line (umbilical or peripheral).
	Administer prophylactic antibiotics.

During Cannulation

Monitor cardiopulmonary status during procedure.	Monitor heart rate and intra-arterial blood pressure continuously.
	Obtain blood gases after paralysis and during cannulation as indicated by the infant's response to the procedure.
Be prepared to administer cardiopulmonary support.	Have available medications and blood products to correct hypovolemia, bradycardia, acidosis, cardiac arrest.
Administer medications.	Give loading dose of heparin systemically when vessels are dissected free and are ready to be cannulated.
	Give paralyzing drug systemically just prior to cannulation of internal jugular vein if infant has not been previously paralyzed.
Reduce ventilator parameters to minimal settings.	Once adequate bypass is achieved, reduce peak inspiratory pressure (PIP) to 16–20 cm H$_2$O, positive end-expiratory pressure (PEEP) to 4 cm H$_2$O, ventilator rate to 10–20 breaths per minute, and FiO$_2$ to 21–30 percent.

collection, administration of fluids and medications, and pulmonary care. The ECMO specialist is responsible for checking and monitoring the circuit, adjusting gas and pump flow, maintaining heparinization, administering appropriate blood products, drawing blood specimens, and documenting data.

The nurse practice acts in many states will not allow the nurse to delegate administration of medications and blood products to non-licensed personnel; hence this responsibility rests with the nurse if the ECMO specialist is not a registered nurse. Tables 4 and 5 outline nursing and ECMO specialist responsibilities and interventions.

Weaning and Decannulation

Signs of improvement and indicators suggesting that the infant is ready to be weaned from ECMO consist of improvement of lung fields as seen on chest films, clinical findings of weight loss, improved aeration via chest aus-

TABLE 4 ▲ Nursing Responsibilities and Interventions for ECMO (continued)

During ECMO Run

Responsibility	Intervention
Monitor and document physiological parameters.	Record hourly: heart rate, blood pressure (systolic, diastolic, mean), respirations, temperature, transcutaneous PO_2, CO_2, oxygen saturation, ACT, ECMO flow.
	Measure hourly accurate intake and output of all body fluids (urine, gastric contents, blood); measure every four hours urine pH, protein, glucose, specific gravity; hematest all stools.
	Assess hourly: color, breath sounds, heart tones, murmurs, cardiac rhythm, arterial pressure wave form (Figure 3), peripheral perfusion.
	Perform hourly neurological check, including fontanel tension, pupil size and reaction, level of consciousness, reflexes, tone, and movement of extremities.
	Record ventilator parameters hourly.
	Assess weight and head circumference daily.
Monitor and document biochemical parameters.	Draw arterial blood gases from umbilical or peripheral line hourly.
	All other blood specimens are drawn from the ECMO circuit by the ECMO specialist: electrolytes, calcium, platelets, Chemstrip, hematocrit every four to eight hours, CBC, PT/PTT, BUN, creatinine, total and direct bilirubin, plasma hemoglobin, fibrinogen, fibrin split products, and daily blood culture as indicated.
Administer medications.	Remove air bubbles and double-check dosages before infusion.
	Administer no medications IM or by venipuncture.
	Place all medications and fluids into the venous side of the ECMO circuit.
	Prepare and administer the arterial line (umbilical or peripheral) infusion.
	Administer parenteral alimentation.
Provide pulmonary support.	Perform endotracheal suctioning based on individual assessment and need.
	Maintain patent airway; be alert to extubation or plugging.
	Obtain daily chest films and tracheal aspirant cultures as indicated.
	Maintain ventilator parameters.
Prevent bleeding.	Avoid all of the following: rectal probes, injections, venipunctures, heel sticks, cuff blood pressures, chest tube stripping, restraints, chest percussion.
	Avoid invasive procedures: Do not change nasogastric tube, urinary catheters, or endotracheal tube unless absolutely necessary, use premeasured endotracheal tube suction technique.
	Observe for blood in the urine, stools, endotracheal or nasogastric tubes.
Maintain excellent infection control.	Change all fluids and tubing daily.
	Change dressings daily and PRN.
	Clean urinary catheter site daily.
	Maintain strict aseptic and handwashing technique.
	Use universal barrier precautions.
Provide physical care.	Keep skin dry, clean, and free from pressure points.
	Give mouth care PRN.
	Provide range of motion as indicated.
	Turn side to side every one to two hours.
Provide pain management, sedation, stress reduction.	Minimize noise level
	Cluster patient care to maximize sleep period
	Administer analgesia: Fentanyl 9–18 µg/kg/hr (increased dosage due to Fentanyl binding to membrane oxygenator) Manage iatrogenic physical dependency by following a dose reduction regime (reduce dose 10 percent every 4 hours)[57]
Be alert to complications and emergencies.	See Tables 2 and 3.

Adapted from: Nugent J: Extracorporeal membrane oxygenation in the neonate, Neonatal Network 4(5), 1986, pp. 34–35. Reprinted with permission.

cultation, rising oxygen pressure (PaO_2), and improved lung compliance. When the infant is initially on bypass, the lungs on x-ray examination appear opaque with variable volume loss; as pulmonary function improves, the lung fields begin to clear. Improvement shown on chest x-

TABLE 5 ▲ ECMO Specialist Responsibilities and Interventions

Responsibility	Intervention
Maintain and monitor ECMO circuit.	Check circuit carefully for air, clots, tightness of connectors, stopcocks.
	Check bladderbox alarm function.
	Monitor pump arterial and venous blood gases each shift to assess oxygenator function. Pump arterial PO_2 less than 100 mmHg, CO_2 retention or leaking membrane indicates oxygenator failure.
Assess infant.	Check cannula placement and stability.
	Assess breath sounds, neurological status.
	Observe volume of fluid and blood drainage.
	Monitor vital signs and lab values.
Maintain prescribed parameters: pH 7.35–7.45 PaO_2 60–80 mmHg $PaCO_2$ 35–45 mmHg MAP 45–55 mmHg HCT 45–55 percent Platelets 70–100,000 SvO_2>70 percent SaO_2>90 percent ACT 180–250 seconds	Maintain infant's systemic arterial blood gases by adjusting sweep gas and pump flow.
	Maintain mean arterial blood pressure (MAP), hematocrit (HCT), and platelets by infusion of appropriate blood products.
	Assess ACT hourly or PRN; titrate heparin infusion to maintain parameters.
Assist nurse in care.	Draw *all* blood samples from circuit except systemic arterial blood gases.
	Coordinate recording of intake and output with nurse.
	Assist in all position changes.
	Administer and monitor all medications, blood products, and fluids placed into the pump circuit.
Be prepared to deal with pump emergencies.	See Tables 2 and 3.

From: Nugent J: Extracorporeal membrane oxygenation in the neonate, Neonatal Network 4(5), 1986, pp. 36. Reprinted with permission.

ray films usually lags behind clinical improvement.[43] Weight loss, which results in a return to baseline, demonstrates a loss of excess extracellular fluid and often heralds improvement in pulmonary function. As the primary pulmonary pathology resolves and pulmonary function improves, oxygenation in that fraction of the cardiac output traversing the lung improves. This is indicated by a rise in the systemic PaO_2.

Recent research has demonstrated that changes in lung compliance can be a sensitive indicator of a neonate's lung improvement while on ECMO. Lotze and associates demonstrated that lung compliance measurements can be used to monitor clinical course and improvement as well as to predict the patient's successful removal from bypass.[44] Employment of sensitive measures of lung function, such as lung compliance, will be very useful in the weaning process and could potentially shorten total time on bypass. This is particularly important when the infant's condition warrants immediate cessation of bypass but arterial blood gas measurements are marginal, as when there is excessive bleeding. Further clinical research in this area is needed.

Once improvement in pulmonary gas exchange has been ascertained, weaning the infant by decreasing the flow rate in small (10–20 cc) increments is begun. Decreasing the flow rate diverts less blood into the extracorporeal circuit and increases blood flow to the infant's lung. The flow is decreased in this manner, usually over a period of days, until extracorporeal support is no longer needed to maintain adequate gas exchange at low ventilator settings.

When the flow rate is decreased to 50 cc/kg/minute, a state of "idling" is achieved. The infant will remain at this lowest possible flow rate for four to eight hours. Heparinization must be maintained for as long as the catheters are in place. During the idling period, the heparin infusion may need to be switched to the patient to maintain appropriate ACT levels. If the infant's condition deteriorates, extracorporeal flow is increased, and support of the infant is resumed.

If improvement in lung function remains stable at low ventilator settings during idling, a test period with the infant off ECMO is attempted. The cannulas are clamped, and the circuit is slowly recirculated via a bridge to prevent stagnation. If it has not already been done during idling, the heparin infusion is now switched to the patient. The gas flow into the oxygenator is discontinued, the heat exchanger temperature is decreased, and all infusions into the ECMO circuit are discontinued and switched to the patient.[30]

Decannulation can proceed if blood gas values remain satisfactory. The same preparation and equipment needed for cannulation are made available. Under local anesthesia, cannulas are removed and vessels are ligated. Until recently, the artery and vein have not been repaired because of significant post-ECMO risk of thrombis formation and embolization at the cannulation site.[34] However, pilot studies indicate that carotid reconstruction can be performed safely with no significant morbidity or mortality in select ECMO patients. Long term follow-up of patients undergoing carotid repair will be needed to determine the efficacy of this procedure.[45,46] Succinylcholine or pancuronium bromide (Pavulon) is given to the infant before decannulation to prevent air embolization. The ventilator settings are increased to compensate for loss of the infant's own ability to ventilate because of drug-induced paralysis.

After decannulation, the infant is weaned as tolerated from mechanical ventilation. Heparin reversal is usually not warranted because heparin is metabolized in a few hours. Once the infant's ACT is within normal limits, routine NICU care can resume. Transfusions to correct anemia are frequently required during the first 24 hours after ECMO. Platelet counts should be followed closely because thrombocytopenia may persist for up to four days following decannulation.[42]

PARENTAL SUPPORT

Support of the family of the infant undergoing ECMO presents some unique challenges. Parents are usually in crisis: Their infant has been critically ill since birth, and they are aware that his chances for survival are poor. Parents are informed that the ECMO procedure itself is a method of last resort with no guarantee of positive outcome. The technical environment is overwhelming. It is not unusual to find the parent grieving and in a state of withdrawal.

Support should be given by listening, communicating, educating, and providing parent-infant and parent-parent support. Parents need continuous communication of concise, accurate information about their child's condition and the required procedures. They should be allowed access to their infant, and the staff should be empathetic and as reassuring as the situation will allow. Parent-to-parent support utilizing parents whose infant has experienced ECMO is efficacious and a positive experience for all involved families. As proficiency with ECMO technology improves, the ECMO candidate has an increasingly better chance for survival, and every effort must be made to encourage parental involvement and bonding.

FOLLOW-UP AND OUTCOME

The survival rate for infants treated with ECMO is steadily improving, and in centers that provide this therapy, it is a feasible life-saving measure for neonates who might otherwise die. The overall survival of infants is 83 percent, the survival for various pathologies are: meconium aspiration 93 percent, RDS 84 percent, congenital diaphragmatic hernia 61 percent, sepsis/pneumonia 77 percent, and persistant pulmonary hypertension of the newborn (PPHN) 88 percent.[26] Critical scrutiny of survivors is essential to properly assess the value and safety of this technique.

Neonatal ECMO survivors are followed closely for possible complications caused by hypoxia and acidosis occurring both before and during the procedure. Survivors are systematically and periodically evaluated for the following parameters: growth and development, cardiorespiratory development, cerebrovascular status, and neurological and psychological functioning.

In early follow-up studies, physical growth and development as well as cardiorespiratory development were reported as normal. All infants have shown evidence of adequate cerebral blood flow to both hemispheres, despite the necessity of carotid artery ligation. Neurological competence appropriate for age was reported in 83 percent of survivors in one study and 75 percent in another.[13,39] In a long-term follow-up study of a group of 18 ECMO survivors aged four to nine years, 13 (72 percent) were basically normal, and 5 (28 percent) had neurologic handicaps.[47] In comparison, follow-up studies of infants surviving respiratory failure and PPHN have reported 0–25 percent incidence of neurologic injury.[48,49]

Schumacker and associates found that right-sided brain abnormalities can exist after ECMO and that carotid artery ligation is not without risk. Eight infants from a group of 59 ECMO survivors demonstrated right-sided brain injury manifested by right hemisphere focal abnormalities or neuromotor abnormalities that were lateralizing in nature. Hypoxic-ischemic brain injury is usually left-sided; the presence of right-sided findings suggests that vessel ligation is a contributing factor in these injuries. The pre-ECMO course of these infants was characterized by severe hypoxia, hypotension, and need for cardiopulmonary resuscitation.[50]

Glass and colleagues, in a recently published study, demonstrated a 90 percent normalcy rate for ECMO survivors at one year of age.

Major morbidity in the form of significant developmental delay or neuromotor abnormality occurred in 10 percent of these survivors. Poor outcome was associated with major intracranial hemorrhage and chronic lung disease. Ligation of the right carotid artery and internal jugular vein was not associated with a consistent lateralizing lesion.[51]

Differentiation between preexisting deficits and those secondary to ECMO manipulations can be difficult. The functional normalcy of the majority of the survivors is encouraging and suggests that ECMO support can be accomplished safely and that subsequent normal development is possible. However, enthusiasm for this procedure must be tempered by careful consideration of the inherent morbidity and mortality risks.

Centers using ECMO must be actively involved in ECMO research if further refinements in technique and reduction of morbidity and mortality are to be forthcoming. Bartlett and associates are seeking ways to eliminate the need for heparinization.[27] This would allow application of the technique to low-birth-weight infants by decreasing the risk of intracranial hemorrhage. Other investigators are testing a double-lumen catheter.[34,52] This would allow blood to be withdrawn and restored to circulation through a single catheter placed in the jugular vein.

Currently, research is under way to substantiate the advantage of initiating ECMO support early in the neonate's disease rather than using it as a last resort.[27] Researchers reason that medical costs could be reduced and cardiorespiratory and neurological outcome improved if intervention were not deferred until 80 percent or greater mortality was predicted.[13]

As the number of ECMO centers escalates, it becomes mandatory to analyze morbidity data as they relate to quality of survival. Enthusiasm for this technique has prompted concern that ECMO centers are being established without a thorough understanding of the complexity, hazards, and uncertainties of this therapy. The American Academy of Pediatrics' Committee on Fetus and Newborn has published recommendations for ECMO centers that describe the rationale for establishing the need for a center as well as required institutional criteria. Regionalization of ECMO centers is recommended to accommodate patient bed needs and provide a milieu of safe and effective ECMO care.[51]

REFERENCES

1. Chatburn R: High frequency ventilation: A report on a state of the art symposium, Respiratory Care 29, 1984, p. 839.

2. Bancalari E, and Goldberg R: High frequency ventilation in the neonate, Clinics in Perinatology 14(581), 1987, p. 97.

3. Krummel T, et al.: Extracorporeal membrane oxygenation in neonatal pulmonary failure, Pediatric Annals 11, 1982, pp. 905–908.

4. Drummond W, et al.: The independent effects of hyperventilation, tolazoline and dopamine on infants with persistent pulmonary hypertension, Journal of Pediatrics, 98, 1981, p. 603.

5. Ormagabal M, Kirkpatrick B, and Muellar D: Alteration of A-aDO$_2$ in response to tolazoline as a predictor of outcome in neonates with persistent pulmonary hypertension, Pediatric Respiration 14, 1980, p. 607.

6. Levin D: Effects of prostaglandin synthesis on fetal development, oxygenation and fetal circulation, Seminars in Perinatology 4, 1980, pp. 35–44.

7. Lyrener RK, et al.: Alkalosis attenuates hypoxic pulmonary vasoconstriction in neonatal lambs, Pediatrics Research 19, 1985, pp. 1268–1271.

8. Ordiz R, Cillery R, and Bartlett R: Extracorporeal membrane oxygenation in pediatric respiratory failure, Pediatric Clinics of North America 34, 1987, pp. 39–46.

9. Rashkind W, et al.: Evaluation of a disposable plastic low flow volume pumpless oxygenator as a lung substitute, Journal of Pediatrics 66, 1965, pp. 94–102.

10. Dorson W, et al.: A perfusion system for infants, Transactions of the American Society for Artificial Organs 15, 1969, pp. 155–157.

11. White J, et al.: Prolonged respiratory support in newborn infants with a membrane oxygenator, Surgery 70, 1971, pp. 288–295.

12. Pyle R, et al.: Clinical use of membrane oxygenation, Archives of Surgery 110, 1975, pp. 996–1002.

13. Bartlett R: Extracorporeal oxygenation in neonates, Hospital Practice, April 1984, pp. 139–151.

14. Kolobow T, Zapol W, and Pierce J: High survival and minimal blood damage in lambs exposed to long term (1 week) veno-venous pumping with a polyurethane chamber roller pump with and without a membrane blood oxygenator, Transactions of the American Society of Artificial Internal Organs 15, 1969, pp. 172–173.

15. Kolobow T, Stood E, and Weathersby P: Superior blood compatibility of silicone rubber free of silicone fiber in membrane lung, Transactions of the American Society of Artificial Organs 20, 1974, pp. 269–270.

16. Kolobow T, Stool E, and Pierce J: Longterm perfusion with the membrane lung in lambs, *in* Zopol W, and Quist J, eds., Artificial Lungs for Acute Respiratory Failure, New York, 1976, Academic Press, pp. 234–242.

17. Bartlett R, et al.: Extracorporeal membrane oxygenation for newborn respiratory failure: Forty-five cases, Surgery 92, 1982, pp. 425–433.

18. Bartlett R, et al.: Extracorporeal circulation in neonatal respiratory failure: A prospective randomized study, Pediatrics 4, 1985, pp. 479–487.

19. Hardesty R, et al.: Extracorporeal membrane oxygenation: Successful treatment of persistent fetal circulation following repair of congenital diaphragmatic hernia, Journal of Thoracic Cardiovascular Surgery 81, 1981, pp. 556–569.

20. Wetmore N, et al.: Defining indications for artificial organ support in respiratory failure, Transactions of the American Society of Artificial Organs 25, 1979, pp. 459–461.

21. Kirkpatrick B, Drummel T, and Mueller D: Use of extracorporeal membrane oxygenation for respiratory failure in term infants, Pediatrics 72, 1983, pp. 872–876.

22. Rapherty R, and Downes J: Congenital diaphragmatic hernia: Prediction of survival, Journal of Pediatric Surgery 8, 1973, pp. 815–818.

23. Paneth N, and Wallenstien S: Extracorporeal membrane oxygenation and the play-the-winner rule, Pediatrics 76, 1985, pp. 622–623.

24. Ware J, and Epstien M: Extracorporeal circulation in respiratory failure, Pediatrics 76, 1985, pp. 849–850.

25. O'Rourke P, et al.: Extracorporeal membrane oxygenation and conventional medical therapy in neonates with persistent pulmonary hypertension of the newborn: A prospective randomized study, Pediatrics 84, 1989, pp. 957–963.

26. Neonatal ECMO Registry Report of the Extracorporeal Life Support Organization, January, 1991.

27. Bartlett R, et al.: Extracorporeal membrane oxygenation (ECMO) in neonatal respiratory failure, Annals of Surgery 204, 1986, pp. 236–245.

28. March D, Wilkerson S, and Cook L: Extracorporeal membrane oxygenation selection criteria: Partial pressure of arterial oxygenation versus alveolar arterial oxygen gradient, Pediatrics 82, 1988, pp. 162–166.

29. Bartlett R, et al.: Extracorporeal membrane oxygenation (ECMO) in the treatment of cardiac and respiratory failure in children, Transactions of the American Society of Artificial Internal Organs 26, 1980, pp. 578–581.

30. Chapman R, Toomasian J, and Bartlett R: Extracorporeal Membrane Oxygenation Technical Specialist Manual, Ann Arbor, Michigan, 1988, University of Michigan Press.

31. Andrews A, et al.: Venovenous extracorporeal membrane oxygenation in neonates with respiratory failure, Journal of Pediatric Surgery 18, 1983, pp. 339–342.

32. Klien M, et al.: Venovenous perfusion in ECMO for newborn respiratory insufficiency, Annals of Surgery 201, 1985, pp. 520–526.

33. Zwischenberger J, et al.: Total respiratory support with single cannula venovenous ECMO: Double lumen continuous flow versus single tidal flow, Transactions of

the American Society of Artificial Internal Organs 31, 1985, pp. 610–615.

34. Andersen HL, et al: Venovenous extracorporeal membrane oxygenation in neonates using the double lumen catheter—summary of 62 cases (abstract), 7th Annual Children's Hospital—National Medical Center—Ecmo Symposium, February, 1991.

35. Bartlett R, and Gazzaniga A: Extracorporeal circulation for cardio-pulmonary failure, Current Problems in Surgery 15, 1978, pp. 1–96.

36. Rivera K, et al.: Maximum flow rates for arterial cannulae used in neonatal ECMO (abstract), 6th Annual Children's Hospital—National Medical Center—ECMO Symposium, February 1990.

37. German J, et al.: Technical aspects in the management of the meconium aspiration syndrome with extracorporeal circulation, Journal of Pediatric Surgery 15, 1980, pp. 378–383.

38. Workman E, and Lentz D: Extracorporeal membrane oxygenation, Association of Operating Room Nurses Journal 45, 1987, pp. 725–739.

39. Krummell T, et al.: The early evaluation of survivors after extracorporeal membrane oxygenation for neonatal pulmonary failure, Journal of Pediatric Surgery 19, 1984, pp. 585–589.

40. Bartlett R, and Gazzaniga A: Physiology and pathophysiology of extracorporeal membrane circulation, *in* Ionesuc M, ed., Technics in Extracorporeal Circulation, Boston, 1980, Butterworths, pp. 1–43.

41. Bartlett R: Respiratory support: Extracorporeal membrane oxygenation in newborn respiratory failure, *in* Welch K, et al., eds., Pediatric Surgery, New York, 1986, Year Book Medical Publishers, pp. 74–77.

42. Anderson H, et al.: Thrombocytopenia in neonates after extracorporeal membrane oxygenation, Transactions of the American Society of Artificial Organs 32, 1986, pp. 534–537.

43. Taylor G, Short B, and Driesmer P: Extracorporeal membrane oxygenation: Radiologic appearance of the neonatal chest, American Journal of Roentgenology 146, 1986, pp. 1257–1259.

44. Lotze A, Short B, and Taylor G: Lung compliance as a measure of lung function in newborns with respiratory failure requiring extracorporeal membrane oxygenation, Critical Care Medicine 15, 1987, pp. 226–229.

45. Riggs P, et al.: Repair following ECMO: Colorflow doppler studies (abstract) 7th Annual Children's Hospital—National Medical Center—ECMO Symposium, February 1991.

46. Spector ML, et al.: Carotid artery reconstruction in the neonate: discharge data and eighteen month followup (abstract) 7th Annual Children's Hospital—National Medical Center—ECMO Symposium, February 1991.

47. Towne B, Lott I, and Hicks D: Long-term follow-up of newborns with persistent pulmonary hypertension in the newborn, Clinics of Perinatology 11, 1984, pp. 410–414.

48. Berbaum J, Russell P, and Sheridan P: Long-term follow-up of newborns with persistent pulmonary hypertension, Critical Care Medicine 12, 1984, pp. 583–5970.

49. Ballard R, and Leonard C: Developmental follow-up of infants with persistent pulmonary hypertension in the newborn, Clinics of Perinatology 11, 1984, pp. 737–755.

50. Schumacker M, et al.: Right-sided brain lesions in infants following extracorporeal membrane oxygenation, Pediatrics 82, 1988, pp. 155–161.

51. Glass P, Miller M, and Short B: Morbidity for survivors of extracorporeal membrane oxygenation: Neurodevelopmental outcome at 1 year of age, Pediatrics 83, 1989, pp. 72–78.

52. Zwischenberger J, et al.: Total respiratory support with single cannula venovenous ECMO: Double lumen continuous flow vs. single lumen tidal flow, Transactions of the American Society of Artificial Internal Organs 31, 1985, pp. 610–614.

53. Committee on Fetus and Newborn: Recommendations on extracorporeal membrane oxygenation, Pediatrics 85, 1990, pp. 618–619.

54. Andrews A, Bartlett R, and Roloff D: Mortality risk graphs for neonates with respiratory distress (abstract), Pediatric Respiration 16, 1982, p. 275A.

55. Beck R, Anderson K, and Pearson G: Criteria for extracorporeal membrane oxygenation in a population of infants with persistent pulmonary hypertension of the newborn, Journal of Pediatric Surgery 21, 1986, pp. 297–302.

56. Bohn D, et al.: Ventilatory predictors of pulmonary hypoplasia in congenital diaphragmatic hernia, confirmed by morphologic assessment, Journal of Pediatrics 111, pp. 423–431.

57. Caron E, and Maguire D: Current management of pain, sedation and narcotic physical dependency of the infant on ECMO, Journal of Perinatal and Neonatal Nursing 4, 1990, pp. 63–74.

Table of Abbreviations

ACT:	Activated clotting time
BPD:	Bronchopulmonary dysplasia
CDP:	Continuous distending pressure
C_L:	Lung compliance
CMT:	Conventional mechanical therapy
CMV:	Conventional mechanical ventilation
CO:	Cardiac output
CPAP:	Continuous positive airway pressure
CVP:	Central venous pressure
D:	Dead space
DNA:	Deoxyribonucleic acid
DPPC:	Dipalmitoyl phosphatidylcholine
ECMO:	Extracorporeal membrane oxygenation
E_T:	Expiratory time
f:	Frequency
FiO_2:	Fraction of inspired oxygen
FRC:	Functional residual capacity
GI:	Gastrointestinal
HFJV:	High-frequency jet ventilation
HFO:	High-frequency oscillation
HFV:	High-frequency ventilation
HFV-A:	High-frequency ventilation–active expiratory flow
HFV-P:	High-frequency ventilation–passive expiratory flow
HMD:	Hyaline membrane disease
Hz:	Hertz (1Hz=1 cycle/second)
I:E ratio:	Inspiratory-to-expiratory time ratio
I_T:	Inspiratory time
IMV:	Intermittent mandatory ventilation
IPPV:	Intermittent positive pressure ventilation
L/S ratio:	Lecithin to sphingomyelin ratio
MAP:	Mean airway pressure
MAS:	Meconium aspiration syndrome
NG:	Nasogastric
NTE:	Neutral thermal environment
OG:	Orogastric
$PaCO_2$:	Partial pressure of carbon dioxide in arterial blood
P_ACO_2:	Alveolar partial pressure of carbon dioxide

PaO_2:   Partial pressure of oxygen in arterial blood

$P\overline{aw}$:   Mean airway pressure

PC: Phosphatidylcholine

PDA: Patent ductus arteriosus

PE: Phosphatidylethanolamine

PEEP: Positive end-expiratory pressure

PG: Phosphatidylglycerol

PI: Phosphatidylinositol

PIE: Pulmonary interstitial emphysema

PIP: Peak inspiratory pressure

PPHN: Persistent pulmonary hypertension of the newborn

PTT: Partial thromboplastin time

$PvCO_2$:   Partial pressure of carbon dioxide in venous blood

PvO_2:   Partial pressure of oxygen in venous blood

PVR: Pulmonary vascular resistance

Q: Perfusion

RDS: Respiratory distress syndrome

REM: Rapid eye movement

RLF: Retrolental fibroplasia

RMSB: Right mainstem bronchus

RNA: Ribonucleic acid

ROP: Retinopathy of prematurity

RPEP: Right ventricular preejection period

RSV: Respiratory syncytial virus

RVET: Right ventricular ejection time

SaO_2:   Arterial oximetry saturation

SI: Sustained inflation or sigh

SpO_2:   Pulse oximetry saturation

$SvCO_2$:   Carbon dioxide saturation of venous blood

SvO_2:   Oxygen saturation of venous blood

$TcPCO_2$:   Transcutaneous carbon dioxide pressure

$TcPO_2$:   Transcutaneous oxygen pressure

TTN: Transient tachypnea of the newborn

$\dot{V}_A/\dot{Q}_C$:   Ventilation-to-perfusion ratio

$\dot{V}_A$:   Ventilation of the alveoli per unit time

VA: Venoarterial

V_D: Respiratory dead space

V_T: Tidal volume

VV: Venovenous

Index

Acute Respiratory Care of the Neonate

TEST DIRECTIONS

1. Please fill out the answer form and include all requested information. We are unable to issue a certificate without complete information.
2. All questions and answers are developed from the information provided in the book. Select the **one best answer** and fill in the corresponding circle on the answer form.
3. Mail the answer form to: NICU INK, 191 Lynch Creek Way, Suite 101, Petaluma, CA 94954-2313 with a check for $50.00 (processing fee) made payable to NICU INK. This fee is non-refundable.
4. Retain the test for your records; we will send you a copy of the correct answers with your results.
5. You will be notified of your results with 6–8 weeks.
6. If you pass the test (70%) you will earn 30 contact hours (3.0 CEUs) for the course. Approved by the California Board of Registered Nursing, provider #06261; Florida Board to Nursing, provider #27I 1040, content code 2505; and Iowa Board to Nursing, provider #189.

COURSE OBJECTIVES

After reading and studying the content, the reader will be able to:

1. Describe physiologic principles of the neonatal respiratory system including: embryologic development, surfactant synthesis, pulmonary and circulatory transitional events.
2. Describe the pathophysiology of specific neonatal respiratory disorders including: respiratory distress syndrome, meconium aspiration, transient tachypnea of the newborn, and persistent pulmonary hypertension of the newborn.
3. Differentiate various modes of neonatal ventilatory support (including positive pressure ventilation, high-frequency jet ventilation, and high-frequency oscillation).
4. Discuss technical aspects of extracorporeal membrane oxygenation.
5. Outline the general care given to infants requiring ventilatory support including: positive pressure ventilation, high-frequency jet ventilation, and high-frequency oscillation.
6. Discuss the general care of infants undergoing the ECMO procedure.
7. Discuss the current status of surfactant replacement therapy.

---

1. The "pseudoglandular" stage of prenatal lung growth encompasses the _____ weeks of gestation.
   a. 1 to 5
   b. 6 to 17
   c. 25 to 30
   d. 32 to 40

2. Lung structures and cells are differentiated to the point that life can be supported around _____ weeks of gestation.
   a. 16–18
   b. 19–20
   c. 22–23
   d. 26–28

3. Gas exchange occurs most rapidly in Type I pneumocytes.
   a. true
   b. false

4. Surfactant is thought to be produced in the :
   a. Type I pneumocyte
   b. Type II pneumocyte
   c. squamous pneumocytes
   d. squamous epithelium

5. The functional development of the lung revolves around:
   a. pulmonary macrophages
   b. pulmonary lyposomes
   c. lamellated bodies
   d. the biochemistry of surfactant

6. The greatest contributor to the composition of surfactant is:
   a. protein
   b. cholesterol
   c. sphingomyelin
   d. phosphatidylcholine

7. Surfactant is first detectable between _____ weeks of gestation:
   a. 18–20
   b. 22–24
   c. 25–30
   d. 35–36

8. The _____ component of surfactant is responsible for decreasing surface tension to zero when compressed during inspiration.
   a. sphingomyelin
   b. phosphatidylcholine
   c. dipalmitoyl phosphatidylcholine
   d. phosphotidylinositol

9. Surfactant stored in lamellar bodies is considered physiologically functional.
   a. true
   b. false

10. As gestation advances the phospholipid content of surfactant:
    a. increases
    b. decreases
    c. remains constant
    d. fluctuates

11. At term, phospholipid concentrations demonstrate:
    a. an increase in phosphatidylglycerol
    b. a decrease in phosphatidylinositol
    c. a & b
    d. none of the above

12. Glucocorticoids _____ the normal pattern of fetal lung development.
    a. retard
    b. have no impact on
    c. accelerate
    d. maintain

13. Thyroid hormones enhance the production of:
    a. phosphatidylglycerol
    b. phosphatidylinositol
    c. phosphatidylcholine
    d. thyroxine

14. Fetal effect(s) of catecholamine is/are to:
    a. stimulate secretion of surfactant
    b. enhance synthesis of phospholipids
    c. inhibit fetal lung fluid secretion
    d. a & c

15. Insulin _____ the development of surfactant.
    a. inhibits
    b. accelerates
    c. has no effect on
    d. has a synergistic effect on

16. The pulmonary artery wall is _____ at birth.
    a. thick
    b. thin
    c. deficient in elastic fibers
    d. none of the above

17. Lung fluid is:
    a. initially secreted in the canalicular stage
    b. derived from alveolar epithelium
    c. not an ultrafiltrate of plasma
    d. all of the above

18. The volume of lung fluid at term is approximately:
    a. 26–30 cc/kg   c. 5–10 cc/kg
    b. 10–25 cc/kg   d. 35–45 cc/kg

19. Alterations in pulmonary fluid dynamics can cause:
    a. lung hypoplasia
    b. lung hyperplasia
    c. functionally immature alveoli
    d. all the above

20. Fetal breathing movements:
    a. occur as early as 11 weeks of gestation
    b. increase in frequency and strength with gestation
    c. are cyclical, increasing during the daytime
    d. all of the above

21. The mechanics of respiratory conversion from fetal to newborn state:
    a. begin with passage of the fetus through the birth canal
    b. are interdependent with the cardiovascular system
    c. require overcoming tissue resistive forces
    d. all of the above

22. The neonatal diaphragm contributes to decreased ventilatory efficiency because of the:
    a. coordination of intercostal and abdominal muscles
    b. lower proportion of fatigue resistant muscle fibers
    c. highly nonpliable neonatal chest wall
    d. none of the above

23. Chest wall compliance affects:
    a. closing pulmonary volume
    b. functional residual capacity
    c. expiratory reserve volume
    d. all of the above

24. Lung resistance:
    a. varies inversely with lung volume
    b. is not affected by the size of airways
    c. decreases with decreasing gestational age
    d. none of the above

25. Lung time constant:
    a. is the time needed for a lung unit to fill completely
    b. depends solely upon compliance
    c. measures lung resistance and compliance
    d. none of the above

26. Physiologic dead space ventilation is:
    a. not related to anatomical dead space
    b. expressed as a fraction of tidal volume
    c. related only to alveolar dead space
    d. none of the above

27. Pleural pressure:
    a. assists in distribution of gases in the lung
    b. increases from apex to the base of the lung
    c. contributes to matching ventilation to perfusion
    d. all of the above

28. Functional residual capacity:
    a. increases the work of breathing
    b. is maintained by the neonate's pliable chest wall
    c. does not change in volume from breath to breath
    d. allows for continuous gas exchange

29. Ventilation-perfusion matching:
    a. contributes to efficient gas exchange
    b. is ideal when the ventilation to perfusion ratio is 1
    c. depends largely on gravity
    d. all of the above

30. When no ventilation takes place during passage of blood through the lungs:
    a. the ventilation to perfusion ratio is zero
    b. the pulmonary capillary blood arrives in the left atrium unoxygenated
    c. a venoarterial shunt may be present
    d. all of the above

31. High ventilation to perfusion ratios:
    a. result from decreased pulmonary dead space
    b. can cause carbon dioxide retention
    c. indicate adequate ventilation
    d. none of the above

32. Low ventilation to perfusion ratios:
    a. are present in alveolar overventilation
    b. are present in airway obstruction diseases
    c. can cause decreased $PaCO_2$
    d. are present in atelectatic diseases

33. In infants with severe RDS a large left-to-right shunt may be present on the first day of life without the characteristic ductal murmur.
    a. true   b. false

34. Which of the following occurs in the recovery phase of RDS?
    a. alveolar aeration decreases
    b. "white-out" effect is seen on x-ray
    c. surfactant production resumes

35. A risk factor for the development of RDS is:
    a. female sex
    b. maternal hypertension
    c. second born twin

36. Antenatal steroid treatment reduces the incidence of RDS in:
    a. singleton females
    b. twins
    c. white males

37. The most distinguishing radiographic feature in infants with RDS is:
    a. bilateral hyperinflation
    b. granularity
    c. peripheral air bronchograms

38. A factor that predisposes the infant to wet lung disease is:
    a. breech delivery
    b. hyperproteinemia
    c. postmaturity

39. The key to diagnosis in transient tachypnea of the newborn is:
    a. route of birth
    b. onset of symptoms
    c. radiographic pattern

40. An infant with pneumonia may not demonstrate pulmonary symptoms.
    a. true   b. false

41. The chest film is the most reliable examination for detecting pneumonia.
    a. true   b. false

42. The most definitive method of diagnosing pneumonia is:
    a. a complete blood count
    b. culture and Gram's stain of pleural fluid
    c. tracheal aspirate obtained at 24 hours

43. The severity of meconium aspiration syndrome is related to the amount of meconium aspirated.
    a. true   b. false

44. The major cause of death in infants with meconium aspiration syndrome is:
    a. cor pulmonale
    b. hypoxemia
    c. respiratory failure

45. Persistent pulmonary hypertension is characterized by:
    a. left-to-right shunting through a patent ductus arteriosus
    b. right-to-left shunt through the foramen ovale and patent ductus
    c. bidirectional shunt through the ductus venosus

46. The key pathophysiologic element in PPHN is:
    a. systemic hypotension
    b. bidirectional shunting through the foramen ovale
    c. elevated pulmonary vascular resistance

47. The presence of a right-to-left shunt may be demonstrated by comparing arterial oxygenation of blood obtained from the:
    a. left radial and umbilical artery
    b. right radial and umbilical artery
    c. right radial and left temporal artery

48. The test used in term infants to differentiate between a fixed right-to-left shunt and a ventilation-perfusion mismatch is:
    a. hyperoxia test
    b. hyperventilation test
    c. contrast echocardiogram

49. In the hypoxemic infant, a PaO_2 difference greater than 15–20 mmHg between preductal and postductal blood samples indicates significant right-to-left shunting at the ductal level.
    a. true   b. false

50. The Apgar score includes evaluation of a newborn's:
    a. blood pressure
    b. heart rate
    c. temperature

51. The main method of heat production in the newborn is:
   a. chemical thermogenesis
   b. involuntary shivering
   c. voluntary muscle activity

52. Heat loss through radiation requires:
   a. air movement
   b. no direct contact
   c. physical contact

53. A newborn who is assessed as small for gestational age is at increased risk for:
   a. birth trauma
   b. congenital infection
   c. respiratory distress syndrome

54. Limited function of the sweat glands in the premature infant increases the risk of:
   a. dehydration
   b. hyperthermia
   c. hypothermia

55. Assessment of gestational age using the criteria defined by Finnstrom utilizes:
   a. physical criteria only
   b. neuromuscular criteria only
   c. both physical and neuromuscular criteria

56. The presence of a metabolic acidosis on an arterial blood gas can be determined by assessing the:
   a. HCO_3^-
   b. $PaCO_2$
   c. PaO_2

57. A respiratory acidosis can be compensated with a:
   a. metabolic acidosis
   b. metabolic alkalosis
   c. respiratory alkalosis

58. Oxygen-hemoglobin affinity is increased by:
   a. alkalosis
   b. hypercapnia
   c. hyperthermia

59. A metabolic alkalosis can result from:
   a. bicarbonate wasting
   b. diuretic therapy
   c. hyperventilation

60. A small cardiac silhouette on a chest x-ray can be the result of:
   a. dehydration
   b. increased venous return
   c. a large thymic shadow

61. An opaque radiographic lung pattern will be seen with:
   a. hyperventilation
   b. pulmonary air leak
   c. pulmonary hemorrhage

62. Insensible water loss is decreased with:
   a. endotracheal intubation
   b. phototherapy
   c. tachypnea

63. Minimal maintenance calories are:
   a. 50 calories/kg/day
   b. 100 calories/kg/day
   c. 150 calories/kg/day

64. A premature may be viewed as a defective infant by his parent(s).
   a. true   b. false

65. Respiratory assessment of the newborn includes:
   a. respiratory rate
   b. symmetry of movement of the chest
   c. auscultation of the chest
   d. all of the above

66. Signs of respiratory distress in the newborn include:
   a. nasal flaring
   b. respiratory rate of 40–60 breaths per minute
   c. grunting
   d. a & c

67. Expiratory grunting in the newborn increases transpulmonary pressure.
   a. true   b. false

68. Retractions occur when the lung is compliant and the chest wall is non-compliant.
   a. true   b. false

69. Flexion of the infant's head moves the endotracheal tube toward the carina, extension of the head moves it toward the glottis.
   a. true   b. false

70. A correctly placed endotracheal tube:
   a. is positioned above the carina at T 2–4
   b. is placed at a depth of 7 cm for a 1 kg infant
   c. a & b
   d. none of the above

71. Intubation has been associated with:
   a. apnea
   b. increased blood pressure
   c. bradycardia
   d. all of the above

72. Observation of fogging or condensation on the endotracheal tube indicates:
   a. the tube is in the trachea
   b. the tube is in the esophagus
   c. the tube is in the oral pharynx
   d. none of the above

73. A right main stem bronchus intubation can clinically mimic a:
   a. right pneumothorax
   b. left pneumothorax
   c. esophageal intubation
   d. none of the above

74. Signs of extubation include:
   a. audible crying
   b. abdominal distention
   c. agitation
   d. all of the above

75. The oxygen-air mixture delivered to an oxgyen hood should:
   a. be warmed and humidified
   b. have the oxygen percentage continuously monitored
   c. have at least a flow of 5–7 liters/minute
   d. all of the above

76. Transcutaneous oxygen monitoring is the measurement of skin oxygen tension rather than arterial oxygen tension.
   a. true
   b. false

77. Skin oxygen tension correlates with arterial oxygen tension when:
   a. the skin is less permeable to oxygen
   b. the oxygen dissociation curve is shifted to the left
   c. there is normal perfusion
   d. all of the above

78. A reading of 159 on a transcutaneous monitor could indicate:
   a. the temperature of the probe is >45°C
   b. the oxygen tension of ambient air
   c. that the infant is lying on the probe
   d. all of the above

79. In suspected cases of right-to-left shunting, $TcPO_2$ readings should be taken at a preductal site such as:
   a. upper right chest wall
   b. upper left chest wall
   c. lower abdomen
   d. none of the above

80. Conditions which could cause inaccurate transcutaneous pulse oximeter readings include:
   a. bright ambient light
   b. poor perfusion
   c. hypothermia
   d. all of the above

81. Components which have been included in the endotracheal suctioning procedure to prevent complications include:
   a. increasing FiO_2
   b. hyperventilation
   c. set catheter-to-endotracheal tube ratio
   d. all of the above

82. The recommended negative pressure used to suction an infant's endotracheal tube is in the range of:
   a. 30–40 mmHg
   b. 75–80 mmHg
   c. 90–100 mmHg
   d. 120–130 mmHg

83. Intermittant bubbling and/or fluctuation of fluid in a chest tube drainage bottle indicates:
   a. the chest tube is outside the chest wall
   b. the tube is patent and functioning
   c. an air leak in the collection tubing
   d. all of the above

84. Research indicates a relationship between pneumothorax and:
   a. intraventricular hemorrhage
   b. gestational age
   c. infants of diabetic mothers
   d. none of the above

85. The first scientist to describe the physiologic phenomena known as surface tension was:
   a. Boyle
   b. Pattle
   c. LaPlace
   d. Von Neergaard

86. The research findings of Avery and Mead (1959) suggested that the etiology of HMD was the presence of hyaline membranes surrounding pulmonary alveolar spaces.
   a. true
   b. false

87. In the 1960s the use of mechanical ventilation was _not_ an accepted method of treatment of RDS because:
   a. it was commonly believed that positive pressure ventilation impeded cardiac return and output
   b. the ability to rapidly evaluate and adjust therapy via blood gas assessment was lacking
   c. exchange of information between clinicians was hampered by inconsistent labeling of RDS
   d. all of the above

88. Neonatal "grunting" does improve the metabolic status of infants with RDS.
   a. true
   b. false

89. Neonatal "grunting" provided the physiologic basis for:
   a. intermittent positive pressure ventilation (IPPV)
   b. positive end-expiratory pressure (PEEP)
   c. continuous positive airway pressure (CPAP)
   d. intermittent mandatory ventilation (IMV)

90. The work of Gregory and associates discounted the theory that positive airway pressure was transmitted to intrathoracic structures thereby impending cardiac return and output.
   a. true
   b. false

91. Adaptation of adult ventilators for neonatal use was unsuccessful because:
    a. continuous flow of gas to the patient was not provided at low ventilatory rates (<20)
    b. small tidal volumes required by infants were difficult to regulate
    c. continuous airway pressure (CPAP) could not be incorporated into the ventilator
    d. all of the above

92. The type of ventilation which best fits neonatal ventilatory needs is:
    a. intermittent positive pressure ventilation
    b. assisted ventilation
    c. intermittent mandatory ventilation
    d. volume-limited ventilation

93. Pressure-limited ventilators end the inspiratory phase:
    a. when a preset volume of gas is delivered
    b. after a preset time has passed
    c. when preset pressure is reached
    d. when the infant begins to exhale

94. CPAP maintains positive airway pressure during expiration and between mandatory breaths of the ventilator.
    a. true   b. false

95. Neonatal IMV ventilators use the _____ to limit the amount of gas delivered during the inspiratory phase.
    a. peak inspiratory pressure (PIP)
    b. PIP and time
    c. PIP and volume
    d. inspiratory time and I:E ratio

96. PIP limits:
    a. maximal airway pressure
    b. maximal continuous airway pressure
    c. maximal airway pressure and volume
    d. maximal airway pressure and inspiratory time

97. The term "ventilation" can refer to carbon dioxide elimination.
    a. true   b. false

98. The lung volume that exists at the end of expiration is:
    a. tidal volume
    b. respiratory dead space
    c. functional residual capacity
    d. vital capacity

99. Alveolar ventilation is equal to the volume of gas inspired with each breath multiplied by the number of breaths per minute.
    a. true   b. false

100. The fourfold increase in surface tension in the alveoli of infants with RDS significantly reduces:
    a. tidal volume
    b. airway resistance
    c. functional residual capacity
    d. vital capacity

101. According to the LaPlace theory, surface tension increases as alveolar radius increases.
    a. true   b. false

102. Lung compliance:
    a. is unaffected by disease states
    b. determines the presence of atelectasis
    c. is the relationship of unit change in volume per unit increase in intrathoracic pressure
    d. is not related to changes in airway resistance

103. As a lung becomes diseased compliance increases.
    a. true   b. false

104. In an infant requiring IMV, unrecognized changes in lung compliance can alter:
    a. tidal volume
    b. vital capacity
    c. functional residual capacity
    d. airway pressure

105. Compliance is greatest when a normal _____ is maintained.
    a. tidal volume
    b. functional residual capacity
    c. alveolar ventilation
    d. inspiratory pressure

106. Compliance is greatest when:
    a. largest change in volume occurs with the least change in pressure
    b. smallest change in volume occurs with the largest change in pressure
    c. largest change in volume occurs with the largest change in pressure

107. If compliance improves and airway pressure remains the same, _____ of the lungs can occur.
    a. atelectasis
    b. underventilation
    c. overdistention
    d. none of the above

108. As compliance improves, chest wall excursion:
    a. decreases
    b. increases
    c. remains unchanged

109. In an infant requiring IMV, undetected changes in compliance can result in overdistention and:
    a. increased cardiac output
    b. decreased cardiac output
    c. atelectasis
    d. increased surfactant production

110. The time constant of the lung is calculated by the following:
    a. resistance × tidal volume
    b. resistance × compliance
    c. compliance × frequency
    d. compliance × tidal volume

111. A pathologic factor which decreases alveolar minute ventilation ($\dot{V}_A$) is:
    a. atelectasis
    b. pulmonary hypoperfusion
    c. pulmonary hyperperfusion
    d. intracardiac shunting of blood

112. A pathologic factor which decreases perfusion (Q_C) is:
    a. extrapulmonary shunting of blood
    b. atelectasis
    c. airway obstruction
    d. apnea

113. Air-trapping in the lung can cause a significant:
    a. rise in PaO_2
    b. rise in $PaCO_2$
    c. decrease in PaO_2
    d. decrease in $PaCO_2$

114. The ventilatory parameter which plays a pivotal role in FRC and V_A during mechanical ventilation is:
    a. PIP
    b. PEEP
    c. $P\bar{a}w$
    d. I:E ratio

115. An example of an atelectatic process is:
    a. RDS
    b. meconium aspiration
    c. BPD
    d. PIE

116. Vasodilators such as tolazoline have been shown to be beneficial to some degree in *all* patients with PPHN.
    a. true   b. false

117. Complications of assisted ventilation include:
    a. infection
    b. intracranial hemorrhage
    c. tracheobronchial injury
    d. all of the above

118. The most common serious complication of assisted ventilation is:
    a. retinopathy of prematurity
    b. pulmonary air leaks
    c. intracranial hemorrhage
    d. infection

119. Gas trapped in the perivascular and connective tissues of the lung results in:
    a. pneumopericardium
    b. pnuemomediastinum
    c. pulmonary interstitial emphysema
    d. tension pneumothorax

120. A pneumothorax occurs when alveoli rupture and air dissects through the:
    a. parietal pleura
    b. pericardial sac
    c. visceral pleura
    d. none of the above

121. Free interstitial air can:
    a. increase lung compliance
    b. impede cardiac output
    c. increase tidal volume
    d. decrease pulmonary vascular resistance

122. In a patient with pulmonary interstitial emphysema (PIE), a pneumothorax:
    a. can decompress PIE
    b. improve patient outcome
    c. a & b
    d. none of the above

123. An infant presenting with sudden cyanosis, hypotension, abdominal distention, and decreased breath sounds may have developed:
    a. pneumomediastinum
    b. pneumoperitoneum
    c. tension pneumothorax
    d. pneumopericardium

124. An infant presenting with inaudible heart sounds, hypotension, decreased pulse pressure, and equal breath sounds may have developed:
    a. pneumopericardium
    b. tension pneumothorax
    c. pneumomediastinum
    d. pneumoperitoneum

125. The appearance of air under the inferior surface of the heart producing a halo around it is diagnostic of:
    a. pneumomediastinum
    b. pneumopericardium
    c. tension pneumothorax
    d. pulmonary interstitial emphysema

126. A pneumoperitoneum can be:
   a. pulmonary or gastrointestinal in origin
   b. associated with pneumomediastinum
   c. only pulmonary in origin
   d. a & b

127. To prevent pulmonary air leaks, inspiratory time should be short and low tidal volumes with fast rates should be used.
   a. true   b. false

128. The most important factor predisposing an infant to bronchopulmonary dysplasia (BPD) is:
   a. small airway reactivity
   b. immature lungs
   c. pulmonary air leaks
   d. patent ductus arteriosus

129. Radiographic findings of hyperinflation, atelectasis, and irregular cysts are characteristic of:
   a. pulmonary interstitial emphysema
   b. bronchopulmonary dysplasia
   c. pneumonitis
   d. none of the above

130. The pathology of BPD includes:
   a. cellular necrosis
   b. edema
   c. fibrosis
   d. all of the above

131. A recommended guideline for weaning an infant with BPD from the ventilator is to allow the $PaCO_2$ to rise as long as the pH is 7.25 and oxygenation is adequate.
   a. true   b. false

132. The nutritional caloric needs of infants with BPD are _____ non-affected infants.
   a. less than
   b. greater than
   c. equal to

133. The diuretic of choice for infants with BPD is:
   a. ethacrynic acid
   b. spironolactone
   c. furosemide
   d. diazide

134. Theophylline is given to infants with BPD:
   a. to assist weaning from the ventilator
   b. for bronchodilation
   c. to increase minute ventilation
   d. all of the above

135. For infants with BPD, monitoring theophylline levels is not indicated for adequate pharmacological management.
   a. true   b. false

136. Hypochloremia as a complication of furosemide therapy can contribute to:
   a. edema
   b. seizures
   c. poor growth
   d. hypokalemia

137. Research indicates that administration of dexamethasone can facilitate weaning ventilator-dependent infants from the ventilator.
   a. true   b. false

138. Vitamin E has been shown to be effective in preventing BPD.
   a. true   b. false

139. Transcutaneous oxygen monitoring is an important adjunct to the care of the infant with BPD.
   a. true   b. false

140. Retinopathy of prematurity (ROP) is solely related to hyperoxia.
   a. true   b. false

141. Factors which predispose infants to ROP include:
   a. blood transfusions
   b. hypercapnia
   c. apnea
   d. all of the above

142. The single greatest risk factor for ROP is:
   a. prematurity
   b. exposure to bright light
   c. exchange transfusions
   d. hyperoxia

143. The most significant pathology in ROP is:
   a. constriction of retinal vessels
   b. vascular proliferation
   c. glaucoma
   d. micro-ophthalmia

144. ROP is now defined in 4 stages and described by zones and clock hours.
   a. true   b. false

145. The technique of cryotherapy in ROP:
   a. reattaches the retina
   b. retards vasoproliferation
   c. prevents glaucoma
   d. none of the above

146. High-frequency jet ventilation (HFJV):
   a. operates at four times the normal neonatal respiratory rate
   b. delivers tidal volumes less than anatomical deadspace
   c. provides gas flow via a flow interrupter system
   d. all of the above

147. HFJV is able to ventilate infants effectively while using less mean airway pressure than conventional mechanical ventilation (CMV).
    a. true   b. false

148. Research demonstrates that gas flow through pneumothoraces _____ during HFJV.
    a. was greater   c. fluctuated
    b. was decreased   d. all of the above

149. HFJV has been found to be the most efficacious in treating pulmonary interstitial emphysema in the _____ weight group of premature infants:
    a. 700–900 gram   c. 1,000–1,500 gram
    b. 900–1,000 gram   d. 2,000–2,500 gram

150. HFJV and CMV differ in:
    a. gas flow
    b. tidal volume
    c. frequency
    d. all of the above

151. In HFJV inhalation is active, exhalation is passive.
    a. true   b. false

152. During HFJV factors which affect carbon dioxide elimination include:
    a. tidal volume
    b. frequency
    c. exhalation time
    d. all of the above

153. During HFJV, air trapping occurs when:
    a. mean airway pressure is decreased
    b. frequency is decreased
    c. expiratory time is shortened
    d. inspiratory time is shortened

154. During HFJV, gas flows:
    a. down the center of the airway and out along the outer walls of the airway
    b. down the outer walls of the airway, out through the center of the airway.
    c. down and out through the center of the airway
    d. none of the above

155. The reported incidence of _____, as a complication of HFJV, is significantly greater in infants treated with HFJV as compared to infants treated with CMV.
    a. pulmonary interstitial emphysema
    b. pneumothorax
    c. pneumopericardium
    d. pneumomediastinum

156. Complications of HFJV include:
    a. necrotizing tracheobronchitis
    b. reactive airway disease
    c. hypotension
    d. all of the above

157. In using HFJV, the "Delta P" is analogous to:
    a. Servo pressure
    b. tidal volume
    c. positive inspiratory pressure
    d. positive end expiratory pressure

158. During HFJV the _____ parameter is controlled by the tandem ventilator.
    a. positive inspiratory pressure
    b. positive end expiratory pressure
    c. tidal volume
    d. Servo pressure

159. During HFJV, the _____ is adjusted internally to maintain PIP.
    a. Servo pressure   c. tidal volume
    b. Delta P   d. positive end-expiratory pressure

160. Changes in Servo pressure may indicate:
    a. extubation   c. atelectasis
    b. pneumothorax   d. all of the above

161. In HFJV, situations which _____ compliance will _____ Servo pressure.
    a. increase, decrease   c. increase, increase
    b. decrease, increase   d. none of the above

162. During HFJV, the jet valve "on/off" light:
    a. flickers at a speed reflecting ventilator rate
    b. is off when the pinch valve is open
    c. is on when the pinch valve is closed
    d. none of the above

163. The amount of humidity in the gas during HFJV is not related to the cartridge temperature.
    a. true   b. false

164. The short green tubing on the HI-LO jet endotracheal tube:
    a. connects to the CMV
    b. allows for monitoring airway pressure
    c. is the jet insufflation lumen
    d. is the port used for suctioning

165. An important and frequently assessed component of the respiratory assessment of an infant requiring HFJV is:
    a. assessment of chest vibrations
    b. assessment of spontaneous aeration
    c. assessment of rales and rhonchi
    d. none of the above

166. The heart rate of an infant on HFJV is best assessed by:
    a. removing infant from HFJV and hand ventilating him
    b. a monitor which determines heart rate from QRS complex and arterial wave form
    c. assessing peripheral pulsations
    d. locating and palpating the point of maximum impulse (PMI)

167. To facilitate ventilation, the green jet line of the jet tracheal tube is placed facing anterior.
   a. true
   b. false

168. When suctioning the endotracheal tube during HFJV, _____ suction is applied:
   a. intermittent
   b. continuous
   c. greater than 80 mmHg
   d. less than 70 mmHg

169. High-frequency oscillation (HFO) is differentiated from other methods of high-frequency ventilation by the nature of expiration.
   a. true
   b. false

170. In high-frequency oscillation _____ occurs:
   a. hypothermia
   b. hypercapnia
   c. active expiration
   d. none of the above

171. Using HFO, adequate ventilation can be achieved using tidal volumes less than anatomical dead space.
   a. true
   b. false

172. Convective dispersion, molecular diffusion, and pendeluft are mechanisms involved in:
   a. gas transport
   b. oscillations
   c. passive expiration
   d. barotrauma

173. Oxygenation and carbon dioxide clearance in HFO are:
   a. secondary to low airway resistance
   b. able to alter lung compliance
   c. manipulated independently
   d. due to reduced turbulent flow

174. Carbon dioxide elimination in HFO is controlled by:
   a. active expiration
   b. tidal volume and frequency
   c. positive end-expiratory pressure
   d. mean airway pressure

175. The ideal frequency used during HFO is:
   a. 10 Hertz
   b. 15 Hertz
   c. 18 Hertz
   d. 20 Hertz

176. During HFO ventilation the continuous vibration of an infant's chest indicates:
   a. a blocked endotracheal tube
   b. a pneumothorax
   c. ventilator failure
   d. adequate oscillated gas flow

177. HFO ventilation can cause:
   a. hypothermia
   b. hypercarbia
   c. hypocarbia
   d. hypoxia

178. The clinical sign(s) of pneumothorax in HFO include:
   1. they are subtle
   2. rise in PCO_2
   3. abrupt deterioration of infant's condition
   4. fall in PaO_2
   a. 1, 2, 4
   b. 3
   c. 2, 3
   d. none of the above.

179. To assess heart tones and breath sounds while treating with HFO, the infant must be:
   a. paralyzed
   b. removed from HFO
   c. placed on a conventional ventilator
   d. positioned prone

180. Viability of the fetus as related to maturation of the pulmonary system is thought to occur at _____ weeks gestation:
   a. 20
   b. 23
   c. 26
   d. 31

181. The exchange of gases in the alveoli occurs by:
   a. active transport
   b. osmosis
   c. diffusion
   d. carrier transport

182. The chemical composition of surfactant is:
   a. 90 percent protein, 10 percent lipid
   b. 10 percent protein, 90 percent lipid
   c. 10 percent cholesterol, 90 percent lipid
   d. 100 percent lipid

183. The major component of surfactant is:
   a. cholesterol
   b. lecithin
   c. phosphatidylglycerol
   d. phosphatidylinositol

184. Sphingomyelin does not lower alveolar surface tension.
   a. true
   b. false

185. Lecithin forms a stable surfactant without the presence of phosphatidylglycerol.
   a. true
   b. false

186. The appearance of _____ marks the absolute maturation of fetal lung surfactant:
   a. phosphatidylcholine
   b. phosphatidylglycerol
   c. phosphatidylinositol
   d. an L/S ratio of 2:1

187. Delayed maturation of the lung may occur in conjunction with which maternal event:
   a. hypertension
   b. prolonged rupture of membranes
   c. degenerative diabetes mellitus
   d. gestational diabetes

188. The clinical picture of an enlarged heart and haziness of lung fields characteristic of a patent ductus arteriosus represents:
    a. right-to-left shunting of blood
    b. left-to-right shunting of blood
    c. decreased pulmonary perfusion
    d. shock lung syndrome

189. Research data suggests that single dose surfactant replacement therapy is as effective as multiple dose therapy.
    a. true   b. false

190. The following are all risks associated with synthetic surfactant therapy except:
    a. mucus plugging of the endotracheal tube
    b. pulmonary hemorrhage
    c. hyperoxia
    d. infectious transmission of disease

191. ECMO:
    1. is an artificial lung
    2. can safely be used for one or two weeks
    3. treats infants with cardiorespiratory failure
    4. is contraindicated when IVH has occurred
    5. diverts blood outside of the body
    a. 1,2,5
    b. 2,3,4
    c. 3,4,5
    d. all of the above

192. Selection criteria for use of ECMO include:
    1. chronic lung pathology
    2. failure to respond to CMV
    3. acute respiratory pathology
    4. severe barotrauma
    5. $AaDO_2$ >620 for 12 hours
    a. 1,2,4,5
    b. 1,4,5
    c. 2,3,4,5
    d. all of the above

193. The oxidation index is used to predict:
    a. 80–90 percent mortality
    b. incidence of bronchopulmonary dysplasia
    c. 50–60 percent mortality
    d. all of the above

194. Indication(s) for ECMO include
    a. meconium aspiration:
    b. cyanotic congenital heart disease
    c. bilateral pulmonary hypoplasia
    d. all of the above

195. Contraindications for ECMO include:
    a. birthweight >2,000 grams
    b. gestational age >34 weeks
    c. chronic lung disease
    d. none of the above

196. Final selection of an ECMO candidate is based on criteria predictive of _____ percent mortality.
    a. 50
    b. 30
    c. 80
    d. 100

197. Intracranial hemorrhage is a contraindication for treatment with ECMO due to:
    a. ligation of the carotid artery
    b. systemic heparinization
    c. compromised cerebral blood flow
    d. all of the above

198. The venoarterial route drains blood from the:
    a. carotid artery   c. internal jugular
    b. aortic arch   d. right atrium

199. The venoarterial route returns blood to the:
    a. carotid artery   c. left ventricle
    b. aortic arch   d. femoral vein

200. A major risk of venoarterial bypass is:
    a. ligation of the internal jugular vein
    b. pneumothorax
    c. air emboli
    d. decompression of the pulmonary circulation

201. A complication of venovenous ECMO is:
    a. a groin infection
    b. carotid artery ligation
    c. femoral artery thrombosis
    d. reduction of pulmonary vascular resistance

202. The venoarterial route of ECMO is the preferred route because:
    a. of shorter stabilization time
    b. total respiratory support can be achieved
    c. of support for heart and lungs
    d. all of the above

203. All medications and parenteral fluids are infused into the arterial side of the ECMO circuit.
    a. true   b. false

204. What percentage of the infant's cardiac output is diverted through the EMCO circuit when on total bypass?
    a. 80   c. 50
    b. 60   d. 100

205. Once the infant is stabilized on ECMO, the ventilator is discontinued.
    a. true   b. false

206. While on ECMO, what parameters need to be assessed
hourly?
1. vital signs
2. head circumference
3. electrolytes
4. neurologic evaluation
5. fluid output
   a. 1,3,5   c. 2,3,5
   b. 1,4,5   d. all of the above

207. When systemic PaO_2 begins to rise at a constant
ECMO flow rate it indicates:
   a. improved pulmonary status
   b. decreased lung compliance
   c. improved cardiac output
   d. ineffective perfusion

208. Causes of inadequate venous return include:
   a. blood loss
   b. pneumothorax
   c. kinking of catheters
   d. all of the above

209. The cellular blood component which demonstrates the
greatest effect of exposure to a foreign surface is:
   a. white blood cells
   b. red blood cells
   c. platelets
   d. hemoglobin

210. During ECMO, total oxygen delivery to the tissues is
equal to extracorporeal oxygen and pulmonary oxygen.
   a. true   b. false

211. An excellent indicator of adequate ECMO flow and
tissue perfusion is:
   a. SvO_2 c. pH
   b. SaO_2 d. PaO_2

ANSWER FORM: Acute Respiratory Care of the Neonate

Please completely fill in the circle of the **one best answer** using a dark pen.

1. a. ○ b. ○ c. ○ d. ○
2. a. ○ b. ○ c. ○ d. ○
3. a. ○ b. ○
4. a. ○ b. ○ c. ○ d. ○
5. a. ○ b. ○ c. ○ d. ○
6. a. ○ b. ○ c. ○ d. ○
7. a. ○ b. ○ c. ○ d. ○
8. a. ○ b. ○ c. ○ d. ○
9. a. ○ b. ○
10. a. ○ b. ○ c. ○ d. ○

11. a. ○ b. ○ c. ○ d. ○
12. a. ○ b. ○ c. ○ d. ○
13. a. ○ b. ○ c. ○ d. ○
14. a. ○ b. ○ c. ○ d. ○
15. a. ○ b. ○ c. ○ d. ○
16. a. ○ b. ○ c. ○ d. ○
17. a. ○ b. ○ c. ○ d. ○
18. a. ○ b. ○ c. ○ d. ○
19. a. ○ b. ○ c. ○ d. ○
20. a. ○ b. ○ c. ○ d. ○

21. a. ○ b. ○ c. ○ d. ○
22. a. ○ b. ○ c. ○ d. ○
23. a. ○ b. ○ c. ○ d. ○
24. a. ○ b. ○ c. ○ d. ○
25. a. ○ b. ○ c. ○ d. ○
26. a. ○ b. ○ c. ○ d. ○
27. a. ○ b. ○ c. ○ d. ○
28. a. ○ b. ○ c. ○ d. ○
29. a. ○ b. ○ c. ○ d. ○
30. a. ○ b. ○ c. ○ d. ○

31. a. ○ b. ○ c. ○ d. ○
32. a. ○ b. ○ c. ○ d. ○
33. a. ○ b. ○
34. a. ○ b. ○ c. ○
35. a. ○ b. ○ c. ○
36. a. ○ b. ○ c. ○
37. a. ○ b. ○ c. ○
38. a. ○ b. ○ c. ○
39. a. ○ b. ○ c. ○
40. a. ○ b. ○

41. a. ○ b. ○
42. a. ○ b. ○ c. ○
43. a. ○ b. ○
44. a. ○ b. ○ c. ○
45. a. ○ b. ○ c. ○
46. a. ○ b. ○ c. ○
47. a. ○ b. ○ c. ○
48. a. ○ b. ○ c. ○
49. a. ○ b. ○
50. a. ○ b. ○ c. ○

51. a. ○ b. ○ c. ○
52. a. ○ b. ○ c. ○
53. a. ○ b. ○ c. ○
54. a. ○ b. ○ c. ○
55. a. ○ b. ○ c. ○
56. a. ○ b. ○ c. ○
57. a. ○ b. ○ c. ○
58. a. ○ b. ○ c. ○
59. a. ○ b. ○ c. ○
60. a. ○ b. ○ c. ○

61. a. ○ b. ○ c. ○
62. a. ○ b. ○ c. ○
63. a. ○ b. ○ c. ○
64. a. ○ b. ○
65. a. ○ b. ○ c. ○ d. ○
66. a. ○ b. ○ c. ○ d. ○
67. a. ○ b. ○
68. a. ○ b. ○
69. a. ○ b. ○
70. a. ○ b. ○ c. ○ d. ○

71. a. ○ b. ○ c. ○ d. ○
72. a. ○ b. ○ c. ○ d. ○
73. a. ○ b. ○ c. ○ d. ○
74. a. ○ b. ○ c. ○ d. ○
75. a. ○ b. ○ c. ○ d. ○
76. a. ○ b. ○
77. a. ○ b. ○ c. ○ d. ○
78. a. ○ b. ○ c. ○ d. ○
79. a. ○ b. ○ c. ○ d. ○
80. a. ○ b. ○ c. ○ d. ○

81. a. ○ b. ○ c. ○ d. ○
82. a. ○ b. ○ c. ○ d. ○
83. a. ○ b. ○ c. ○ d. ○
84. a. ○ b. ○ c. ○ d. ○
85. a. ○ b. ○ c. ○ d. ○
86. a. ○ b. ○
87. a. ○ b. ○ c. ○ d. ○
88. a. ○ b. ○
89. a. ○ b. ○ c. ○ d. ○
90. a. ○ b. ○

91. a. ○ b. ○ c. ○ d. ○
92. a. ○ b. ○ c. ○ d. ○
93. a. ○ b. ○ c. ○ d. ○
94. a. ○ b. ○
95. a. ○ b. ○ c. ○ d. ○
96. a. ○ b. ○ c. ○ d. ○
97. a. ○ b. ○
98. a. ○ b. ○ c. ○ d. ○
99. a. ○ b. ○
100. a. ○ b. ○ c. ○ d. ○

101. a. ○ b. ○
102. a. ○ b. ○ c. ○ d. ○
103. a. ○ b. ○
104. a. ○ b. ○ c. ○ d. ○
105. a. ○ b. ○ c. ○ d. ○
106. a. ○ b. ○ c. ○
107. a. ○ b. ○ c. ○ d. ○
108. a. ○ b. ○ c. ○ d. ○
109. a. ○ b. ○ c. ○ d. ○
110. a. ○ b. ○ c. ○ d. ○

111. a. ○ b. ○ c. ○ d. ○
112. a. ○ b. ○ c. ○ d. ○
113. a. ○ b. ○ c. ○ d. ○
114. a. ○ b. ○ c. ○ d. ○
115. a. ○ b. ○ c. ○ d. ○
116. a. ○ b. ○
117. a. ○ b. ○ c. ○ d. ○
118. a. ○ b. ○ c. ○ d. ○
119. a. ○ b. ○ c. ○ d. ○
120. a. ○ b. ○ c. ○ d. ○

[illegible] b. ○ c. ○ d. ○
122. a. ○ b. ○ c. ○ d. ○
123. a. ○ b. ○ c. ○ d. ○
124. a. ○ b. ○ c. ○ d. ○
125. a. ○ b. ○ c. ○ d. ○
126. a. ○ b. ○ c. ○ d. ○
127. a. ○ b. ○
128. a. ○ b. ○ c. ○ d. ○
129. a. ○ b. ○ c. ○ d. ○
130. a. ○ b. ○ c. ○ d. ○

131. a. ○ b. ○
132. a. ○ b. ○ c. ○
133. a. ○ b. ○ c. ○ d. ○
134. a. ○ b. ○ c. ○ d. ○
135. a. ○ b. ○
136. a. ○ b. ○ c. ○ d. ○
137. a. ○ b. ○
138. a. ○ b. ○
139. a. ○ b. ○
140. a. ○ b. ○

141. a. ○ b. ○ c. ○ d. ○
142. a. ○ b. ○ c. ○ d. ○
143. a. ○ b. ○ c. ○ d. ○
144. a. ○ b. ○
145. a. ○ b. ○ c. ○ d. ○
146. a. ○ b. ○ c. ○ d. ○
147. a. ○ b. ○
148. a. ○ b. ○ c. ○ d. ○
149. a. ○ b. ○ c. ○ d. ○
150. a. ○ b. ○ c. ○ d. ○

151. a. ○ b. ○
152. a. ○ b. ○ c. ○ d. ○
153. a. ○ b. ○ c. ○ d. ○
154. a. ○ b. ○ c. ○ d. ○
155. a. ○ b. ○ c. ○ d. ○
156. a. ○ b. ○ c. ○ d. ○
157. a. ○ b. ○ c. ○ d. ○
158. a. ○ b. ○ c. ○ d. ○
159. a. ○ b. ○ c. ○ d. ○
160. a. ○ b. ○ c. ○ d. ○

161. a. ○ b. ○ c. ○ d. ○
162. a. ○ b. ○ c. ○ d. ○
163. a. ○ b. ○
164. a. ○ b. ○ c. ○ d. ○
165. a. ○ b. ○ c. ○ d. ○
166. a. ○ b. ○ c. ○ d. ○
167. a. ○ b. ○
168. a. ○ b. ○ c. ○ d. ○
169. a. ○ b. ○
170. a. ○ b. ○ c. ○ d. ○

171. a. ○ b. ○
172. a. ○ b. ○ c. ○ d. ○
173. a. ○ b. ○ c. ○ d. ○
174. a. ○ b. ○ c. ○ d. ○
175. a. ○ b. ○ c. ○ d. ○
176. a. ○ b. ○ c. ○ d. ○
177. a. ○ b. ○ c. ○ d. ○
178. a. ○ b. ○ c. ○ d. ○
179. a. ○ b. ○ c. ○ d. ○
180. a. ○ b. ○ c. ○ d. ○

181. a. ○ b. ○ c. ○ d. ○
182. a. ○ b. ○ c. ○ d. ○
183. a. ○ b. ○ c. ○
184. a. ○ b. ○
185. a. ○ b. ○
186. a. ○ b. ○ c. ○ d. ○
187. a. ○ b. ○ c. ○ d. ○
188. a. ○ b. ○ c. ○ d. ○
189. a. ○ b. ○
190. a. ○ b. ○ c. ○ d. ○

191. a. ○ b. ○ c. ○ d. ○
192. a. ○ b. ○ c. ○ d. ○
193. a. ○ b. ○ c. ○ d. ○
194. a. ○ b. ○ c. ○ d. ○
195. a. ○ b. ○ c. ○ d. ○
196. a. ○ b. ○ c. ○ d. ○
197. a. ○ b. ○ c. ○ d. ○
198. a. ○ b. ○ c. ○ d. ○
199. a. ○ b. ○ c. ○ d. ○
200. a. ○ b. ○ c. ○ d. ○

201. a. ○ b. ○ c. ○ d. ○
202. a. ○ b. ○ c. ○ d. ○
203. a. ○ b. ○
204. a. ○ b. ○ c. ○ d. ○
205. a. ○ b. ○
206. a. ○ b. ○ c. ○ d. ○
207. a. ○ b. ○ c. ○ d. ○
208. a. ○ b. ○ c. ○ d. ○
209. a. ○ b. ○ c. ○ d. ○
210. a. ○ b. ○

211. a. ○ b. ○ c. ○ d. ○

Acute Respiratory Care of the Neonate

Name ____________________________
Please Print

Address ____________________________

City ____________________ State __________ Zip __________

Nursing License # ________________ State(s) of License ________________

Social Security # ________________ required for Alabama participants only.

Mail with a $50.00 processing fee to
NICU INK, 191 Lynch Creek Way, Suite 101, Petaluma, CA 94954-2313.
Please make check payable to NICU INK.
Foreign Participants: International Money Order drawn on U.S. Bank only. Thank you.

FOR OFFICE USE ONLY

RECEIVED ______

CHECK ______

GRADE ______

PASSED / FAILED

CERTIFICATE ISSUED ______

MAIL DATE IF DIFFERENT ______

REFERENCE # ______

TELEPHONE ______